Polycystic Kidney Disease

Benjamin D. Cowley, Jr. • John J. Bissler
Editors

Polycystic Kidney Disease

Translating Mechanisms into Therapy

Springer

Editors
Benjamin D. Cowley, Jr.
John Gammill Professor in Polycystic Kidney Disease
Chief, Section of Nephrology and Hypertension
Department of Medicine
University of Oklahoma Health Sciences Center
Oklahoma City, OK, USA

John J. Bissler
Federal Express Chair of Excellence
Chief, Division of Nephrology
Department of Pediatrics
Director, Tuberous Sclerosis Center of Excellence at Le Bonheur Children's Hospital
Medical Director, Nephrology
St. Jude Children's Research Hospital
University of Tennessee Health Science Center
Children's Foundation Research Center
Memphis, TN, USA

ISBN 978-1-4939-7782-6 ISBN 978-1-4939-7784-0 (eBook)
https://doi.org/10.1007/978-1-4939-7784-0

Library of Congress Control Number: 2018938827

Printed on acid-free paper

This Springer imprint is published by the registered company Springer Science+Business Media, LLC part of Springer Nature.
The registered company address is: 233 Spring Street, New York, NY 10013, U.S.A.

This book is dedicated to the memory of
Jared James Grantham, M.D.,
who was an inspiration to us all.

Preface

Polycystic kidney disease exists in many forms, with different onset patterns, inheritance, and renal survival times. A common theme binding all these diseases together is the suffering experienced by patients and their families. Empathy has made this group of affected people even larger, by recruiting our mentors, colleagues, and friends. Knowledge in the field of polycystic kidney disease has grown rapidly, so much so that the American Society of Nephrology, supported by the Polycystic Kidney Disease Foundation, hosted this topic in their early programs four times in the last decade. This book is in many ways an extension of those programs. When the Polycystic Kidney Research Foundation (now the Polycystic Kidney Disease Foundation) was founded over 35 years ago, very little was known about the mechanisms of disease initiation and progression. The concept of developing therapies was only an aspirational goal. Since that time, many bright, talented, and dedicated individuals have expanded our knowledge of disease mechanisms, making this book possible. What we hope to achieve is a summary to help center the reader and identify areas in need of further research. Experts in the field have generously provided chapters with the intent of including critical information regarding basic and translational science, clinical features, and care of patients with polycystic kidney disease in one place to bring clinicians, researchers, and other interested individuals up to date. The editors thank our patients, the Polycystic Kidney Disease Foundation, our expert friends who wrote chapters, the leaders and mentors in the field who have inspired us, the participants in the early programs over the years, and our families for supporting us in this effort to help all those affected by polycystic kidney disease.

Oklahoma City, OK, USA — Benjamin D. Cowley, Jr.
Memphis, TN, USA — John J. Bissler

Contents

Contributors

Ahsan Alam, MD, MS, FRCPC Division of Nephrology, Department of Medicine, McGill University Health Centre, Royal Victoria Hospital, Montreal, QC, Canada

Osama W. Amro, MD, MS Swedish Center for Comprehensive Care, Swedish Medical Center, Seattle, WA, USA

Moumita Barua, MD Divisions of Nephrology and Genomic Medicine, University Health Network and University of Toronto, Toronto, ON, Canada

Harpreet Bhutani, MD Department of Medicine, Emory University School of Medicine, Atlanta, GA, USA

John J. Bissler, MD, FAAP, FASN Federal Express Chair of Excellence, Chief of the Division of Nephrology, Department of Pediatrics, Director, Tuberous Sclerosis Center of Excellence at Le Bonheur Children's Hospital, Medical Director, Nephrology at St. Jude Children's Research Hospital, University of Tennessee Health Science Center, Children's Foundation Research Center, Memphis, TN, USA

Arlene Chapman, MD Department of Medicine, Emory University School of Medicine, Atlanta, GA, USA

Fouad T. Chebib, MD Mayo Medical School, Division of Nephrology & Hypertension, Department of Internal Medicine, Mayo Clinic, Rochester, MN, USA

Emilie Cornec-Le Gall, MD, PhD Department of Nephrology, European University of Brittany, Brest, Brittany, France

Peter G. Czarnecki, MD Brigham & Women's Hospital, Harvard Medical School, Boston, MA, USA

Charles L. Edelstein, MD, PhD, FAHA Division of Renal Diseases and Hypertension, University of Colorado at Denver, Aurora, CO, USA

Pranav S. Garimella, MD, MPH Division of Nephrology, Department of Medicine, Tufts Medical Center, Boston, MA, USA

Alison Grazioli, MD Department of Medicine, Division of Nephrology, University of Maryland School of Medicine, Baltimore, MD, USA

James C. Harms, MD Division of Nephrology, Department of Medicine, University of Alabama at Birmingham, Birmingham, AL, USA

Peter C. Harris, PhD Division of Nephrology and Hypertension, Mayo Clinic, Rochester, MN, USA

Scott J. Henke, BA Department of Cell, Developmental and Integrative Biology, University of Alabama at Birmingham Medical School, Birmingham, AL, USA

Marie C. Hogan, MD, PhD Mayo Medical School, Division of Nephrology & Hypertension, Department of Internal Medicine, Mayo Clinic, Rochester, MN, USA

Young-Hwan Hwang, MD, PhD Department of Medicine, Eulji General Hospital, Seoul, South Korea

Divisions of Nephrology and Genomic Medicine, University Health Network and University of Toronto, Toronto, ON, Canada

Maria V. Irazabal, MD Division of Nephrology and Hypertension, Mayo Clinic, Rochester, MN, USA

Nicholas Katsanis, PhD Center for Human Disease Modeling, Duke University School of Medicine, Durham, NC, USA

Korosh Khalili, MD Department of Medical Imaging, University Health Network and University of Toronto, Toronto, ON, Canada

Ahd Al Khunaizi, MD McGill University Health Centre, Montreal, QC, Canada

Dawn E. Landis, PhD Department of Cell, Developmental and Integrative Biology, University of Alabama at Birmingham Medical School, Birmingham, AL, USA

Yangfan P. Liu, PhD Center for Human Disease Modeling, Duke University School of Medicine, Durham, NC, USA

Anna McNaught, MD Department of Medical Imaging, University Health Network and University of Toronto, Toronto, ON, Canada

Dana C. Miskulin, MD, MS Division of Nephrology, Department of Medicine, Tufts Medical Center, Boston, MA, USA

Ankush Mittal, BS Department of Medicine, Emory University School of Medicine, Atlanta, GA, USA

Michal Mrug, MD Division of Nephrology, Department of Medicine, University of Alabama at Birmingham, Birmingham, AL, USA

Department of Veterans Affairs Medical Center, Birmingham, AL, USA

Patricia Outeda, PhD Department of Medicine, Division of Nephrology, University of Maryland School of Medicine, Baltimore, MD, USA

York Pei, MD Divisions of Nephrology and Genomic Medicine, University Health Network and University of Toronto, Toronto, ON, Canada

Ronald D. Perrone, MD CTRC, Tufts University CTSI, Tufts University School of Medicine, Boston, MA, USA

Division of Nephrology, Department of Medicine, Tufts Medical Center, Boston, MA, USA

Frederic Rahbari-Oskoui, MD, MS Department of Medicine, Emory University School of Medicine, Atlanta, GA, USA

Cristian Riella, MD Beth Israel Deaconess Medical Center, Harvard Medical School, Boston, MA, USA

Cheng Jack Song, BS Department of Cell, Developmental and Integrative Biology, University of Alabama at Birmingham, Birmingham, AL, USA

Theodore I. Steinman, MD Beth Israel Deaconess Medical Center and Brigham & Women's Hospital, Harvard Medical School, Boston, MA, USA

Vicente E. Torres, MD, PhD Division of Nephrology and Hypertension, Mayo Clinic, Rochester, MN, USA

Terry Watnick, MD Department of Medicine, Division of Nephrology, University of Maryland School of Medicine, Baltimore, MD, USA

Olubunmi Williams, MD, MPH Department of Medicine, Emory University School of Medicine, Atlanta, GA, USA

Bradley K. Yoder, PhD Department of Cell, Developmental and Integrative Biology, University of Alabama at Birmingham Medical School, Birmingham, AL, USA

Part I

PKD: Genes and Proteins

Classical Polycystic Kidney Disease: Gene Structures and Mutations and Protein Structures and Functions

1

Emilie Cornec-Le Gall and Peter C. Harris

For the purposes of this chapter, classical forms of PKD are defined as ones where the phenotypes resulting in morbidity and mortality are mainly limited to the kidney and the liver. The diseases defined in this category are autosomal dominant polycystic kidney disease (ADPKD) and autosomal recessive polycystic kidney disease (ARPKD). Other syndromic diseases, where PKD is just one of a range of pleotropic phenotypes, will be addressed separately, in Chaps. 2 and 3.

Autosomal Dominant Polycystic Kidney Disease (ADPKD)

Introduction to Autosomal Dominant Polycystic Kidney Disease (ADPKD)

ADPKD (incidence 1/500–1000) is an inherited nephropathy where the typical presentation is progressive cyst development and enlargement that results in bilateral renal expansion and often in end-stage renal disease (ESRD) [1, 2]. Cysts develop as outpouchings from the normally developed tubules, with only a fraction of tubules developing cysts that eventually bud off from the tubules but continue growing. Some cysts develop in utero but likely new cysts develop and grow throughout the patient's life [3]. Kidney expansion occurs in an exponential fashion but is much more heterogeneous at the level of the individual cyst [4, 5]. A measurable decline in renal function typically only occurs a dozen years or so before ESRD. The process by which cyst expansion results in destruction of normal tubules is poorly defined but likely involves mechanical damage through cystic expansion, development of fibrosis, and the effects of paracrine factors [6]. The typical age at ESRD is related to gene and mutation type (see section "Genotype/Phenotype Studies"). Major extrarenal phenotypes of clinical significance are polycystic liver disease and vascular abnormalities (see Chaps. 10 and 11 for details). The majority of patients have a parent diagnosed with ADPKD, although not necessarily reaching ESRD. However, at least 10% of families appear to have a negative family history within the traceable period of the family [7].

The ADPKD Genes

PKD1

The first defined ADPKD gene, *PKD1*, was linked to the tip of chromosome 16 (16p13.3), ~5 cM from the α-globin locus, in 1985 [8].

E. Cornec-Le Gall, MD, PhD
Department of Nephrology, European University of Brittany, Brest, Brittany, France
e-mail: emilie.cornec-legall@chu-brest.fr

P. C. Harris, PhD (✉)
Division of Nephrology and Hypertension, Mayo Clinic, Rochester, MN, US
e-mail: harris.peter@mayo.edu

B. D. Cowley, Jr., J. J. Bissler (eds.), *Polycystic Kidney Disease*,
https://doi.org/10.1007/978-1-4939-7784-0_1

Employing positional cloning, *PKD1* was identified in 1994 through analysis of a patient with a chromosomal translocation disrupting the gene [9]. Due to much of *PKD1* lying in a segmentally duplicated region of the genome (Fig. 1.1), the full extent of the *PKD1* coding region and predicted protein structure were not revealed until the following year [10, 11]. The longest defined coding region is 12,909 bp with 5′ and 3′ untranslated regions (UTR) of 211 bp and 1018 bp, respectively, making a total transcript size of 14,138 bp. *PKD1* contains 46 exons and lies in a region of the genome enriched for cytosine and guanine bases (GC rich), and, characteristic of such genes, the genomic structure is compact with a total genomic size of ~49.5 kb. Of note, exon size varies considerably from the very large exon 15 (3620 bp) to exon 32 of 53 bp. Interestingly, and reflecting the compact genomic structure, the smallest intron is only 66 bp, barely larger than required for efficient excision. Examples of alternative splicing have been suggested, but the only substantiated case is an alternately included codon at the start of exon 32, explaining the difference between the two described sizes of the coding region, 12,906 bp and 12,909 bp. *PKD1* encodes the protein polycystin-1 (PC1).

The 5′ region of *PKD1*, from 1376 bp 5′ to the start codon to nucleotide position 10,304 in exon 33 (genomic region of ~42 kb), lies within an intrachromosomal duplicated region, with six pseudogenes *(PKD1P1–P6)* defined that are localized more proximally on 16p [9, 12] (Fig. 1.1). *PKD1* is localized ~2.19–2.14 Mb from the 16p telomere, while the pseudogenes are spread over ~3.5 Mb in 16p13.1: *PKD1P1* (~16.31–16.35 Mb), *PKD1P2* (~16.35–16.38 Mb), *PKD1P3* (~14.91–14.94 Mb), *PKD1P4* (~18.36–18.33 Mb), *PKD1P5* (~18.40–18.37 Mb), and *PKD1P6* (~15.15–15.12 Mb). All the pseudogenes have a common 3′ sequence, with major differences from *PKD1* shown in Fig. 1.1. Many of the pseudogenes are expressed since for *PKD1P1*, *P3*, *P5*, and *P6*, the promoter region is also duplicated. But due to a frameshifting duplication in exon 1 (found in *PKD1P1*, *P3*, and *P5*) and frameshifting deletion in exon 7 for

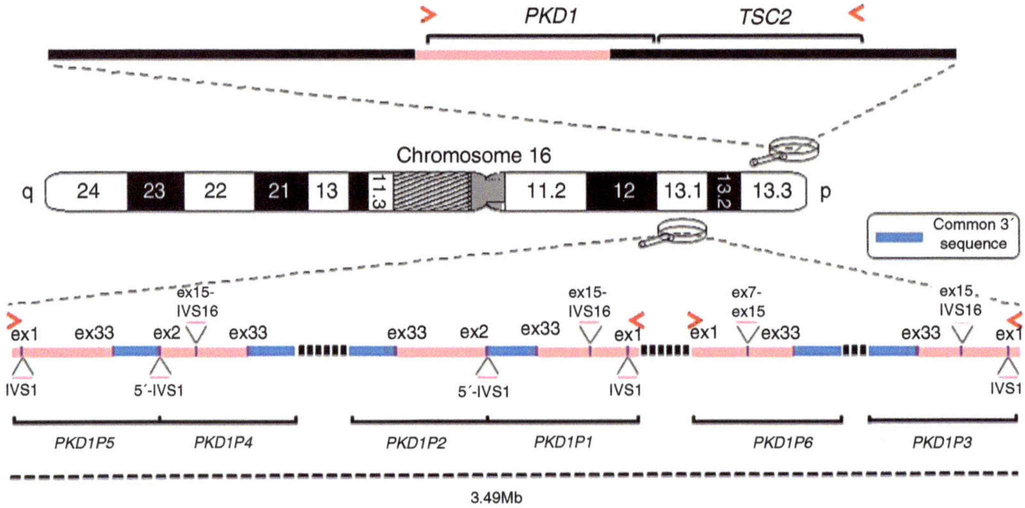

Fig. 1.1 Structures of the *PKD1* pseudogenes. At the top is shown the PKD1 gene lying in a tail-to-tail orientation with the tuberous sclerosis gene, *TSC2*. Most of *PKD1* lies in a segmentally duplicated region (*pink*), including the promoter region. At the bottom are shown the structures of the six *PKD1* pseudogenes (*PKD1P1–PKD1P6*). The middle region shows the relative location of *PKD1* (16p13.3) and the pseudogenes (16p13.1) on chromosome 16. Pink areas of the pseudogenes show areas of homology with *PKD1*, while a common pseudogene 3′ region is shown in blue. Promoters and transcriptional direction are shown with red arrows, and regions deleted relative to *PKD1* are shown above and below the pseudogene structure

PKD1P6, the pseudogenes are not predicted to generate long protein products. The duplication occurred during the evolution of the great apes (within the last 10Myr), and consequently sequence similarity between the pseudogenes and *PKD1* is very high (~98%). Therefore, locus-specific enrichment methods are needed to screen *PKD1* for mutations [7, 13].

PKD2

Before *PKD1* was identified, locus heterogeneity was noted with families unlinked to the *PKD1* region, and a second locus, *PKD2,* was identified linked to chromosome 4q22.1 in 1993 [14, 15]. Employing a positioned cloning approach and taking advantage of a region of homology between PC1 and the PKD2 protein, PC2, *PKD2* was identified in 1996 [16]. In contrast to the complexity of *PKD1*, *PKD2* is a more conventional gene with a coding region of 2904 bp, a 5′UTR of 67 bp, and a substantial 3′UTR (2081 bp), resulting in a messenger RNA (mRNA) of ~5050 bp. *PKD2* has 15 exons and a genomic size of 70.1 kb.

Further ADPKD Genetic Heterogeneity?

During the 1990s, five families apparently unlinked to *PKD1* or *PKD2* were described, suggesting further genetic heterogeneity [17–21]. Recently, these families were screened for mutations in the ADPKD genes, and in three families a *PKD1* mutation was found, a *PKD2* mutation in one family, with no mutation in the fifth [22]. The unresolved family was atypical for ADPKD, with atrophy of a kidney in one of the two affected individuals. The reasons for lack of linkage include false-positive diagnoses by ultrasound in three cases and sample mix-ups in three families. A de novo mutation, a subject with a few simple cysts, and a possible weak allele explain the lack of linkage in the fourth family. Overall, this study is not supportive of further genetic heterogeneity in ADPKD. However, since mutations are not detected in a significant proportion of ADPKD patients (see section "Mutation Analysis of the ADPKD Genes") and because there is some overlap between ADPKD and other cystic phenotypes (see section "What Types of Mutations Cause ADPKD?" and Chap. 3), the question of further genetic heterogeneity in ADPKD remains unresolved. Since the initial preparation of this chapter, a third ADPKD gene, *GANAB*, that is also associated with autosomal dominant polycystic liver disease (ADPLD), has been identifed [23, 24].

Mutation Analysis of the ADPKD Genes

Screening Approaches

The segmental duplication of the 3′ ~80% of the *PKD1* transcript limited initial descriptions of mutations to the 3′ single copy region (exons 33–46). However, locus-specific enrichment methods were soon developed for *PKD1* including long-range (LR) polymerase chain reaction (PCR) with a primer anchored in the single copy region and locus-specific LR-PCR exploiting the rare mismatches between *PKD1* and all six pseudogenes [7, 13, 25]. A variety of methods were employed to screen *PKD1* and *PKD2*, including single-strand conformation polymorphism (SSCP) analysis, heteroduplex analysis, denaturing gradient gel electrophoresis (DGGE), protein truncation testing (PTT), and denaturing high-performance liquid chromatography (DHPLC), but up until recently, Sanger sequencing of exonic amplicons from the locus-specific LR-PCR (duplicated region) or directly (rest of *PKD1* and *PKD2*) has been the method of choice [26, 27].

Recently next-generation sequencing (NGS) methods have been used to screen the ADPKD genes [28, 29]. To analyze *PKD1* specifically, methods have employed direct NGS of the locus-specific LR-PCR products, plus LR-PCR products covering the rest of *PKD1* and *PKD2.* Hybridization capture methods also capture the pseudogenes so whole exome sequencing is not a reliable means to screen the duplicated portion of *PKD1*. Two recent studies described targeted capture of *PKD1* and *PKD2* and then NGS, with a variety of bioinformatics methods and segregation employed to detect mutations in the duplicated *PKD1* region [30, 31]. However, the sensitivity and the specificity of these methods have not been rigorously tested, and locus-specific enrichment and Sanger or NGS sequencing is employed for some clinical molecular testing.

Larger rearrangements are not detected by the sequencing approaches, and such mutations in the duplicated part of *PKD1* are not readily detected by global methods to detect larger rearrangements, such as array CGH or microarrays. Specific, multiplex ligation-dependent probe amplification (MLPA) methods have been developed to screen the ADPKD genes (including the duplicated region of *PKD1*) to detect multi-exon deletions and duplications [32].

What Types of Mutations Cause ADPKD?

Two large and comprehensive mutation screens of the ADPKD genes have been completed by Sanger sequencing that provide a clear view of the mutational pattern in ADPKD; 202 families from the CRISP study [26] and 519 from the French, Genkyst cohort were screened [27, 33]. The level of PKD1 families in mutation resolved cases was 85.6% [26, 32] and 80.5% [27, 33]. There is some evidence that the level of PKD2 may be higher in geographic populations not focused on patients with renal insufficiency, and in patient populations enriched for milder disease [34]. No mutation was detected (NMD) in 8.4% [26, 32], 10.1% [27], and 6.3% of families [33]. These NMD families likely reflect missed mutations at the existing loci, including detected variants (and variant combinations) not recognized as pathogenic, deep intronic cryptic splicing changes, and promoter and 3′UTR (miR binding site) mutations that were not screened in these studies. Some mutations are also likely not detected because of mosaicism (see section "Mosaicism in ADPKD"), while mutations in other PKD genes such as the renal cysts and diabetes (RCAD) syndrome gene, *HNF1B*, and the polycystic liver disease (without PKD; PCLD) genes (*SEC63*, *PRKCSH*, *GANAB*, *SEC61B*, *ALG8* and *LRP5*) can occasionally present with an ADPKD-like phenotype [23, 24, 35–40]. However, further genetic heterogeneity cannot be ruled out.

Mutations can be considered as definite where the change is predicted to truncate the protein (frameshifting deletions and insertions [indels], including larger rearrangements and large inframe mutations, nonsense mutations, and typical splicing changes), while for non-truncating mutations (missense, small inframe indels, and atypical splicing events), further scoring is required to determine if a mutation is likely pathogenic. Bioinformatics methods judging the significance of amino acid substitutions based on conservation in a multi-sequence alignment of orthologous proteins, the strength of the chemical change of a substitution (including through the use of mutation assessment programs, such as SIFT, PolyPhen2, Align GVGD, and MutationTaster), plus conservation in domains, segregation in the family, and other contextual information about the mutation have been employed to determine if non-truncating mutations are pathogenic [26, 27, 33, 41, 42].

The frequencies of specific types of *PKD1* and *PKD2* truncation/non-truncating mutations determined from the CRISP and the Genkyst population are shown in Table 1.1 [26, 27, 32, 33]. This shows that more *PKD1* mutations are non-truncating (~30–35%) than in *PKD2* (6–18%). The most frequent single mutation group in *PKD1* is frameshifting mutations, whereas nonsense mutations are most common for *PKD2*. The ADPKD Mutation Database (PKDB) [43] collects data on published and unpublished mutations and contains records on a total of 2323 different *PKD1* and 278 *PKD2* variants. A large number of these variants are predicted as neutral in *PKD1* (857), while this number is lower in *PKD2* [44]. In the PKDB there are a total of 1273 different pathogenic *PKD1* mutations listed, accounting for 1895 families, while there are 202 different pathogenic *PKD2* mutations from 438 families. The number of mutations found recurrently is significant, with 28.1% for *PKD1* and 40.7% for *PKD2* in the CRISP study, while in the Genkyst study, 20.8% of mutations were found in more than one pedigree, with 18.8% of *PKD1* and 33.3% *PKD2* mutations previously described [26, 27, 33]. No single mutation accounts for as much as 2% of all

Table 1.1 Breakdown of mutation types associated with ADPKD in the CRISP and Genkyst cohorts

Gene	Mutation type	Crisp (%)	Genkyst (%)
PKD1	*Truncating*	*70.2*	*65.1*
	Frameshifting	28.7	33.2
	Nonsense	24.2	22.9
	Splicing	10.2	8.2
	Large rearrangements	5.1	0.8
	Non-truncating	*29.8*	*34.9*
	Missense	26.1	28
	Inframe	5.7	6.9
PKD2	*Truncating*	*81.5*	*93.7*
	Frameshifting	25.9	13.7
	Nonsense	33.3	43.1
	Splicing	22.2	21.1
	Large rearrangements	0	15.8
	Non-truncating	*18.5*	*6.3*
	Missense	11.1	6.3
	Inframe	7.4	0.0

ADPKD families with c.5014_5015delAG (43 families; 1.9%) the most common *PKD1* mutation recorded in PKDB [43] and p.E2771K (29 families; 1.3%) the most common missense change. In *PKD2* the most common mutations are two nonsense variants, p.R872X (21 families; 0.9%) and p.R306X (18 families; 0.8%).

The large number of different *PKD1* and *PKD2* mutations of various types that are spread throughout the genes indicates that any mutation that completely inactivates an ADPKD allele results in PKD. This lack of specificity of the mutation and the observation that only a single mutation is required for pathogenesis probably explain why ADPKD is such a common disease, rather than the genes being particularly mutagenic. The large number of different mutations, even within specific racial/ethnic groups, indicates that new mutations are occurring at a significant rate, consistent with the level of families with a negative family history (>10%) that has been noted [7].

One unusual form of mutation that has been described in the duplicated region of *PKD1* is gene conversions, where sequence from one of the pseudogenes converts a part of *PKD1* to contain the pseudogene sequence. The best-characterized gene conversion event, studied by NGS, extended ~8.5 kb from exon 28 to IVS32 and is due to a gene conversion by *PKD1P6* [28]. Other possible gene conversions have been described in exon 23 [45]. This mutation type is not a common cause of ADPKD, but because of the locus-specific amplification approaches employed to identify *PKD1*, they may be under-detected with existing screening methodologies.

Mosaicism in ADPKD

As indicated earlier, de novo mutations are relatively common in ADPKD and have been demonstrated molecularly in a few cases [9]. If the de novo mutation occurs in the germ cell, the patient offspring will have the mutation in all cells. However, more rarely, the mutation occurs in the embryo at a few cell stage in which case the patient will be a chimeric (a mosaic) where some cells in the patient have the mutation and others do not. Mosaicism has been described in ADPKD, which may or may not be associated with a milder disease outcome, likely depending on the level of the cells containing the mutation in the kidney [32, 46, 47]. Mosaicism can also occur at the level of the germ cells, so that, for instance, some sperm have the mutation and some do not. In this case, siblings with the same ADPKD gene haplotype can be affected or unaffected, depending on whether the mutation is present, confounding linkage-based diagnostics [48]. Mosaicism is difficult to detect by Sanger sequencing, and so the number of cases is probably greatly underestimated in de novo cases.

Genotype/Phenotype Studies

Genic Effects

Studies extending from before the *PKD2* gene was identified indicated that PKD1 was a more severe disease in terms of renal severity. The study of Hateboer [49] of a linkage determined population found the median age at the onset of ESRD was 54.3 years in PKD1 and 74.0 years in PKD2. More recent data from Genkyst shows a median age at ESRD of 58.1 years in PKD1 and 79.7 years in PKD2, indicating that many PKD2 patients do not experience ESRD [33]. The median age at onset of hypertension is also earlier in PKD1 (38.6 years) than PKD2 (48.6 years). For extrarenal manifestations, intracranial aneurysms (ICA) are found in both diseases, and the proportion of families with at least one patient with an ICA is about as expected given the gene frequencies [50]. Recent data indicates that severe PLD is as common in PKD2 as PKD1 [51, 52]. Overall, the clinical phenotypes are similar for PKD1 and PKD2 but with significantly more severe renal disease in PKD1.

Allelic Effects

Early studies of *PKD1* reported different renal disease severity in different families but did not identify differences in renal disease severity in *PKD1* populations based on the type of mutation (truncating or non-truncating) [53]. However, a modest difference was found associated with the position of the mutation in *PKD1*, with 5′ mutations associated with more severe renal disease [53]. A similar association was found between 5′ mutations and the development of ICA, which was seen especially in families with more than one ICA case and early rupture [50]. However, analysis of the larger Genkyst *PKD1* population study did not find an association between mutation position and severity of renal disease [33]. Analysis of a *PKD2* population did not find a correlation between mutation type or position and severity of renal disease [54].

The recent Genkyst study found a strong association between renal disease severity and the type of mutation [33]. Patients with truncating mutations in *PKD1* had an average age at onset of ESRD of 55.6 years, whereas those with non-truncating mutations reached ESRD at 67.9 years, approximately midway between that for truncating *PKD1* mutations and *PKD2* patients. This data strongly indicates that a significant proportion of non-truncating *PKD1* mutations are incompletely penetrant (hypomorphic); the mutant protein has some residual function. However, not all non-truncating *PKD1* mutations are hypomorphic; a gradation from fully inactivating mutations to ones associated with very mild PKD not resulting in renal failure likely describes this population [55]. A recent Canadian study also found that *PKD1* patients with non-truncating mutations had later ESRD and smaller kidneys than *PKD1* patients with truncating mutations [34]. An unresolved problem in using this allelic information prognostically is reliably identifying hypomorphic alleles and determining the relative level of residual activity of each allele, with family and cellular studies likely to be helpful. However, a simple approach (the PROPKD Score) of rating patients dependent on gene/allele type (*PKD1* truncating or non-truncating or *PKD2*), gender, early hypertension, and early urologic event has been used to predict renal survival [56].

Recessive Inheritance of ADPKD Alleles and Early-Onset ADPKD

Consistent with ADPKD being a dominant disease and studies of mouse models (see section "ADPKD Rodent Models"), no patient with two inactivating *PKD1* or *PKD2* mutations has been described; a family with two affected parents and multiple miscarriages also hinted at embryonic lethality [57]. Therefore, two families with moderate to severe PKD associated with homozygosity of a *PKD1* variant were of particular interest [41]. In a consanguineous US family of French origin, two patients with ESRD at 62 years and

75 years were homozygous for the *PKD1* variant p.R3277C, while heterozygotes developed a few cysts. In a second consanguineous family, two patients with childhood onset PKD and the father with PKD were homozygous for the variant *PKD1*: p.N3188S. Both of these variants are at well-conserved sites in PC1, but the viable phenotypes suggest they are hypomorphic variants.

Occasionally in families with otherwise typical ADPKD, PKD is diagnosed in utero with enlarged and echogenic kidneys, which can result in death in the perinatal period with a phenotype of oligohydramnios and Potter' sequence, similar to severe cases of ARPKD [58]. Analysis of a French family showed that co-inheritance of the familial *PKD1* inactivating mutation in trans with the putative hypomorphic allele, *PKD1*: p.R3277C, resulted in very early-onset disease [41]. The hypomorphic nature of p.R3277C (RC) has been proven by making a knock-in mouse mimicking this allele (see section "ADPKD Rodent Models") [59]. A combination of hypomorphic alleles in trans was also found in two ARPKD-like families with early-onset PKD and a negative family history [42]. In addition, a recent French study found a second *PKD1* allele predicted to be pathogenic in 15 prenatal onset *PKD1* cases [60]. One hypomorphic allele has been described in PKD2, where a patient with early-onset renal disease was homozygous for the missense variant, *PKD2*: p.L656W, that arose through uniparental disomy [61]. There is additional evidence that mutant variants in other cystogenes may cause early-onset disease in combination with a *PKD1* mutation, with *HNF1B* alleles the most compelling [62].

ADPKD Digenic Inheritance

One family with more than the expected numbers of affected individuals was found to have both a *PKD1* and *PKD2* mutation [44]. In this family, since the *PKD1* mutation was hypomorphic, there was considerable phenotypic overlap in terms of renal disease severity in the family [63]. However, the two digenic patients had more severe disease, with ESRD ~20 years before other family members with either the *PKD1* or *PKD2* mutation alone. Other studies employing hypomorphic and hypermutable mouse models have shown that digenic, *PKD1/PKD2* animals have appreciably more severe disease than the monogenic equivalents [64].

Contiguous Deletion of PKD1 and TSC2 Results in Early-Onset PKD

The tuberous sclerosis (TSC) gene, *TSC2*, lies immediately 3′ of *PKD1*, with their 3′ ends just 63 bp apart [65]. TSC is a dominant disease associated with the development of benign tumors throughout the body, including angiomyolipoma and sometimes cysts in the kidney (see Chap. 3 for details). Patients with large deletions that disrupt the coding regions of both genes (the *TSC2/PKD1* contiguous gene syndrome, CGS) typically have infantile or childhood onset PKD with enlarged kidneys, as well as various features of TSC [66]. The average age at ESRD is ~20 years [67]. De novo, mosaic cases are common and the severity of renal disease in these cases is much more variable. It is not clear if the *TSC2* mutation enhances the renal phenotype because of direct interaction of PC1 with the TSC2 (tuberin) protein, through common signaling pathways, or additive effects through different pathways [68, 69].

Molecular Diagnostics in ADPKD

Diagnosing an at-risk ADPKD adult family member can normally be performed by renal imaging (see Chaps. 7 and 8). However, when the imaging data is equivocal, especially when a definite diagnosis is required, such as in the case of evaluating a living-related kidney donor, molecular testing can be helpful [70]. Molecular testing can also provide a definite diagnosis in patients with a negative family history, ones with mild disease and those with an asymmetric presentation. In early-onset ADPKD, molecular analysis of the *PKD1* and *PKD2* genes can help understand the etiology, especially if a modifying allele can also be identified (see section "Recessive Inheritance of ADPKD Alleles and Early-Onset

ADPKD"). Mutation data may also be of prognostic value [56].

In the past, linkage studies have been employed to provide presymptomatic diagnoses, but because of the significant level of de novo mutations and mosaicism in ADPKD, this method is no longer recommended. Due to the genetic and extreme allelic heterogeneity in ADPKD, mutation screening of all exons of both the *PKD1* and *PKD2* gene by Sanger or NGS with locus-specific amplification of the duplicated region of *PKD1*, and MLPA to screen for larger rearrangements, is recommended for clinical and research testing. When testing a living-related kidney donor, the mutation should first be defined in an affected family member before the donor is tested for the mutation. Single exon analysis for the familial mutation can be performed in all family members of a mutation characterized case. Complications from molecular testing include that no mutation is detected in ~8% of cases, plus uncertainty whether some non-truncating variants are pathogenic, and their level of penetrance. Consulting the PKDB, bioinformatics analysis and segregation can help evaluate the likelihood of pathogenicity. As well as presymptomatic testing, prenatal diagnosis has occasionally been employed in ADPKD, with particular relevance in families with an early-onset case [71]. Recently, there has been increased interest in preimplantation genetic diagnosis (PGD) in ADPKD. In this case, following in vitro fertilization, a cell is removed from the embryo at a few cells stage, and the familial mutation (or employing gene flanking markers) is screened for and only negative embryos are implanted [72, 73]. For prenatal diagnosis and PGD, the familial disease gene and mutation need to be known in the family before testing is performed.

ADPKD Rodent Models

Pkd1$^{-/-}$ and *Pkd2*$^{-/-}$ mice develop cystic kidneys and pancreas from embryonic age E12.5 and typically die by ~E14.5, showing that ADPKD is a loss of function disease [74, 75]. Heterozygous animals develop very few kidney and liver cysts even if maintained to 24 months [76]. These models are therefore of limited value for preclinical testing. The *Pkd2*^{WS25} hypermutable allele in combination with a null *PKD2* allele results in progressive cyst development in the kidney and liver and has been extensively used for drug testing [77, 78]. Inducible, conditional models have also provided important insights into the processes of cystogenesis in ADPKD. Interestingly, the timing of loss of the second allele in the kidney significantly influences the phenotype. Before P13 (while the kidney is still developing) loss results in rapidly progressive cystogenesis, while complete loss after this time results in slowly progressive disease [79, 80]. These results indicate changing roles for PC1/PC2 and/or an altered environment in the kidneys at this time, possibly associated with the reduction in proliferation after kidney development. By careful use of specific Cre transgenics and by altering the time of polycystin loss, models mimicking adult onset ADPKD have been developed and employed for preclinical testing [81]. A low level of induced deletion of the normal allele during adulthood results in slow cyst development with later cyst clustering around early ones, possibly due to paracrine cystogenic factors [82]. Interaction studies between conditional mouse models of *Pkd1*, *Pkd2*, *Sec63*, *Prkcsh* and inactivation of the ARPKD gene (*Pkhd1*) in many cases showed enhanced cystic phenotypes in digenic animals with *Pkd1*, in particular, suggesting PC1 as the rate-limiting component in cystogenesis [83].

Other rodent models that have advanced the understanding of pathogenesis and mimic human ADPKD are hypomorphic models. Lowering the level of functional *PKD1* to 13–20% of normal by inducing splicing defects results in rapidly progressive ADPKD that causes increasing fibrosis and reduction of kidney size starting at about P30 [84–86]. Mimicking the human *PKD1* hypomorphic allele, p.R3277C (RC), has also generated an interesting model where homozygotes develop slowly progressive disease with cystic expansion over 9 months, with increasing fibrosis occurring thereafter [59]. This model, therefore, mimics cyst development in human ADPKD (but on a faster scale), and, hence, the model is valuable for preclinical testing [87]. *Pkd1*$^{RC/-}$ mice develop rapidly progressive disease, such that ~25% of body weight is accounted for by kidney weight at P25. These animals live on average to P28 but there is variability with a few animals, living to adulthood. This model shows that the level of reduction of functional PC1 is associated with the severity of disease.

The Mutational Mechanism in ADPKD

For the past ~30 years, there has been debate about how mutation to just a single *PKD1* or *PKD2* allele results in the development of the innumerable cysts that are characteristic of ADPKD. The classical view, as first enunciated in 1992, is that ADPKD is a two-hit disease and that cyst initiation requires inactivation of the "normal" allele by somatic mutation [88]. Consistent with this theory, analysis of cystic epithelia from single cysts has shown somatic mutations resulting in loss of heterozygosity or base-pair changes in large kidney and liver cysts [89–91]. In addition, cysts have been proposed to be clonal and, hence, derived from a single cell. Other evidence comes from hypermutable and conditional mouse models (see section "ADPKD Rodent Models"). The need for a somatic mutation for cyst initiation could also explain the focal nature of the disease. Using this rationale, *PKD1* may be a more common disease than *PKD2* since *PKD1* is a larger mutational target. Of interest, fewer cysts are found in PKD2, but both diseases have a similar kidney growth rate [92].

However, there has been some doubt about the two-hit theory since the number of individual cysts (1000s in a *PKD1* kidney) would suggest a very high level of somatic mutation. More recent data employing mouse models and ADPKD families (see sections "ADPKD Rodent Models" and "Recessive Inheritance of ADPKD Alleles and Early-Onset ADPKD") show that cysts can develop even if some PC1 is present [84, 85] and that the severity of biallelic disease is related to the penetrance of the alleles [59]. Analysis of cysts in chimeric mice shows that cysts are dynamic at early stages containing PC1-positive and PC1-negative cells but that the PC1-negative cells over time become the dominant form [93]. Similarly, somatic mutation to *PKD2* in *PKD1* cysts and vice versa indicates complexity in cyst development [94, 95].

Taken together, a threshold hypothesis now seems most likely to explain cystogenesis in ADPKD [59, 96, 97]. In this case, cyst development can occur when the level of functional PC1 (or PC2) falls below a certain threshold (Fig. 1.2). In mice, slowly progressive cyst development occurs when the level of functional PC1 is ~40% of normal and is rapidly progressive with ~20% functional PC1 [59, 84, 85]. In patients with a 50% reduction of functional PC1 or PC2 (typical patients with one fully inactivating mutation), cysts can occur if the level of PC1 falls below the cystogenic threshold. This may occur by somatic mutation to the other allele, but mutations to other cystogenes and stochastic variability in expression levels may also determine if a cyst develops. Once initiated, further genetic events at the disease locus, other cystogenes, and elsewhere, similar to tumor development in cancer, likely favor cyst growth and survival. Environmental influences, like a response to kidney damage resulting in proliferation, may also influence cystogenesis [98, 99]. Identification of genetic modifiers of ADPKD will help understand the cystogenic process. DKK3, a negative regulator of Wnt signaling, has been suggested to be a modifier from a candidate screen [100], but genome-wide approaches may be more powerful.

ADPKD Proteins: Structure of the Polycystins

Identification and sequencing of the ADPKD genes have enabled the structure of PC1 and PC2 to be predicted. In addition, analyses with antibodies, tagged constructs, and other approaches have enabled questions about expression, processing, and localization to be explored.

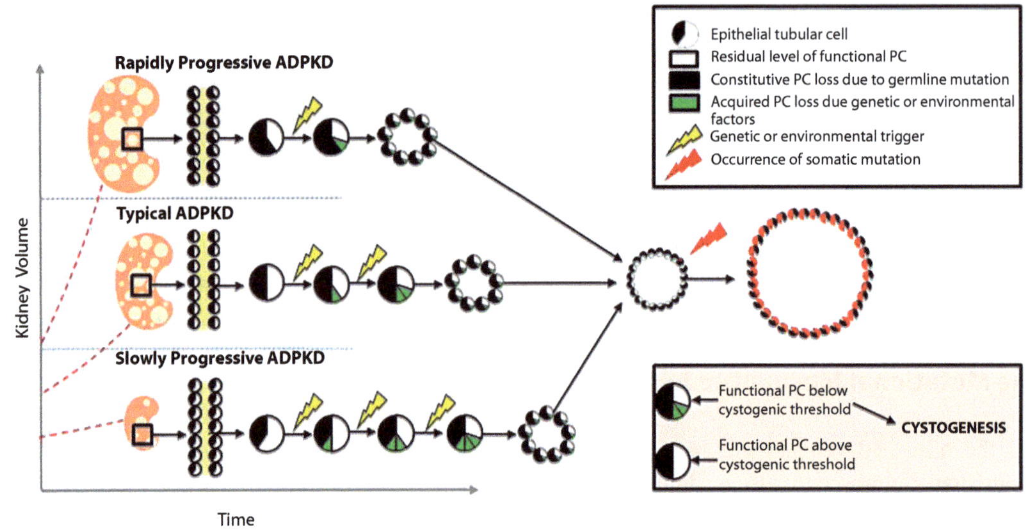

Fig. 1.2 Pathogenesis of ADPKD and illustration of the threshold hypothesis. To trigger cystogenesis, the residual level of PC1 and PC2 is reduced below a critical threshold. In the slowly progressive example, the initial level of PC conferred by the "normal" and the mutant allele (in this case a hypomorphic allele) is far above the critical threshold, and a succession of secondary events (either environmental factors or genetic events, including somatic mutations at the disease locus and elsewhere, and stochastic events) are needed to trigger cystogenesis, accounting for the low cyst number and late-onset and slow disease progression. In the typical case, the residual level of PC results from the expression of the "normal allele" only (the mutation is fully inactivating). Acquired PC loss sufficient to trigger cystogenesis is therefore more likely to occur than in the slowly progressive case. Lastly, the rapidly progressive case has co-inherited a hypomorphic allele with a null allele, resulting in a PC level constitutively low and close to the critical threshold. In this case, minimal secondary events will be sufficient to trigger cystogenesis resulting in an early-onset form of the disease. In addition, somatic mutations acquired in rapidly dividing cystic cells can secondarily provide the cyst a growth or survival advantage

Polycystin-1 (PC1)

PC1 is predicted to be a large, membrane-associated protein with a cleavable signal peptide and topology with the N-terminus extracellular and C-terminus cytoplasmic (Fig. 1.3). It consists of 4303 amino acids (460 kDa peptide backbone, ~600 kDa glycosylated) with an ectodomain of ~3000aa, 11 transmembrane domains, and a short carboxy-terminal intracellular portion, including a coil-coiled domain that mediates binding to PC2 [10, 101]. The three-dimensional structure of PC1 remains largely unknown, although recent atomic force microscopy suggests that the N-terminal domains and the transmembrane region form globular structures that are linked by a string consisting of the PKD repeats [102]. More detailed information about the structure and roles of a significant number of domains have steadily been unraveled since the identification of the protein [103]. The ectodomain consists of a number of regions involved in protein-protein (e.g., LRR domain) and protein-carbohydrate (e.g., C-type lectin and WSC domain) interactions, and the region of 16 PKD repeats with an immunoglobulin domain-like conformation has been shown to have mechanical stability properties that may also be the case for repeats in the REJ region [104–106]. The PLAT domain is conserved in a wide range of different proteins and has a beta sandwich structure [107]. Recent NMR studies of the human domain show binding to specific acidic phospholipids and calcium; it may function as a lipid/protein domain.

A major processing event that gives rise to functional PC1 is cis-autoproteolysis cleavage at the GPS domain, yielding a large N-terminal (NT) and a transmembrane C-terminal (CT) product [108, 109]. The products are thought to usually remain tethered and functionally act

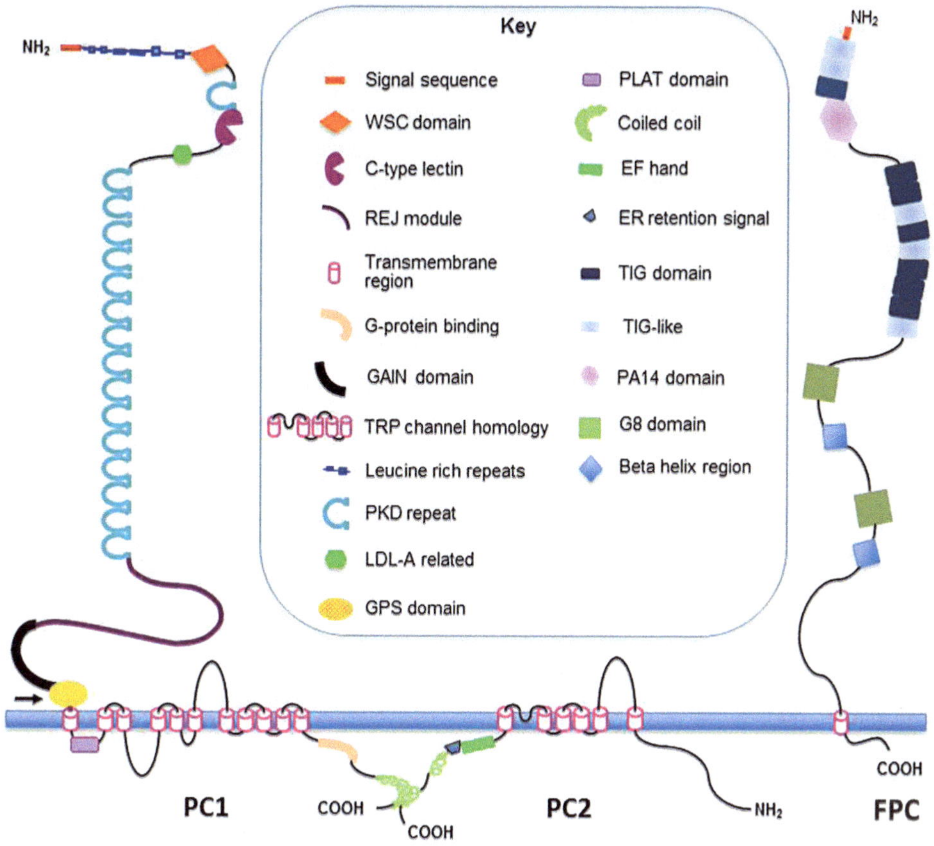

Fig. 1.3 Structures of the ADPKD proteins, polycystin-1 (PC1) and polycystin-2 (PC2), and the ARPKD protein, fibrocystin/polyductin (FPC). Details of domains and conserved motifs found in these proteins are shown in the key

together, although separate functions of the NT and CT products have recently been proposed [110]. The GPS cleavage event is important for PC1 folding, maturation, and surface localization [64, 111]. The GAIN regulatory domain, located immediately before the first transmembrane helix, is a highly conserved 320-residue region, including the GPS motif, that mediates PC1 cleavage [112]. A handful of *PKD1* missense mutations disrupting cleavage have been shown to be likely fully penetrant mutations in cellular systems [59, 108, 109]. Uncleaved PC1 may play a critical role during development, as a *PKD1* cleavage mouse mutant escapes embryonic lethality but develops rapidly progressive PKD [109]. Additional C-tail cleavage has been suggested, generating products that translocate to the nucleus and act as coactivators of several transcriptional pathways [113, 114].

Polycystin-2 (PC2)

PC2 is a protein of 968aa (~110 kDa) that comprises two intracytoplasmic extremities and six transmembrane domains [16] (Fig. 1.3). The transmembrane region of PC2 has homology with the last six transmembrane domain region of PC1. The C-terminal tail has a number of recognized domains and motifs, including an EF hand with a standard calcium-binding pocket [115], an ER-retention signal, and two coiled-coil domains [116]. The C-terminal coiled-coil domain (CC2) has been implicated in homotypic interactions and heterotypic interactions with PC1, although the precise structure of the PC1/PC2 complex is unresolved [117, 118]. A number of phosphorylation sites in the N and C terminal regions have also been identified [119]. PC2, also known as TRPP2, has been defined as a member of the transient receptor potential (TRP) family of calcium-responsive cation channels and has been shown to function as a high-conductance, nonselective, calcium-permeable channel [16, 120, 121]. Recently the structure of a homotetrameric PC2 complex has been resolved by cryo-EM [122–124]. This shows that the large extracellular loop between transmembrane domains 1 and 2, the polycystin or TOP domain, may play a role in gating the channel.

Localization and Trafficking of the Polycystins

Expression studies have shown that *PKD1* and *PKD2* are widely expressed at the mRNA level [16, 125] and immunolocalization indicates widespread expression of the proteins [126, 127].

Subcellular Localization

In renal and biliary epithelial cells, the primary cilium, a sensory organelle, is found on the apical surface. Consistent with the description of ADPKD as a cilia-related disease (a ciliopathy) [128] (see Chap. 5), PC1 and PC2 form a complex and are localized to the primary cilia membrane [129]. However, it is likely that PC1 has other subcellular localizations, including on the plasma membrane [64], with specific localization suggested at tight junctions of the lateral membrane and desmosomes [130]. PC1 is secreted from cells with the protein likely associated with specific extracellular vesicles (exosomes) [131]. PC2 is mainly localized in the endoplasmic reticulum (ER), where it is thought to play a role as a nonselective calcium channel in replenishing ER calcium stores and interacts with both the ryanodine receptor (RyR) and the inositol-1,4,5-triphosphate receptor (IP3R) [132–134].

Cilia/Plasma Membrane (PM) Trafficking

Recent data have shed light on PC1 and PC2 interdependence for maturation and trafficking, with interaction of these proteins occurring in the ER before GPS cleavage [129, 64]. Characterization of different PC1 glycoforms has helped to understand this process with two N-terminal GPS cleavage products, defined by endoglycosidase H (EndoH) treatment: mature (trafficking through the trans-Golgi) and sensitive (ER localized) [59, 64]. Data indicates that PC2 is not required for PC1 cleavage (although it may make it more efficient), but is absolutely required for PC1 maturation and trafficking to the PM and cilia, in a dose-dependent manner [64]. This study did not find an EndoH mature form of PC2, suggesting that cilia trafficking may occur separately for the two proteins. However, a second study found an EndoH-resistant form of PC2 in a cilia fraction, suggesting co-trafficking of the proteins for cilia localization [129]. A Rabep1/GGA1/Arl3-dependent mechanism has been proposed to facilitate this trafficking.

Functions of the Polycystins

A wide body of evidence, much from syndromic forms of PKD (Chaps. 2 and 5), strongly link ciliary signaling defects and PKD [128]. Unlike many of these syndromic PKD proteins that regulate protein trafficking to cilia, the PC complex is thought to have a sensory/mechanosensory role on the cilium. Generally ciliary defects have not been associated with ADPKD mutations (in contrast with syndromic disorders); however, the observation of longer cilia in the $Pkd1^{RC}$ model is interesting and may be a compensatory response to reduced cilia signaling [59]. The role of PC2 as a calcium channel suggests that calcium transport through the PC complex, with PC1 regulating PC2, is the basic defect in ADPKD. Cilia movement (mechanically or by flow) is associated with a calcium influx, and analysis of *PKD1* null cells suggested that the PC complex acts as a ciliary flow receptor, with the calcium influx required to maintain the normal epithelial differentiated state [135, 136]. However, there is controversy over whether the PC1/PC2 complex regulates the level of ciliary calcium (see also section "Polycystin Paralogs") [137]. Further controversy over the exact role of the PC complex and cilia comes from a study showing in conditional *Pkd1* or *Pkd2* knockout models that disruption of the cilia by inactivation of genes essential to its formation (*Kif3a* or *Ift20*) attenuate the cystic phenotype [138]. Based on these unexpected findings, the authors suggest that the polycystins may act as a regulator of a yet-unidentified cilia-dependent proliferative pathway. One other mechanism of how the PCs could alter ciliary signaling is by PC-bearing exosomes interacting and fusing with cilia downstream in the nephron from where the exosomes are shed, triggering a signaling reaction or by transferring a protein or miR cargo [131, 139].

ER localized PC1 and PC2 are thought to regulate intracellular Ca^{2+} homeostasis by interacting with other calcium channels and sensor proteins, such as IP3R and STIM1 (stromal interaction molecule 1) for PC1, and IP3R, RyR, and several other TRP channels for PC2 [140]. Hence, the PC complex might enhance the cilia calcium signal, through calcium-induced calcium release [136]. However, this model has been challenged by the observation that ciliary calcium stores may be too low to trigger any response from the ER PC2 [137], suggesting that other intermediate steps may be involved. Recently, other studies have shown a cellular response to a ciliary calcium signal [141]. PKD proteins have also been implicated in other key functions such as maintenance of planar cell polarity [142], although the significance to ADPKD is questioned [143], cell cycle regulation through JAK2/STAT signaling [144], and regulation of cell-cell or cell-matrix interactions [145]. For more details on PC functions, including downstream signaling pathways, readers are referred to Chaps. 4 and 5.

Polycystin Paralogs

Several polycystin-like proteins have been described that potentially provide further insight into this protein family. The highest degree of similarity between PC1 paralogs is in the transmembrane regions, while the structure of PC2 paralogs (PKD2L1, PKD2L2) is closely similar to PC2. PKD1L1, in association with PC2, senses nodal flow during embryonic development, with disruption of these proteins associated with laterality defects [146, 147], while PKD1L1 and PKD2L1 have recently been described to regulate calcium levels in cilia [137]. PKDREJ is expressed just in the testis, and possible acting with PKD2L2 is a mediator of the sperm acrosome reaction [148, 149]. PKD1L3, in combination with PKD2L1, acts as the sour (H^+) taste detector [150]. The role of PKD1L2 is still unknown, but its upregulation in mice results in chronic neuromuscular impairment [151].

Autosomal Recessive Polycystic Kidney Disease

Introduction to ARPKD

Autosomal recessive polycystic kidney disease (ARPKD) is a severe, early-onset cystic kidney disease, with an estimated Caucasian prevalence of 1 in 20,000 live births [152], corresponding to a carrier frequency of 1:70 in non-isolated populations. First symptoms of the disease typically arise during pregnancy or in the neonatal period, with greatly enlarged, hyperechogenic kidneys. The most extreme cases are associated with the Potter type I sequence, which includes pulmonary hypoplasia, spine and limb abnormalities, and characteristic facies. In up to 30% of cases, ARPKD results in neonatal demise, mainly due to respiratory insufficiency. The majority of surviving children develop hypertension and chronic kidney disease in early childhood, with 50% of them reaching ESRD in the first decade of life [152]. Congenital hepatic fibrosis (CHF) due to ductal plate malformation represents the most common liver involvement and often results in portal hypertension (i.e., splenomegaly with hypersplenism, varices at risk of bleeding, abdominal ascites). In addition, bile duct dilatation (Caroli disease) can result in cholangitis [153]. ARPKD is marked by significant phenotypic variability with later-presenting cases in adolescence or even adulthood more frequent than once thought, which most often exhibit predominant liver involvement [154].

Identification of the ARPKD Gene, *PKHD1*

The ARPKD gene locus was first mapped to chromosome 6p21 in 1994 [155], and the region involved successively refined [156–159] through the 1990s. Positional cloning approaches, including study of a recessively inherited rat model of PKD, PCK, led finally to the identification of the disease gene, *PKHD1*, in 2002 [160, 161]. The region of the PCK gene, on rat chromosome 9, was mapped in a cohort of F2 rats, which appeared to be syntenic to the human chromosome 6 interval containing *PKHD1*. Using a RT-PCR approach linking predicted exons, *PKHD1* was successfully cloned and mutations initially identified in 11 pedigrees [160].

Mutation Analysis of *PKHD1*

PKHD1 is a large gene covering more than 472 kb of genomic DNA and comprising 67 exons, 66 coding. The canonical transcript is 16,235 bp with a coding region of 12,222 bp, a 5′UTR of 276 bp and a 3′UTR of 3634 bp. A complex splicing pattern for *PKHD1* has been described [161–164], although for diagnostic testing generally just the canonical gene is screened. Analysis of the PKHD1 protein, fibrocystin, also termed polyductin (hence FPC), also questions the importance of the detected alternatively spliced forms [139].

Apart from the large gene size, other factors hampering routine molecular diagnostic testing in ARPKD include the high levels of allelic heterogeneity; half of the identified mutations are private to a single pedigree. In addition, ~60% of mutations are missense (with ~40% truncating), and as is typical for novel missense variants, pathogenicity is difficult to prove [165–168]. Over 700 different mutations have been inventoried on the ARPKD/*PKHD1* mutation database (http://www.humgen.rwth-aachen.de). A minority of recurrent mutations have been described, some specific for certain populations [166], and most notably the missense mutation p.T36M that accounts for approximately 20% of all European pathogenic alleles, and likely has a common ancestral origin [169, 170]. Although there are no evident mutational hot spots, an uneven distribution of mutations, partly due to the locations of recurrent/ancestral mutations, has led to the cost-effectiveness proposition of incremental analysis of exons [169, 171]. However, since it is important to identify all variants in *PKHD1* to understand the phenotype, complete analysis by sequencing of the 66 coding exons and flanking intronic regions is typically performed. Current overall mutation detection rates in cases with strong clinical evidence for ARPKD approached 90% [172], although this may be less in patients with just CHF [154]. Increasingly, next-generation sequencing approaches are being employed for routine screening, either of *PKHD1* alone, as part of a ciliopathy disease panel, or by whole exome sequencing [173, 174].

Genotype-Phenotype Studies

Several studies have underlined that the presence of at least one non-truncating (missense) variant is needed to escape embryonic lethality, indicating that many missense variants are incompletely penetrant (hypomorphic) alleles that still generate some functional protein [165–168, 175, 176]. However, it is worth noting that many missense variants are likely fully inactivating; hence some lethal cases have two missense mutations, and there are exceptional cases of patients with nonlethal ARPKD harboring two truncating mutations [164]. Due to the difficulty of predicting the penetrance of *PKHD1* missense variants, analysis for prognostic purposes should be exercised with caution. This is amplified by the findings in 126 sibships of the occurrence of significant intrafamilial variability, suggesting the role of additional genetic modifying factors [176]. In the future, insights from large international cohorts, such as the recently launched ARegPKD initiative, may enhance our understanding of clinical variability of the disease [177].

Molecular Diagnosis in ARPKD

Molecular analysis in ARPKD may be discussed in different contexts.

Confirm or Establish the Diagnosis in a Proband

The diagnosis of ARPKD usually relies on typical findings on renal imaging (increased renal size from antenatal period to childhood, increased echogenicity, poor corticomedullary differentiation) and one or more of the following: imaging findings of biliary ductal ectasia, clinical or biologic signs of portal hypertension, pathologic findings demonstrating CHF (especially in adolescent or young adults), or pathologic or genetic diagnosis of ARPKD in an affected sib [178]. Ultrasound examinations should be obtained in both parents to confirm the absence of cystic kidney disease. However, liver or kidney cysts detected in ~10% of *PKHD1* mutation carriers complicates this analysis [24, 179]. Recommendations recently issued by an international group of experts have underlined that given the technical difficulties of *PKHD1* analysis and the high number of differential diagnoses of ARPKD, "single gene analysis should not been considered as a first line diagnostic approach for infant and children presenting with an ARPKD-like phenotype" [152].

However, clinical diagnostic criteria may not be met in some patients, and genetic testing may therefore allow a firm diagnosis of ARPKD to be made. The testing strategy is usually to sequence the entire coding region of ARPKD and secondarily to search for deletion or duplication if two mutations are not identified [180]. While the identification of two pathogenic mutations allow a firm diagnosis of ARPKD to be made, physicians and patients should keep in mind that the absence of mutations does not exclude the diagnosis, as the overall mutation detection rate is <90% [178]. Also, some missense variants of unknown pathogenicity may be difficult to interpret. In addition, several other cystic diseases can phenocopy ARPKD, such as severe forms of ADPKD [42, 60], RCAD due to mutations of *HNF1B*, as well as rare hepatorenal fibrocystic diseases, including nephronophthisis, Joubert syndrome, and the related disorders of Bardet-Biedl and Meckel syndrome [172, 181, 182] (see Chap. 2).

Prenatal Diagnostics

In families with a previous child affected by ARPKD where the pathogenic alleles have been identified, prenatal genetic testing can provide an earlier diagnosis than ultrasound screening, as echographic abnormalities may arise only at the end of the second trimester or beyond. Molecular prenatal diagnostics is usually done after chorionic villus sampling between 10 and 12 weeks of pregnancy. In the past, haplotype-based linkage analysis was performed for ARPKD prenatal diagnosis, but given the existence of phenocopies and the possibility of further genetic heterogeneity, it is no longer a method of choice [152], and sequencing of *PKHD1* should have previously been conducted to identify the mutated alleles unequivocally. In the future, a harmless – yet challenging – alternative may be the development of noninvasive prenatal testing of the cell-free DNA in the mother's plasma.

Preimplantation Diagnosis (PGD)

PGD can be considered as a valuable alternative especially for couples having already experienced fetal loss or with an infant with the severe form of the disease [183, 184], provided that the mutations involved have previously been identified.

ARPKD Rodent Models

The PCK rat model is the rodent model most closely resembling human ARPKD, although the renal disease is progressive (ADPKD-like) and cysts as well as fibrosis are found in the liver [185, 186]. This model has been widely employed for preclinical testing in PKD [185]. A number of knockout mouse models of ARPKD have been described with a variety of *Pkhd1* mutations [139, 187–190]. All of the mouse models develop biliary dysgenesis and fibrosis, similar to human ARPKD, but the kidney disease is generally mild and late-onset compared to severe human ARPKD. Pancreatic cysts, including grossly enlarged pancreatic cystic disease, can occur. In contrast to ADPKD, abnormal ciliary structures have been described in several rodent models [187, 191]. A mouse generating tagged FPC has been helpful for analysis of the expression and processing of the protein, plus analysis of FPC containing exosomes [139].

Structure and Processing of Fibrocystin (FPC)

FPC is a large (4074aa) (447 kDa unglycosylated, ~550 kDa glycosylated) type I integral membrane protein. The large ectodomain of FPC contains 12 TIG/IPT domains (immunoglobulin-like fold shared by plexins and transcription factors), which is reminiscent of the above-described PKD1 repeats (Fig. 1.3) [160]. In addition in the extracellular region, a PA14 domain with a beta-barrel architecture that may be involved in carbohydrate binding, two G8 domains, and a region of 120aa that is glycine rich and composed of five β-strand pairs, plus two right-hand β-helical regions, have been defined [160, 161, 192–194]. At the C-terminus is a cytoplasmic tail of 192aa, which carries an 18-residue ciliary targeting signal [160, 161, 192, 193]. The protein is thought to be cleaved at a pro-protein convertase site between residues 3617 and 3620, with the extracellular region shed into the urine [195]. More controversially, cleavage of the C-tail has been suggested that is transported to the nucleus where it may activate transcription [195, 196].

Localization and Function of FPC

Unlike *PKD1* and *PKD2*, *PKHD1*/*Pkhd1* has a restricted expression pattern in the kidney, liver, pancreas, and lung [160]. Studies with a *Pkhd1*$^{lacZ/+}$ model showed expression in the renal collecting ducts, proximal tubules, Bowman's capsule, and pancreatic ducts, and regions of the *Pkhd1* promoter have been used to drive renal-specific expression of other genes, like *PKD1* [190, 197]. Antibody studies have localized FPC to the cortical and medullary collecting ducts and thick ascending limbs of the loop of Henle and in the biliary and pancreatic tracts [198]. At a subcellular level, FPC has been localized to the shaft of the cilium, to the basal body as well as to the mitotic spindle [198–200]. Like the polycystins, high quantities of mature FPC are found in exosomes [131, 139].

The precise function of fibrocystin is at present unknown, but it may mediate its activity through PC2 [201, 202], with which it is thought to interact through its C-terminal tail, regulating its expression and function. FPC has also been implicated in the maintenance of planar cell polarity (see Chap. 5), with disruption of FPC causing loss of oriented cell division [142].

Fibrocystin Paralog

A FPC paralog, fibrocystin-L, has sequence homolog with FPC throughout its length but, in contrast to FPC, is widely expressed in most tissues and conserved to fish (FPC is only conserved to frog [203]). The function of fibrocystin-L is unknown.

Acknowledgments These studies are supported by funding from the NIDDK (DK058816, DK059597, DK079856, and the Mayo Translational PKD Center: DK090728), the PKD Foundation, the Zell Family Foundation, Robert M. and Billie Kelley Pirnie, and the Mayo Clinic. ECLG is a recipient of an ASN Kidney Research Fellowship.

References

1. Torres VE, Harris PC, Pirson Y. Autosomal dominant polycystic kidney disease. Lancet. 2007;369(9569):1287–301.
2. Harris P, Torres VE. Polycystic kidney disease, autosomal dominant. GeneReviews [Internet]; Genetic Disease Online Reviews at GeneTests-GeneClinics (University of Washington, Seattle) http://www.

genetests.org/ 2015 [updated 2015]; Available from: httw://www.geneclinics.org.

3. Reeders ST, Zerres K, Gal A, Hogenkamp T, Propping P, Schmidt W, et al. Prenatal diagnosis of autosomal dominant polycystic kidney disease with a DNA probe. Lancet. 1986;ii:6–8.
4. Grantham JJ, Torres VE, Chapman AB, Guay-Woodford LM, Bae KT, King BF Jr, et al. Volume progression in polycystic kidney disease. N Engl J Med. 2006;354:2122–30.
5. Bae K, Park B, Sun H, Wang J, Tao C, Chapman AB, et al. Segmentation of individual renal cysts from MR images in patients with autosomal dominant polycystic kidney disease. Clin J Am Soc Nephrol: CJASN. 2013;8(7):1089–97.
6. Grantham JJ, Mulamalla S, Swenson-Fields KI. Why kidneys fail in autosomal dominant polycystic kidney disease. Nat Rev Nephrol. 2011;7(10):556–66.
7. Rossetti S, Strmecki L, Gamble V, Burton S, Sneddon V, Peral B, et al. Mutation analysis of the entire PKD1 gene: genetic and diagnostic implications. Am J Hum Genet. 2001;68(1):46–63.
8. Reeders ST, Breuning MH, Davies KE, Nicholls RD, Jarman AP, Higgs DR, et al. A highly polymorphic DNA marker linked to adult polycystic kidney disease on chromosome 16. Nature. 1985;317:542–4.
9. Consortium EPKD. The polycystic kidney disease 1 gene encodes a 14 kb transcript and lies within a duplicated region on chromosome 16. Cell. 1994;77(6):881–94.
10. Hughes J, Ward CJ, Peral B, Aspinwall R, Clark K, San Millán JL, et al. The polycystic kidney disease 1 (*PKD1*) gene encodes a novel protein with multiple cell recognition domains. Nat Genet. 1995;10(2):151–60.
11. International Polycystic Kidney Disease Consortium. Polycystic kidney disease: the complete structure of the *PKD1* gene and its protein. Cell. 1995;81(2):289–98.
12. Loftus BJ, Kim U-J, Sneddon VP, Kalush F, Brandon R, Fuhrmann J, et al. Genome duplications and other features in 12 Mbp of DNA sequence from human chromosome 16p and 16q. Genomics. 1999;60:295–308.
13. Phakdeekitcharoen B, Watnick T, Germino GG. Mutation analysis of the entire replicated portion of *PKD1* using genomic DNA samples. J Am Soc Nephrol. 2001;12:955–63.
14. Kimberling WJ, Fain PR, Kenyon JB, Goldgar D, Sujansky E, Gabow PA. Linkage heterogeneity of autosomal dominant polycystic kidney disease. N Engl J Med. 1988;319:913–8.
15. Peters DJM, Spruit L, Saris JJ, Ravine D, Sandkuijl LA, Fossdal R, et al. Chromosome 4 localization of a second gene for autosomal dominant polycystic kidney disease. Nat Genet. 1993;5:359–62.
16. Mochizuki T, Wu G, Hayashi T, Xenophontos SL, Veldhusien B, Saris JJ, et al. PKD2, a gene for polycystic kidney disease that encodes an integral membrane protein. Science. 1996;272(5266):1339–42.
17. Daoust MC, Reynolds DM, Bichet DG, Somlo S. Evidence for a third genetic locus for autosomal dominant polycystic kidney disease. Genomics. 1995;25:733–6.
18. de Almeida S, de Almeida E, Peters D, Pinto JR, Távora I, Lavinha J, et al. Autosomal dominant polycystic kidney disease: evidence for the existence of a third locus in a Portuguese family. Hum Genet. 1995;96:83–8.
19. Bogdanova N, Dworniczak B, Dragova D. Genetic heterogeneity of polycystic kidney disease in Bulgaria. Hum Genet. 1995;95:645–50.
20. Turco AE, Clementi M, Rossetti S, Tenconi R, Pignatti PF. An Italian family with autosomal dominant polycystic kidney disease unlinked to either the PKD1 or PKD2 gene. Am J Kidney Dis. 1996;28(5):759–61.
21. Ariza M, Alvarez V, Marin R, Aguado S, Lopez-Larrea C, Alvarez J, et al. A family with a milder form of adult dominant polycystic kidney disease not linked to the PKD1 (16p) or PKD2 (4q) genes. J Med Genet. 1997;34(7):587–9.
22. Paul BM, Consugar MB, Ryan Lee M, Sundsbak JL, Heyer CM, Rossetti S, et al. Evidence of a third ADPKD locus is not supported by re-analysis of designated PKD3 families. Kidney Int. 2014;85(2):383–92.
23. Porath B, Gainullin VG, Cornec-Le Gall E, Dillinger EK, Heyer CM, Hopp K, Edwards ME, Madsen CD, Mauritz SR, Banks CJ, Baheti S, Reddy B, Herrero JI, Banales JM, Hogan MC, Tasic V, Watnick TJ, Chapman AB, Vigneau C, Lavainne F, Audrezet MP, Ferec C, Le Meur Y, Torres VE, Genkyst Study Group HPoPKDG, Consortium for Radiologic Imaging Studies of Polycystic Kidney D, Harris PC. Mutations in GANAB, Encoding the Glucosidase IIalpha Subunit, Cause Autosomal-Dominant Polycystic Kidney and Liver Disease. Am J Hum Genet. 2016;98:1193–207.
24. Besse W, Dong K, Choi J, Punia S, Fedeles SV, Choi M, Gallagher AR, Huang EB, Gulati A, Knight J, Mane S, Tahvanainen E, Tahvanainen P, Sanna-Cherchi S, Lifton RP, Watnick T, Pei YP, Torres VE, Somlo S. Isolated polycystic liver disease genes define effectors of polycystin-1 function. J Clin Invest. 2017;127:1772–85.
25. Rossetti S, Chauveau D, Walker D, Saggar-Malik A, Winearls CG, Torres VE, et al. A complete mutation screen of the ADPKD genes by DHPLC. Kidney Int. 2002;61(5):1588–99.
26. Rossetti S, Consugar MB, Chapman AB, Torres VE, Guay-Woodford LM, Grantham JJ, et al. Comprehensive molecular diagnostics in autosomal dominant polycystic kidney disease. J Am Soc Nephrol. 2007;18(7):2143–60.
27. Audrezet MP, Cornec-Le Gall E, Chen JM, Redon S, Quere I, Creff J, et al. Autosomal dominant polycystic kidney disease: comprehensive mutation analysis of PKD1 and PKD2 in 700 unrelated patients. Hum Mutat. 2012;33(8):1239–50.

28. Rossetti S, Hopp K, Sikkink RA, Sundsbak JL, Lee YK, Kubly V, et al. Identification of gene mutations in autosomal dominant polycystic kidney disease through targeted resequencing. J Am Soc Nephrol. 2012;23(5):915–33.
29. Tan AY, Michaeel A, Liu G, Elemento O, Blumenfeld J, Donahue S, et al. Molecular diagnosis of autosomal dominant polycystic kidney disease using next-generation sequencing. J Mol Diagn. 2014;16(2):216–28.
30. Trujillano D, Bullich G, Ossowski S, Ballarin J, Torra R, Estivill X, et al. Diagnosis of autosomal dominant polycystic kidney disease using efficient PKD1 and PKD2 targeted next-generation sequencing. Mol Genet Genomic Med. 2014;2(5):412–21.
31. Yang T, Meng Y, Wei X, Shen J, Zhang M, Qi C, et al. Identification of novel mutations of PKD1 gene in Chinese patients with autosomal dominant polycystic kidney disease by targeted next-generation sequencing. Clin Chim Acta. 2014;433:12–9.
32. Consugar MB, Wong WC, Lundquist PA, Rossetti S, Kubly V, Walker DL, et al. Characterization of large rearrangements in autosomal dominant polycystic kidney disease and the *PKD1/TSC2* contiguous gene syndrome. Kidney Int. 2008;74(11):1468–79.
33. Cornec-Le Gall E, Audrezet MP, Chen JM, Hourmant M, Morin MP, Perrichot R, et al. Type of PKD1 mutation influences renal outcome in ADPKD. J Am Soc Nephrol. 2013;24(6):1006–13.
34. Hwang YH, Conklin J, Chan W, Roslin NM, Liu J, He N, et al. Refining genotype-phenotype correlation in autosomal dominant polycystic kidney disease. J Am Soc Nephrol. 2016;27(6):1861–8.
35. Drenth JP, Te Morsche RH, Smink R, Bonifacino JS, Jansen JB. Germline mutations in *PRKCSH* are associated with autosomal dominant polycystic liver disease. Nat Genet. 2003;33:345–7.
36. Li A, Davila S, Furu L, Qian Q, Tian X, Kamath PS, et al. Mutations in *PRKCSH* cause isolated autosomal dominant polycystic liver disease. Am J Hum Genet. 2003;72:691–703.
37. Davila S, Furu L, Gharavi AG, Tian X, Onoe T, Qian Q, et al. Mutations in *SEC63* cause autosomal dominant polycystic liver disease. Nat Genet. 2004;36(6):575–7.
38. Heidet L, Decramer S, Pawtowski A, Moriniere V, Bandin F, Knebelmann B, et al. Spectrum of *HNF1B* mutations in a large cohort of patients who harbor renal diseases. Clin J Am Soc Nephrol. 2010;5(6):1079–90.
39. Cnossen WR, Te Morsche RH, Hoischen A, Gilissen C, Chrispijn M, Venselaar H, et al. Whole-exome sequencing reveals LRP5 mutations and canonical Wnt signaling associated with hepatic cystogenesis. Proc Natl Acad Sci U S A. 2014;111(14):5343–8.
40. Cnossen WR, Te Morsche RH, Hoischen A, Gilissen C, Venselaar H, Mehdi S, et al. LRP5 variants may contribute to ADPKD. Eur J Hum Genet. 2016;24:237–42.
41. Rossetti S, Kubly V, Consugar MB, van't Hoff WG, Niaduet WP, Torres VE, et al. Incompletely penetrant *PKD1* alleles associated with mild, homozygous or in utero onset PKD. J Am Soc Nephrol. 2009;18:848–55.
42. Vujic M, Heyer CM, Ars E, Hopp K, Markoff A, Orndal C, et al. Incompletely penetrant *PKD1* alleles mimic the renal manifestations of ARPKD. J Am Soc Nephrol. 2010;21(7):1097–102.
43. Autosomal dominant polycystic kidney disease mutation database [database on the Internet] 2015 [accessed October 2015]. Available from: http://pkdb.mayo.edu.
44. Pei Y, Paterson AD, Wang KR, He N, Hefferton D, Watnick T, et al. Bilineal disease and trans-heterozygotes in autosomal dominant polycystic kidney disease. Am J Hum Genet. 2001;68:355–63.
45. Watnick TJ, Gandolph MA, Weber H, Neumann HPH, Germino GG. Gene conversion is a likely cause of mutation in *PKD1*. Hum Mol Genet. 1998;7:1239–43.
46. Tan AY, Blumenfeld J, Michaeel A, Donahue S, Bobb W, Parker T, et al. Autosomal dominant polycystic kidney disease caused by somatic and germline mosaicism. Clin Genet. 2015;87(4):373–7.
47. Reiterova J, Stekrova J, Merta M, Kotlas J, Elisakova V, Lnenicka P, et al. Autosomal dominant polycystic kidney disease in a family with mosaicism and hypomorphic allele. BMC Nephrol. 2013;14:59.
48. Connor A, Lunt PW, Dolling C, Patel Y, Meredith AL, Gardner A, et al. Mosaicism in autosomal dominant polycystic kidney disease revealed by genetic testing to enable living related renal transplantation. Am J Transplant. 2008;8(1):232–7.
49. Hateboer N, van Dijk MA, Bogdanova N, Coto E, Saggar-Malik AK, San Millan JL, et al. Comparison of phenotypes of polycystic kidney disease types 1 and 2. Lancet. 1999;353:103–7.
50. Rossetti S, Chauveau D, Kubly V, Slezak J, Saggar-Malik A, Pei Y, et al. Association of mutation position in polycystic kidney disease 1 (PKD1) gene and development of a vascular phenotype. Lancet. 2003;361:2196–201.
51. Bozza A, Aguiari G, Scapoli C, Scalia P, Perini L, De Paoli VE, et al. Autosomal dominant polycystic kidney disease linked to PKD2 locus in a family with severe extrarenal manifestations. Am J Nephrol. 1997;17(5):458–61.
52. Chebib FT, Jung Y, Heyer CM, Irazabal MV, Hogan MC, Harris PC, Torres VE, El-Zoghby ZM. Effect of genotype on the severity and volume progression of polycystic liver disease in ADPKD. Nephrol Dial Transplant. 2016;31:952–60.
53. Rossetti S, Burton S, Strmecki L, Pond GR, San Millán JL, Zerres K, et al. The position of the polycystic kidney disease 1 (PKD1) gene mutation correlates with the severity of renal disease. J Am Soc Nephrol. 2002;13(5):1230–7.

54. Magistroni R, He N, Wang K, Andrew R, Johnson A, Gabow P, et al. Genotype-renal function correlation in type 2 autosomal dominant polycystic kidney disease. J Am Soc Nephrol. 2003;14(5):1164–74.
55. Harris PC, Hopp K. The mutation, a key determinant of phenotype in ADPKD. J Am Soc Nephrol. 2013;24(6):868–70.
56. Cornec-Le Gall E, Audrezet MP, Rousseau A, Hourmant M, Renaudineau E, Charasse C, et al. The PROPKD score: a new algorithm to predict renal survival in autosomal dominant polycystic kidney disease. J Am Soc Nephrol. 2016;27(3):942–51.
57. Paterson AD, Wang KR, Lupea D, St George-Hyslop P, Pei Y. Recurrent fetal loss associated with bilineal inheritance of type 1 autosomal dominant polycystic kidney disease. Am J Kidney Dis. 2002;40(1):16–20.
58. Zerres K, Rudnik-Schöneborn S, Deget F. German working group on paediatric nephrology. Childhood onset autosomal dominant polycystic kidney disease in sibs: clinical picture and recurrence risk. J Med Genet. 1993;30(7):583–8.
59. Hopp K, Ward CJ, Hommerding CJ, Nasr SH, Tuan HF, Gainullin VG, et al. Functional polycystin-1 dosage governs autosomal dominant polycystic kidney disease severity. J Clin Invest. 2012;122(11):4257–73.
60. Audrezet MP, Corbiere C, Lebbah S, Moriniere V, Broux F, Louillet F, et al. Comprehensive PKD1 and PKD2 mutation analysis in prenatal autosomal dominant polycystic kidney disease. J Am Soc Nephrol. 2016;27(3):722–9.
61. Losekoot M, Ruivenkamp CA, Tholens AP, Grimbergen JE, Vijfhuizen L, Vermeer S, et al. Neonatal onset autosomal dominant polycystic kidney disease (ADPKD) in a patient homozygous for a PKD2 missense mutation due to uniparental disomy. J Med Genet. 2012;49(1):37–40.
62. Bergmann C, von Bothmer J, Ortiz Bruchle N, Venghaus A, Frank V, Fehrenbach H, et al. Mutations in multiple PKD genes may explain early and severe polycystic kidney disease. J Am Soc Nephrol. 2011;22(11):2047–56.
63. Pei Y, Lan Z, Wang K, Garcia-Gonzalez M, He N, Dicks E, et al. A missense mutation in PKD1 attenuates the severity of renal disease. Kidney Int. 2012;81(4):412–7.
64. Gainullin VG, Hopp K, Ward CJ, Hommerding CJ, Harris PC. Polycystin-1 maturation requires polycystin-2 in a dose-dependent manner. J Clin Invest. 2015;125(2):607–20.
65. Harris PC, Ward CJ, Peral B, Hughes J. Autosomal dominant polycystic kidney disease: molecular analysis. Hum Mol Genet. 1995;4:1745–9.
66. Brook-Carter PT, Peral B, Ward CJ, Thompson P, Hughes J, Maheshwar MM, et al. Deletion of the *TSC2* and *PKD1* genes associated with severe infantile polycystic kidney disease – a contiguous gene syndrome. Nat Genet. 1994;8:328–32.
67. Sampson JR, Maheshwar MM, Aspinwall R, Thompson P, Cheadle JP, Ravine D, et al. Renal cystic disease in tuberous sclerosis: role of the polycystic kidney disease 1 gene. Am J Hum Genet. 1997;61:843–51.
68. Kleymenova E, Ibraghimov-Beskrovnaya O, Kugoh H, Everitt J, Xu H, Kiguchi K, et al. Tuberin-dependent membrane localization of polycystin-1: a functional link between polycystic kidney disease and the TSC2 tumor suppressor gene. Mol Cell. 2001;7:823–32.
69. Shillingford JM, Murcia NS, Larson CH, Low SH, Hedgepeth R, Brown N, et al. The mTOR pathway is regulated by polycystin-1, and its inhibition reverses renal cystogenesis in polycystic kidney disease. Proc Natl Acad Sci U S A. 2006;103(14):5466–71.
70. Harris PC, Rossetti S. Molecular diagnostics for autosomal dominant polycystic kidney disease. Nat Rev Nephrol. 2010;6(4):197–206.
71. MacDermot KD, Saggar-Malik AK, Economides DL, Jeffery S. Prenatal diagnosis of autosomal dominant polycystic kidney disease (PKD1) presenting in utero and prognosis for very early onset disease. J Med Genet. 1998;35:13–6.
72. Zeevi DA, Renbaum P, Ron-El R, Eldar-Geva T, Raziel A, Brooks B, et al. Preimplantation genetic diagnosis in genomic regions with duplications and pseudogenes: long-range PCR in the single-cell assay. Hum Mutat. 2013;34(5):792–9.
73. De Rycke M, Georgiou I, Sermon K, Lissens W, Henderix P, Joris H, et al. PGD for autosomal dominant polycystic kidney disease type 1. Mol Hum Reprod. 2005;11(1):65–71.
74. Lu W, Peissel B, Babakhanlou H, Pavlova A, Geng L, Fan X, et al. Perinatal lethality with kidney and pancreas defects in mice with a targeted *PKD1* mutation. Nat Genet. 1997;17(2):179–81.
75. Wu G, Somlo S. Molecular genetics and mechanism of autosomal dominant polycystic kidney disease. Mol Genet Metab. 2000;69:1–15.
76. Lu W, Fan X, Basora N, Babakhanlou H, Law T, Rifai N, et al. Late onset of renal and hepatic cysts in *Pkd1*-targeted heterozygotes. Nat Genet. 1999;21:160–1.
77. Wu G, D'Agati V, Cai Y, Markowitz G, Park JH, Reynolds DM, et al. Somatic inactivation of *PKD2* results in polycystic kidney disease. Cell. 1998;93(2):177–88.
78. Torres VE, Wang X, Qian Q, Somlo S, Harris PC, Gattone VH. Effective treatment of an orthologous model of autosomal dominant polycystic kidney disease. Nat Med. 2004;10:363–4.
79. Piontek K, Menezes LF, Garcia-Gonzalez MA, Huso DL, Germino GG. A critical developmental switch defines the kinetics of kidney cyst formation after loss of Pkd1. Nat Med. 2007;13(12):1490–5.
80. Lantinga-van Leeuwen IS, Leonhard WN, van der Wal A, Breuning MH, de Heer E, Peters DJ. Kidney-specific inactivation of the PKD1 gene induces rapid cyst formation in developing kidneys and a slow onset of disease in adult mice. Hum Mol Genet. 2007;16(24):3188–96.

81. Shillingford JM, Piontek KB, Germino GG, Weimbs T. Rapamycin ameliorates PKD resulting from conditional inactivation of *Pkd1*. J Am Soc Nephrol. 2010;21(3):489–97.
82. Leonhard WN, Zandbergen M, Veraar K, van den Berg S, van der Weerd L, Breuning M, et al. Scattered deletion of PKD1 in kidneys causes a cystic snowball effect and recapitulates polycystic kidney disease. J Am Soc Nephrol: JASN. 2015;26(6):1322–33.
83. Fedeles SV, Tian X, Gallagher AR, Mitobe M, Nishio S, Lee SH, et al. A genetic interaction network of five genes for human polycystic kidney and liver diseases defines polycystin-1 as the central determinant of cyst formation. Nat Genet. 2011;43(7):639–47.
84. Lantinga-van Leeuwen IS, Dauwerse JG, Baelde HJ, Leonhard WN, van de Wal A, Ward CJ, et al. Lowering of PKD1 expression is sufficient to cause polycystic kidney disease. Hum Mol Genet. 2004;13(24):3069–77.
85. Jiang ST, Chiou YY, Wang E, Lin HK, Lin YT, Chi YC, et al. Defining a link with autosomal-dominant polycystic kidney disease in mice with congenitally low expression of *Pkd1*. Am J Pathol. 2006;168(1):205–20.
86. Happe H, van der Wal AM, Salvatori DC, Leonhard WN, Breuning MH, de Heer E, et al. Cyst expansion and regression in a mouse model of polycystic kidney disease. Kidney Int. 2013;83(6):1099–108. https://doi.org/10.1038/ki2013132013.
87. Hopp K, Hommerding CJ, Wang X, Ye H, Harris PC, Torres VE. Tolvaptan plus Pasireotide shows enhanced efficacy in a PKD1 model. J Am Soc Nephrol. 2014;26(1):39–47.
88. Reeders ST. Multilocus polycystic disease. Nat Genet. 1992;1:235–7.
89. Qian F, Watnick TJ, Onuchic LF, Germino GG. The molecular basis of focal cyst formation in human autosomal dominant polycystic kidney disease type I. Cell. 1996;87(6):979–87.
90. Brasier JL, Henske EP. Loss of the polycystic kidney disease (*PKD1*) region of chromosome 16p13 in renal cyst cells supports a loss-of-function model for cyst pathogenesis. J Clin Invest. 1997;99:194–9.
91. Watnick TJ, Torres VE, Gandolph MA, Qian F, Onuchic LF, Klinger KW, et al. Somatic mutation in individual liver cysts supports a two-hit model of cystogenesis in autosomal dominant polycystic kidney disease. Mol Cell. 1998;2:247–51.
92. Harris PC, Bae K, Rossetti S, Torres VE, Grantham JJ, Chapman A, et al. Cyst number but not the rate of cystic growth is associated with the mutated gene in ADPKD. J Am Soc Nephrol. 2006;17(11): 3013–9.
93. Nishio S, Hatano M, Nagata M, Horie S, Koike T, Tokuhisa T, et al. PKD1 regulates immortalized proliferation of renal tubular epithelial cells through p53 induction and JNK activation. J Clin Invest. 2005;115(4):910–8.
94. Watnick T, He N, Wang K, Liang Y, Parfrey P, Hefferton D, et al. Mutations of *PKD1* in ADPKD2 cysts suggest a pathogenic effect of trans-heterozygous mutations. Nat Genet. 2000;25:143–4.
95. Koptides M, Mean R, Demetriou K, Pierides A, Deltas CC. Genetic evidence for a trans-heterozygous model for cystogenesis in autosomal dominant polycystic kidney disease. Hum Mol Genet. 2000;9(3):447–52.
96. Gallagher AR, Germino GG, Somlo S. Molecular advances in autosomal dominant polycystic kidney disease. Adv Chronic Kidney Dis. 2010;17(2):118–30.
97. Cornec-Le Gall E, Audrezet M, Le Meur Y, Chen J, Ferec C. Genetics and pathogenesis of autosomal dominant polycystic kidney disease: 20 years on. Hum Mutat. 2014. 2014;35(12):1393–406.
98. Takakura A, Contrino L, Zhou X, Bonventre JV, Sun Y, Humphreys BD, et al. Renal injury is a third hit promoting rapid development of adult polycystic kidney disease. Hum Mol Genet. 2009;18(14):2523–31.
99. Happé H, Leonhard WN, van der Wal A, van de Water B, Lantinga-van Leeuwen IS, Breuning MH, et al. Toxic tubular injury in kidneys from *Pkd1*-deletion mice accelerates cystogenesis accompanied by dysregulated planar cell polarity and canonical Wnt signaling pathways. Hum Mol Genet. 2009;18(14):2532–42.
100. Liu X-G, Shi S, Senthilnathan S, Yu J, Wu E, Bergmann C, et al. Genetic variation of DKK3 may modify renal disease severity in PKD1. J Am Soc Nephrol. 2010;21:1510–20.
101. Qian F, Germino FJ, Cai Y, Zhang X, Somlo S, Germino GG. PKD1 interacts with PKD2 through a probable coiled-coil domain. Nat Genet. 1997;16(2):179–83.
102. Oatley P, Stewart AP, Sandford R, Edwardson JM. Atomic force microscopy imaging reveals the domain structure of polycystin-1. Biochemistry. 2012;51(13):2879–88.
103. Ong AC, Harris PC. A polycystin-centric view of cyst formation and disease: the polycystins revisited. Kidney Int. 2015;88(4):699–710.
104. Forman JR, Qamar S, Paci E, Sandford RN, Clarke J. The remarkable mechanical strength of polycystin-1 supports a direct role in mechanotransduction. J Mol Biol. 2005;349(4):861–71.
105. Qian F, Wei W, Germino G, Oberhauser A. The nanomechanics of polycystin-1 extracellular region. J Biol Chem. 2005;280(49):40723–30.
106. Xu M, Ma L, Bujalowski PJ, Qian F, Sutton RB, Oberhauser AF. Analysis of the REJ module of polycystin-1 using molecular modeling and force-spectroscopy techniques. J Biophys. 2013;2013:525231.
107. Xu Y, Streets AJ, Hounslow AM, Tran U, Jean-Alphonse F, Needham AJ, et al. The polycystin-1, lipoxygenase, and alpha-toxin domain regulates polycystin-1 trafficking. J Am Soc Nephrol. 2016;27:1159–73.
108. Qian F, Boletta A, Bhunia AK, Xu H, Liu L, Ahrabi AK, et al. Cleavage of polycystin-1 requires the

receptor for egg jelly domain and is disrupted by human autosomal-dominant polycystic kidney disease 1- associated mutations. Proc Natl Acad Sci U S A. 2002;99(26):16981–6.
109. Yu S, Hackmann K, Gao J, He X, Piontek K, Garcia-Gonzalez MA, et al. Essential role of cleavage of polycystin-1 at G protein-coupled receptor proteolytic site for kidney tubular structure. Proc Natl Acad Sci U S A. 2007;104(47):18688–93.
110. Kurbegovic A, Kim H, Xu H, Yu S, Cruanes J, Maser RL, et al. Novel functional complexity of polycystin-1 by GPS cleavage in vivo: role in polycystic kidney disease. Mol Cell Biol. 2014;34(17):3341–53.
111. Chapin HC, Rajendran V, Caplan MJ. Polycystin-1 surface localization is stimulated by polycystin-2 and cleavage at the G protein-coupled receptor proteolytic site. Mol Biol Cell. 2010;21(24):4338–48.
112. Arac D, Boucard AA, Bolliger MF, Nguyen J, Soltis SM, Sudhof TC, et al. A novel evolutionarily conserved domain of cell-adhesion GPCRs mediates autoproteolysis. EMBO J. 2012;31(6):1364–78.
113. Chauvet V, Tian X, Husson H, Grimm DH, Wang T, Hieseberger T, et al. Mechanical stimuli induce cleavage and nuclear translocation of the polycystin-1 C terminus. J Clin Invest. 2004;114(10):1433–43.
114. Low SH, Vasanth S, Larson CH, Mukherjee S, Sharma N, Kinter MT, et al. Polycystin-1, STAT6, and P100 function in a pathway that transduces ciliary mechanosensation and is activated in polycystic kidney disease. Dev Cell. 2006;10(1):57–69.
115. Allen MD, Qamar S, Vadivelu MK, Sandford RN, Bycroft M. A high-resolution structure of the EF-hand domain of human polycystin-2. Protein Sci. 2014;23(9):1301–8.
116. Celic A, Petri ET, Demeler B, Ehrlich BE, Boggon TJ. Domain mapping of the polycystin-2 C-terminal tail using de novo molecular modeling and biophysical analysis. J Biol Chem. 2008;283(42): 28305–12.
117. Giamarchi A, Feng S, Rodat-Despoix L, Xu Y, Bubenshchikova E, Newby LJ, et al. A polycystin-2 (TRPP2) dimerization domain essential for the function of heteromeric polycystin complexes. EMBO J. 2010;29(7):1176–91.
118. Yu Y, Ulbrich MH, Li MH, Buraei Z, Chen XZ, Ong AC, et al. Structural and molecular basis of the assembly of the TRPP2/PKD1 complex. Proc Natl Acad Sci U S A. 2009;106(28):11558–63.
119. Streets AJ, Wessely O, Peters DJ, Ong AC. Hyperphosphorylation of polycystin-2 at a critical residue in disease reveals an essential role for polycystin-1-regulated dephosphorylation. Hum Mol Genet. 2013;22(10):1924–39.
120. Gonzalez-Perrett S, Kim K, Ibarra C, Damiano AE, Zotta E, Batelli M, et al. Polycystin-2, the protein mutated in autosomal dominant polycystic kidney disease (ADPKD), is a Ca^{2+}-permeable nonselective cation channel. Proc Natl Acad Sci U S A. 2001;98(3):1182–7.
121. Koulen P, Cai Y, Geng L, Maeda Y, Nishimura S, Witzgall R, et al. Polycystin-2 is an intracellular calcium release channel. Nat Cell Biol. 2002;4:191–7.
122. Shen PS, Yang X, DeCaen PG, Liu X, Bulkley D, Clapham DE, Cao E. The Structure of the Polycystic Kidney Disease Channel PKD2 in Lipid Nanodiscs. Cell, 167. 2016;e711:763–73.
123. Grieben M, Pike AC, Shintre CA, Venturi E, El-Ajouz S, Tessitore A, Shrestha L, Mukhopadhyay S, Mahajan P, Chalk R, Burgess-Brown NA, Sitsapesan R, Huiskonen JT, Carpenter EP. Structure of the polycystic kidney disease TRP channel Polycystin-2 (PC2). Nat Struct Mol Biol. 2017;24:114–22.
124. Wilkes M, Madej MG, Kreuter L, Rhinow D, Heinz V, De Sanctis S, Ruppel S, Richter RM, Joos F, Grieben M, Pike AC, Huiskonen JT, Carpenter EP, Kuhlbrandt W, Witzgall R, Ziegler C. Molecular insights into lipid-assisted Ca2+ regulation of the TRP channel Polycystin-2. Nat Struct Mol Biol. 2017;24:123–30.
125. The polycystic kidney disease 1 gene encodes a 14 kb transcript and lies within a duplicated region on chromosome 16. The European Polycystic Kidney Disease Consortium. Cell. 1994;77(6):881–94.
126. Markowitz GS, Cai YQ, Li L, Wu GQ, Ward LC, Somlo S, et al. Polycystin-2 expression is developmentally regulated. Am J Physiol – Renal Fluid Electro Physiol. 1999;46(1):F17–25.
127. Ward CJ, Turley H, Ong ACM, Comley M, Biddolph S, Chetty R, et al. Polycystin, the polycystic kidney disease 1 protein, is expressed by epithelial cells in fetal, adult and polycystic kidney. Proc Natl Acad Sci U S A. 1996;93:1524–8.
128. Hildebrandt F, Benzing T, Katsanis N. Ciliopathies. New Eng J Med. 2011;364(16):1533–43.
129. Kim H, Xu H, Yao Q, Li W, Huang Q, Outeda P, et al. Ciliary membrane proteins traffic through the Golgi via a Rabepl/GGA1/Arl3-dependent mechanism. Nat Commun. 2014;5:5482.
130. Scheffers MS, van der Bent P, Prins F, Spruit L, Breuning MH, Litvinov SV, et al. Polycystin-1, the product of the polycystic kidney disease 1 gene, co-localizes with desmosomes in MDCK cells. Hum Mol Genet. 2000;9(18):2743–50.
131. Hogan MC, Manganelli L, Woollard JR, Masyuk AI, Masyuk TV, Tammachote R, et al. Characterization of PKD protein-positive exosome-like vesicles. J Am Soc Nephrol. 2009;20(2):278–88.
132. Cai Y, Maeda Y, Cedzich A, Torres VE, Wu G, Hayashi T, et al. Identification and characterization of polycystin-2, the PKD2 gene product. J Biol Chem. 1999;274:28557–65.
133. Anyatonwu GI, Estrada M, Tian X, Somlo S, Ehrlich BE. Regulation of ryanodine receptor-dependent calcium signaling by polycystin-2. Proc Natl Acad Sci U S A. 2007;104(15):6454–9.
134. Li Y, Wright JM, Qian F, Germino GG, Guggino WB. Polycystin 2 interacts with type I inositol 1,4,5-trisphosphate receptor to modulate

intracellular Ca^{2+} signaling. J Biol Chem. 2005;280(50):41298–306.
135. Praetorius HA, Spring KR. Bending the MDCK cell primary cilium increases intracellular calcium. J Membr Biol. 2001;184(1):71–9.
136. Nauli SM, Alenghat FJ, Luo Y, Williams E, Vassilev P, Li X, et al. Polycystins 1 and 2 mediate mechanosensation in the primary cilium of kidney cells. Nat Genet. 2003;33(2):129–37.
137. Delling M, DeCaen PG, Doerner JF, Febvay S, Clapham DE. Primary cilia are specialized calcium signalling organelles. Nature. 2013;504(7479):311–4.
138. Ma M, Tian X, Igarashi P, Pazour GJ, Somlo S. Loss of cilia suppresses cyst growth in genetic models of autosomal dominant polycystic kidney disease. Nat Genet. 2013;45(9):1004–12.
139. Bakeberg JL, Tammachote R, Woollard JR, Hogan MC, Tuan H, van Deursen JM, et al. Epitope-tagged Pkhd1 tracks the processing, secretion, and localization of fibrocystin. J Am Soc Nephrol. 2011;22(12):2266–77.
140. Chebib FT, Sussman CR, Wang X, Harris PC, Torres VE. Vasopressin and disruption of calcium signalling in polycystic kidney disease. Nat Rev Nephrol. 2015;11(8):451–64.
141. Yuan S, Zhao L, Brueckner M, Sun Z. Intraciliary calcium oscillations initiate vertebrate left-right asymmetry. Curr Biol. 2015;25(5):556–67.
142. Fischer E, Legue E, Doyen A, Nato F, Nicolas JF, Torres V, et al. Defective planar cell polarity in polycystic kidney disease. Nat Genet. 2006;38(1):21–3.
143. Nishio S, Tian X, Gallagher AR, Yu Z, Patel V, Igarashi P, et al. Loss of oriented cell division does not initiate cyst formation. J Am Soc Nephrol. 2010;21(2):295–302.
144. Bhunia AK, Piontek K, Boletta A, Liu L, Qian F, Xu PN, et al. *PKD1* induces $p21^{waf1}$ and regulation of the cell cycle via direct activation of the JAK-STAT signaling pathway in a process requiring *PKD2*. Cell. 2002;109(2):157–68.
145. Streets AJ, Newby LJ, O'Hare MJ, Bukanov NO, Ibraghimov-Beskrovnaya O, Ong AC. Functional analysis of PKD1 transgenic lines reveals a direct role for polycystin-1 in mediating cell-cell adhesion. J Am Soc Nephrol. 2003;14:1804–15.
146. Field S, Riley KL, Grimes DT, Hilton H, Simon M, Powles-Glover N, et al. Pkd1l1 establishes left-right asymmetry and physically interacts with Pkd2. Development. 2011;138(6):1131–42.
147. Kamura K, Kobayashi D, Uehara Y, Koshida S, Iijima N, Kudo A, et al. Pkd1l1 complexes with PKD2 on motile cilia and functions to establish the left-right axis. Development. 2011;138(6):1121–9.
148. Sutton KA, Jungnickel MK, Ward CJ, Harris PC, Florman HM. Functional characterization of PKDREJ, a male germ cell-restricted polycystin. J Cell Physiol. 2006;209(2):493–500.
149. Chen Y, Zhang Z, Lv XY, Wang YD, Hu ZG, Sun H, et al. Expression of Pkd2l2 in testis is implicated in spermatogenesis. Biol Pharm Bull. 2008;31(8):1496–500.
150. Ishimaru Y, Inada H, Kubota M, Zhuang H, Tominaga M, Matsunami H. Transient receptor potential family members PKD1L3 and PKD2L1 form a candidate sour taste receptor. Proc Natl Acad Sci U S A. 2006;103(33):12569–74.
151. Mackenzie FE, Romero R, Williams D, Gillingwater T, Hilton H, Dick J, et al. Upregulation of PKD1L2 provokes a complex neuromuscular disease in the mouse. Hum Mol Genet. 2009;18(19):3553–66.
152. Guay-Woodford LM, Bissler JJ, Braun MC, Bockenhauer D, Cadnapaphornchai MA, Dell KM, et al. Consensus expert recommendations for the diagnosis and management of autosomal recessive polycystic kidney disease: report of an international conference. J Pediatr. 2014;165(3):611–7.
153. Shneider BL, Magid MS. Liver disease in autosomal recessive polycystic kidney disease. Pediatr Transplant. 2005;9(5):634–9.
154. Adeva M, El-Youssef M, Rossetti S, Kamath PS, Kubly V, Consugar M, et al. Clinical and molecular characterization defines a broadened spectrum of autosomal recessive polycystic kidney disease (ARPKD). Medicine. 2006;85(1):1–21.
155. Zerres K, Mücher G, Bachner L, Deschennes G, Eggermann T, Kääriäinen H, et al. Mapping of the gene for autosomal recessive polycystic kidney disease (ARPKD) to chromosome 6p21-cen. Nat Genet. 1994;7:429–32.
156. Guay-Woodford LM, Muecher G, Hopkins SD, Avner ED, Germino GG, Guillot AP, et al. The severe perinatal form of autosomal recessive polycystic kidney disease maps to chromosome 6p21.1-p12: implications for genetic counseling. Am J Hum Genet. 1995;56:1101–7.
157. Lens XM, Onuchic LF, Wu G, Hayashi T, Daoust M, Mochizuki T, et al. An integrated genetic and physical map of the autosomal recessive polycystic kidney disease region. Genomics. 1997;41(3):463–6.
158. Mücher G, Becker J, Knapp M, Büttner R, Moser M, Rudnik-Schöneborn S, et al. Fine mapping of the autosomal recessive polycystic kidney disease locus (PKHD1) and the genes MUT, RDS, CSNK2β, and GSTA1 at 6p21.2-p12. Genomics. 1998;48:40–5.
159. Park JH, Dixit MP, Onuchic LF, Wu G, Goncharuk AN, Kneitz S, et al. A 1-Mb BAC/PAC-based physical map of the autosomal recessive polycystic kidney disease gene (*PKHD1*) region on chromosome 6. Genomics. 1999;57(2):249–55.
160. Ward CJ, Hogan MC, Rossetti S, Walker D, Sneddon T, Wang X, et al. The gene mutated in autosomal recessive polycystic kidney disease encodes a large, receptor-like protein. Nat Genet. 2002;30(3):259–69.
161. Onuchic LF, Furu L, Nagasawa Y, Hou X, Eggermann T, Ren Z, et al. *PKHD1*, the polycystic kidney and hepatic disease 1 gene, encodes a novel large protein containing multiple immunoglobulin-like plexin-transcription-factor domains and parallel beta-helix 1 repeats. Am J Hum Genet. 2002;70(5):1305–17.

162. Bergmann C, Frank V, Kupper F, Schmidt C, Senderek J, Zerres K. Functional analysis of PKHD1 splicing in autosomal recessive polycystic kidney disease. J Hum Genet. 2006;51(9):788–93.
163. Boddu R, Yang C, O'Connor AK, Hendrickson RC, Boone B, Cui X, et al. Intragenic motifs regulate the transcriptional complexity of Pkhd1/PKHD1. J Mol Med (Berl). 2014;92(10):1045–56.
164. Frank V, Zerres K, Bergmann C. Transcriptional complexity in autosomal recessive polycystic kidney disease. Clin J Am Soc Nephrol. 2014;9(10):1729–36.
165. Bergmann C, Senderek J, Sedlacek B, Pegiazoglou I, Puglia P, Eggermann T, et al. Spectrum of mutations in the gene for autosomal recessive polycystic kidney disease (ARPKD/PKHD1). J Am Soc Nephrol. 2003;14(1):76–89.
166. Rossetti S, Torra R, Coto E, Consugar M, Kubly V, Malaga S, et al. A complete mutation screen of *PKHD1* in autosomal recessive polycystic kidney pedigrees. Kidney Int. 2003;64:391–403.
167. Furu L, Onuchic LF, Gharavi AG, Hou X, Esquivel EL, Nagasawa Y, et al. Milder presentation of recessive polycystic kidney disease requires presence of amino acid substitution mutations. J Am Soc Nephrol. 2003;14:2004–14.
168. Sharp AM, Messiaen LM, Page G, Antignac C, Gubler MC, Onuchic LF, et al. Comprehensive genomic analysis of *PKHD1* mutations in ARPKD cohorts. J Med Genet. 2005;42(4):336–49.
169. Bergmann C, Kupper F, Dornia C, Schneider F, Senderek J, Zerres K. Algorithm for efficient *PKHD1* mutation screening in autosomal recessive polycystic kidney disease (ARPKD). Hum Mutat. 2005;25(3):225–31.
170. Consugar MB, Anderson SA, Rossetti S, Pankratz VS, Ward CJ, Torra R, et al. Haplotype analysis improves molecular diagnostics of autosomal recessive polycystic kidney disease. Am J Kidney Dis. 2005;45:77–87.
171. Krall P, Pineda C, Ruiz P, Ejarque L, Vendrell T, Camacho JA, et al. Cost-effective PKHD1 genetic testing for autosomal recessive polycystic kidney disease. Pediatr Nephrol. 2014;29(2):223–34.
172. Hartung EA, Guay-Woodford LM. Autosomal recessive polycystic kidney disease: a hepatorenal fibrocystic disorder with pleiotropic effects. Pediatrics. 2014;134(3):e833–45.
173. Tavira B, Gomez J, Malaga S, Santos F, Fernandez-Aracama J, Alonso B, et al. A labor and cost effective next generation sequencing of PKHD1 in autosomal recessive polycystic kidney disease patients. Gene. 2015;561(1):165–9.
174. Eisenberger T, Decker C, Hiersche M, Hamann RC, Decker E, Neuber S, et al. An efficient and comprehensive strategy for genetic diagnostics of polycystic kidney disease. PLoS One. 2015;10(2):e0116680.
175. Denamur E, Delezoide AL, Alberti C, Bourillon A, Gubler MC, Bouvier R, et al. Genotype-phenotype correlations in fetuses and neonates with autosomal recessive polycystic kidney disease. Kidney Int. 2010;77(4):350–8.
176. Bergmann C, Senderek J, Windelen E, Kupper F, Middeldorf I, Schneider F, et al. Clinical consequences of *PKHD1* mutations in 164 patients with autosomal-recessive polycystic kidney disease (ARPKD). Kidney Int. 2005;67(3):829–48.
177. Ebner K, Feldkoetter M, Ariceta G, Bergmann C, Buettner R, Doyon A, et al. Rationale, design and objectives of ARegPKD, a European ARPKD registry study. BMC Nephrol. 2015;16:22.
178. Sweeney WE, Avner ED. Polycystic kidney disease, autosomal recessive. In: Pagon RA, Adam MP, Ardinger HH, Bird TD, Dolan CR, Fong CT, et al., editors. GeneReviews(R). Seattle: University of Washington, Seattle; 2014. Internet. http://www.ncbi.nlm.nih.gov/pubmed/20301501.
179. Gunay-Aygun M, Turkbey BI, Bryant J, Daryanani KT, Gerstein MT, Piwnica-Worms K, Choyke P, Heller T, Gahl WA. Hepatorenal findings in obligate heterozygotes for autosomal recessive polycystic kidney disease. Mol Genet Metab. 2011;104:677–81.
180. Zvereff V, Yao S, Ramsey J, Mikhail FM, Vijzelaar R, Messiaen L. Identification of PKHD1 multi-exon deletions using multiplex ligation-dependent probe amplification and quantitative polymerase chain reaction. Genet Test Mol Biomarkers. 2010;14(4):505–10.
181. Gunay-Aygun M, Parisi MA, Doherty D, Tuchman M, Tsilou E, Kleiner DE, et al. MKS3-related ciliopathy with features of autosomal recessive polycystic kidney disease, nephronophthisis, and Joubert Syndrome. J Pediatr. 2009;155(3):386–92 e1.
182. Bergmann C. ARPKD and early manifestations of ADPKD: the original polycystic kidney disease and phenocopies. Pediatr Nephrol. 2015;30:15–30.
183. Gigarel N, Frydman N, Burlet P, Kerbrat V, Tachdjian G, Fanchin R, et al. Preimplantation genetic diagnosis for autosomal recessive polycystic kidney disease. Reprod Biomed Online. 2008;16(1):152–8.
184. Lau EC, Janson MM, Roesler MR, Avner ED, Strawn EY, Bick DP. Birth of a healthy infant following preimplantation *PKHD1* haplotyping for autosomal recessive polycystic kidney disease using multiple displacement amplification. J Assist Reprod Genet. 2010;27(7):397–407.
185. Gattone VH 2nd, Wang X, Harris PC, Torres VE. Inhibition of renal cystic disease development and progression by a vasopressin V2 receptor antagonist. Nature Med. 2003;9(10):1323–6.
186. Lager DJ, Qian Q, Bengal RJ, Ishibashi M, Torres VE. The pck rat: a new model that resembles human autosomal dominant polycystic kidney and liver disease. Kidney Int. 2001;59(1):126–36.
187. Woollard JR, Punyashtiti R, Richardson S, Masyuk TV, Whelan S, Huang BQ, et al. A mouse model of autosomal recessive polycystic kidney disease with biliary duct and proximal tubule dilatation. Kidney Int. 2007;72(3):328–36.

188. Garcia-Gonzalez MA, Menezes LF, Piontek KB, Kaimori J, Huso DL, Watnick T, et al. Genetic interaction studies link autosomal dominant and recessive polycystic kidney disease in a common pathway. Hum Mol Genet. 2007;16(16):1940–50.
189. Gallagher AR, Esquivel EL, Briere TS, Tian X, Mitobe M, Menezes LF, et al. Biliary and pancreatic dysgenesis in mice harboring a mutation in Pkhd1. Am J Pathol. 2008;172(2):417–29.
190. Williams SS, Cobo-Stark P, James LR, Somlo S, Igarashi P. Kidney cysts, pancreatic cysts, and biliary disease in a mouse model of autosomal recessive polycystic kidney disease. Pediatr Nephrol. 2008;23(5):733–41.
191. Masyuk TV, Huang BQ, Ward CJ, Masyuk AI, Yuan D, Splinter PL, et al. Defects in cholangiocyte fibrocystin expression and ciliary structure in the PCK rat. Gastroenterology. 2003;125:1303–10.
192. Follit JA, Li L, Vucica Y, Pazour GJ. The cytoplasmic tail of fibrocystin contains a ciliary targeting sequence. J Cell Biol. 2010;188:21–8.
193. He QY, Liu XH, Li Q, Studholme DJ, Li XW, Liang SP. G8: a novel domain associated with polycystic kidney disease and non-syndromic hearing loss. Bioinformatics. 2006;22(18):2189–91.
194. Rigden DJ, Mello LV, Galperin MY. The PA14 domain, a conserved all β–domain in bacterial toxins, enzymes, adhesins and signaling molecules. Trends Biochem Sci. 2004;29(7):335–9.
195. Kaimori JY, Nagasawa Y, Menezes LF, Garcia-Gonzalez MA, Deng J, Imai E, et al. Polyductin undergoes notch-like processing and regulated release from primary cilia. Hum Mol Genet. 2007;16(8):942–56.
196. Hiesberger T, Gourley E, Erickson A, Koulen P, Ward CJ, Masyuk TV, et al. Proteolytic cleavage and nuclear translocation of fibrocystin is regulated by intracellular Ca2+ and activation of protein kinase C. J Biol Chem. 2006;281(45):34357–64.
197. Williams SS, Cobo-Stark P, Hajarnis S, Aboudehen K, Shao X, Richardson JA, et al. Tissue-specific regulation of the mouse Pkhd1 (ARPKD) gene promoter. Am J Physiol Renal Physiol. 2014;307(3): F356–68.
198. Ward CJ, Yuan D, Masyuk TV, Wang X, Punyashthiti R, Whelan S, et al. Cellular and subcellular localization of the ARPKD protein; fibrocystin is expressed on primary cilia. Hum Mol Genet. 2003;12: 2703–10.
199. Wang S, Luo Y, Wilson PD, Witman GB, Zhou J. The autosomal recessive polycystic kidney disease protein is localized to primary cilia, with concentration in the basal body area. J Am Soc Nephrol. 2004;15(3):592–602.
200. Zhang J, Wu M, Wang S, Shah JV, Wilson PD, Zhou J. Polycystic kidney disease protein fibrocystin localizes to the mitotic spindle and regulates spindle bipolarity. Hum Mol Genet. 2010;19(17):3306–19.
201. Wang S, Zhang J, Nauli SM, Li X, Starremans PG, Luo Y, et al. Fibrocystin/polyductin, found in the same protein complex with polycystin-2, regulates calcium responses in kidney epithelia. Mol Cell Biol. 2007;27(8):3241–52.
202. Kim I, Fu Y, Hui K, Moeckel G, Mai W, Li C, et al. Fibrocystin/polyductin modulates renal tubular formation by regulating polycystin-2 expression and function. J Am Soc Nephrol. 2008;19(3):455–68.
203. Hogan MC, Griffin MD, Rossetti S, Torres VE, Ward CJ, Harris PC. *PKHDL1*, a homolog of the autosomal recessive polycystic kidney disease gene, encodes a receptor with inducible T lymphocyte expression. Hum Mol Genet. 2003;12:685–9.

Bardet-Biedl Syndrome

2

Yangfan P. Liu and Nicholas Katsanis

Introduction

Bardet-Biedl syndrome (BBS, MIM#209900) is a rare genetic disease with an estimated prevalence that ranges from 1:160,000 in northern Europeans [1, 2] to 1:13,500 in the Bedouin population of Kuwait [3, 4]. Interest in BBS started with the discovery of a wide spectrum of phenotypes including birth defects and metabolic disorders [2, 5–7]. These phenotypes can be attributed to mutations in two alleles of one single causal gene, but the penetrance and expressivity of phenotypes can vary within and between families due to the presence of a third allele on a second locus [8–11]. The primary cellular mechanism underlying Bardet-Biedl syndrome is the dysfunction of the basal body/cilium, which groups BBS with a spectrum of cilium-related disorders named ciliopathies [12]. Here we summarize the clinical features and the molecular genetics of BBS and provide an overview of BBS proteins in regulating specific developmental events and disease states.

Y. P. Liu, PhD · N. Katsanis, PhD (✉)
Center for Human Disease Modeling, Duke University School of Medicine, Durham, NC, USA
e-mail: nicholas.katsanis@duke.edu

Clinical Features of Bardet-Biedl Syndrome

The diagnosis of BBS as a clinically discrete entity is based on the presence of a characteristic combination of multiple symptoms. Here, we have listed the clinical phenotypes of BBS, separated by major and minor symptoms according to prevalence among affected individuals, and summarized the diagnostic criteria.

Major Symptoms

Retinal Degeneration

Retinitis pigmentosa, a hallmark of BBS, is an atypical pigmentary retinal dystrophy of rod and cone photoreceptors with early maculopathy, which affects more than 90% of BBS children as early as 7–8 years old [13]. Extinguished rod and cone electroretinography are observed before the occurrence of black pigment in the peripheral retina (Fig. 2.1a) [19]. By the end of the second decade, almost all patients manifest night blindness, followed by loss of peripheral vision. In advanced disease cases, central vision may deteriorate over time [20, 21].

Obesity (Fig. 2.1b)

Another major symptom observed in 72–96% of BBS patients is obesity [22]. Despite normal birth weight, obesity begins at about 1 or

B. D. Cowley, Jr., J. J. Bissler (eds.), *Polycystic Kidney Disease*,
https://doi.org/10.1007/978-1-4939-7784-0_2

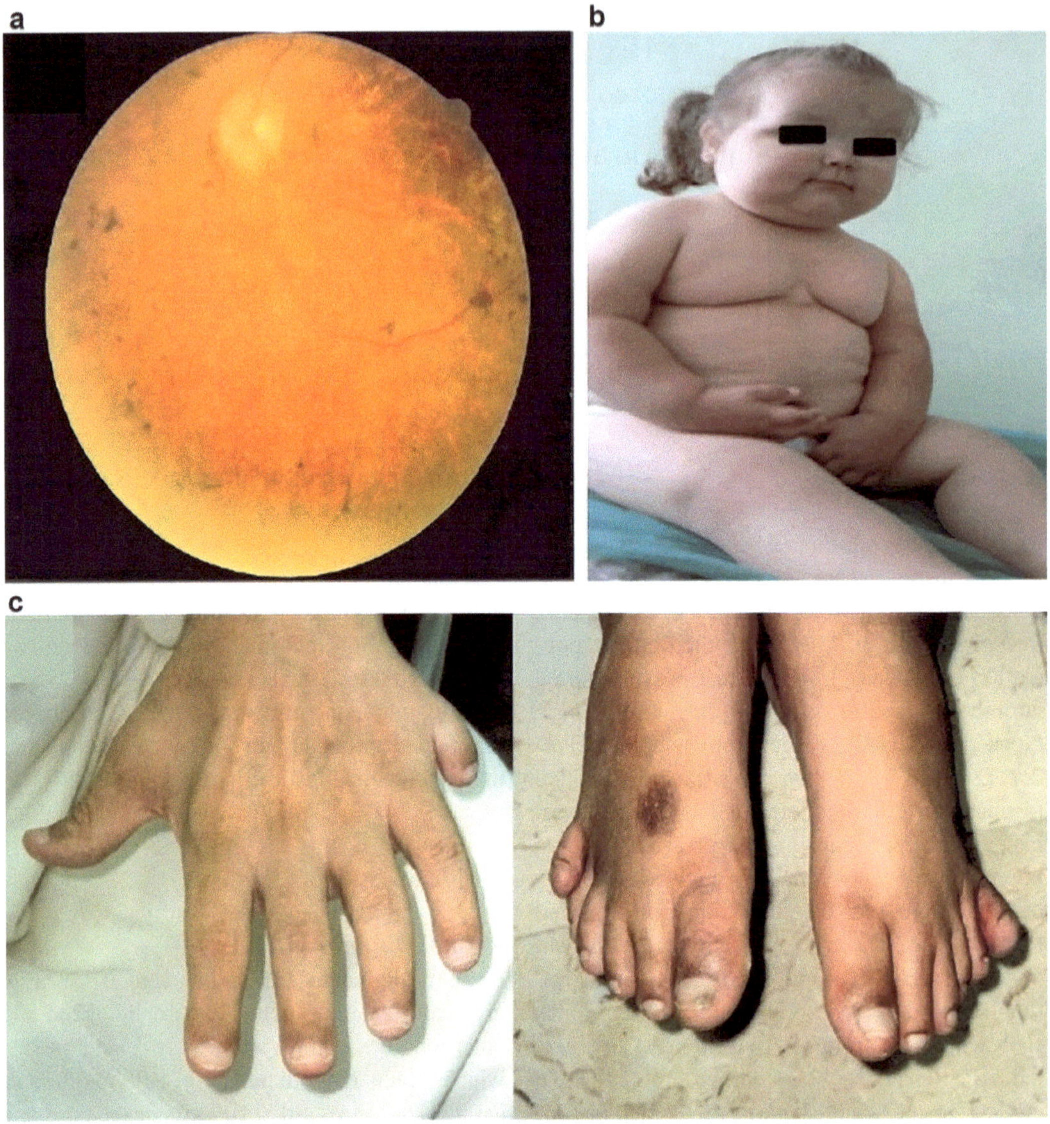

Fig. 2.1 Bardet-Biedl syndrome symptoms. (**a**) Retinitis pigmentosa: a speckling of the retinal pigment epithelium with bone spicule pigmentation, optic nerve pallor, and retinal arteriolar attenuation (Reprinted from Al-Adsani and Gader [14], https://www.ncbi.nlm.nih.gov/pmc/articles/PMC2850186/. Copyright © Annals of Saudi Medicine). (**b**) Central obesity (From Pasinska et al. [15], https://www.omicsonline.com/open-access/prenatal-and-postnatal-diagnostics-of-a-child-with-bardetbiedl-syndromecase-study-1747-0862-1000189.php?aid=65495. Copyright © 2015 Pasińska et al.). (**c**) Postaxial polydactyly of hand and foot (Reprinted from Al-Adsani and Gader [14], https://www.ncbi.nlm.nih.gov/pmc/articles/PMC2850186/. Copyright © Annals of Saudi Medicine). (**d**) Micropenis and absence of secondary sexual characters (Reprinted from Chakravarti et al. [16] by permission of Oxford University Press). (**e**) Hematoxylin and eosin stain of cystic kidney (Reprinted from Karmous-Benailly et al. [17] with permission from Elsevier). (**f**) Characterized facial features of BBS patients include downward palpebral fissures, a long philtrum, a thin upper lip, and micrognathia (Reproduced from Beales et al. [13] with permission from BMJ Publishing Group LTD). (**g**) MRI shows cerebral and cerebellar atrophy in a BBS patient compared to control (Reproduced from Baker et al. [18] with permission from John Wiley and Sons)

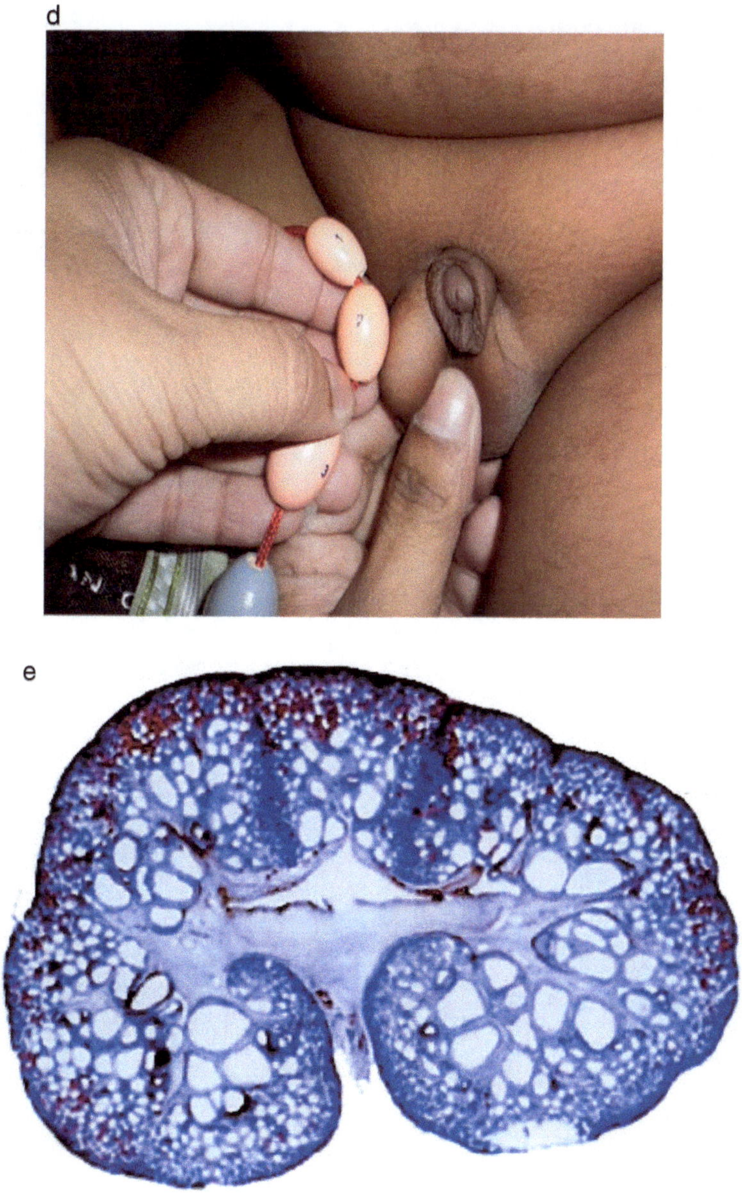

Fig. 2.1 (continued)

f

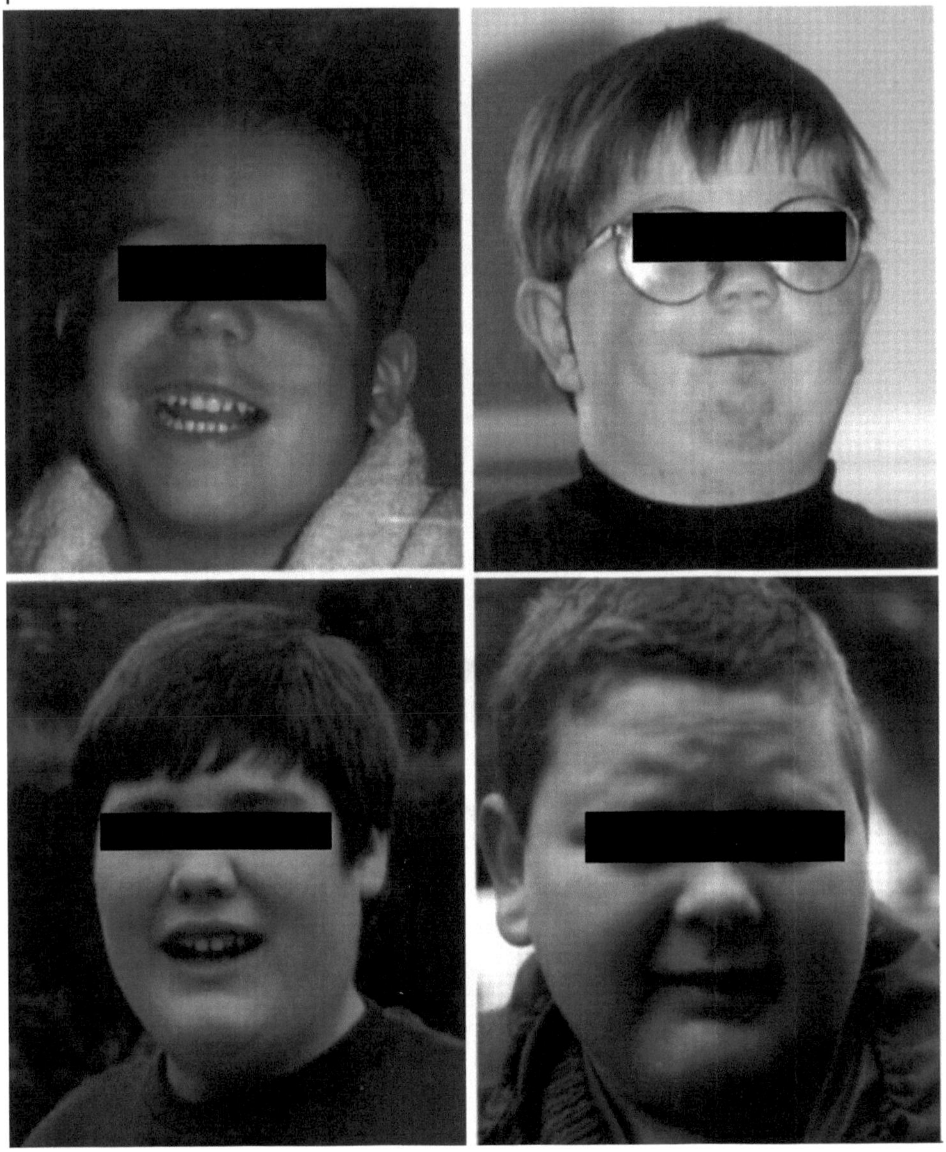

Fig. 2.1 (continued)

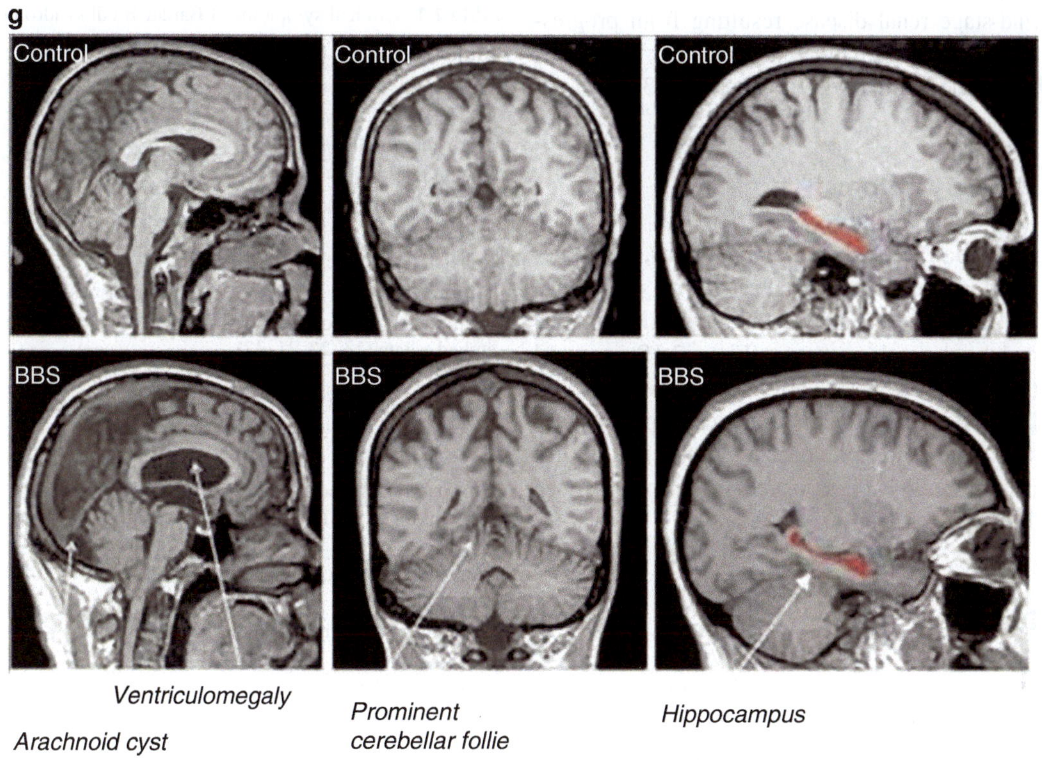

Fig. 2.1 (continued)

2 years of age, and the body mass index can reach 40 kg/m^2 in adulthood [13]. The distribution of adipose tissue changes with age and progresses from a global distribution to an accumulation in the trunk and proximal limbs during adulthood [19].

Limb Abnormalities (Fig. 2.1c)

Postaxial polydactyly is observed in 58–69% of patients. Accessory digits can be found on only one limb or up to all four limbs [13, 23]. In addition, other limb deformities, such as brachydactyly, partial syndactyly, fifth finger clinodactyly, and "sandal gap," have been reported at lower prevalences of 8–46% [13, 19].

Intellectual Disability

About 62% of BBS patients have significant learning disabilities during childhood. Although impaired vision may contribute to these conditions, IQ tests have confirmed deficiencies in mental faculties in 40% of cases [13, 22, 24].

Genital Abnormalities

Genital abnormalities in BBS females include hydrometrocolpos, uterine and ovarian hypoplasia, and absence of vaginal and/or urethral orifices [25–27]. Hypogenitalism in about 50% of male patients [28] is characterized by a small penile shaft and/or testes (Fig. 2.1d). In spite of genital abnormalities, there are several reports of BBS females giving birth and two reports of affected males fathering children [13].

Renal Abnormalities (Fig. 2.1e)

Both structural and functional renal abnormalities are observed in BBS patients, although most anatomical abnormalities (in 46% BBS patients) are present without the manifestation of physiological symptoms (in 5% BBS patients) [13, 29]. Anatomical abnormalities include fetal lobulation, calyceal clubbing or calyceal cysts, cortical scarring, and polycystic kidney disease. Physiological symptoms include polyuria, polydipsia, renal tubular acidosis, anemia, and hypertension.

End-stage renal disease resulting from progressive renal abnormalities accounts for most morbidity and mortality in BBS patients [30].

Minor Symptoms

In addition to the six major symptoms, other phenotypes are observed at a lower prevalence (<50%). These include abnormalities in the facial skeletal system (Fig. 2.1f), central (Fig. 2.1g) and peripheral nervous system, teeth, heart, liver, metabolism (diabetes, hypertension), sensation (anosmia, hearing deficit), left/right patterning, as well as psychiatric problems (see Table 2.1 for details).

Table 2.1 Clinical symptoms of Bardet-Biedl syndrome

Major symptoms [13]	
Retinitis pigmentosa	
Obesity	
Limb abnormalities	
Mental retardation	
Hypogenitalism and genital abnormalities	
Renal abnormalities	
Minor symptoms	**Tissues**
Craniofacial dysmorphism, high-arched palate [13, 22, 31, 32]	Skeletal system
Structural cerebral abnormalities (hydrocephalus) [33], developmental delay, speech disorder/delay, ataxia, poor coordination, imbalance [13]	Central nervous system
Hirschsprung's disease [31, 34, 35], mild spasticity [13]	Peripheral nervous system
Strabismus, cataracts, glaucoma, astigmatism [13]	Eye
Dental crowding, hypodontia, small roots [13]	Tooth
Left ventricular hypertrophy, congenital heart disease [36]	Heart
Hepatic fibrosis [37]	Liver
Diabetes mellitus [5], hypertension [38]	Metabolism
Anosmia [39, 40], hearing deficit [41]	Sensation
Situs inversus [35, 42]	Left/right patterning
Anxiety, depression, autism, bipolar disorder, obsessive compulsive behavior [22]	Psychiatric problems

Diagnosis

Diagnosis of BBS can be challenging, because of the incomplete manifestation of symptoms until the age of about 9 [13], the intrafamilial as well as interfamilial variability in penetrance and expressivity, and the phenotypic overlap with other genetic disorders, most of which are now understood to share the same organellar etiopathology (see subsequent section on "Ciliopathies"). To resolve this issue, Schachat and Maumenee (1982) compared BBS to other syndromes with similar symptoms and proposed that the detection of four of the five major symptoms would suffice to make a diagnosis [43]. Renal abnormalities were not considered in early studies and were later added as a sixth major symptom [5]. Beales et al. (1999) further refined these criteria based on a survey describing the prevalence of the major and minor features in 109 BBS patients and their families [13]. The new "4 or 3+2" criterion proposed by Beales et al. (1999) is utilized for the diagnosis of BBS today, which requires a minimum of four major symptoms or three major symptoms plus two minor symptoms.

Upon clinical diagnosis based on phenotypic criteria, genetic tests can confirm a molecular diagnosis of BBS, and determine the causal genes and mutations in each family. Resequencing the exons of all *BBS* genes can also detect both novel and previously reported point mutations and small insertions/deletions (several base pairs), but this method is costly and time-consuming. Genotyping for targeted mutations is more efficient and cost-effective, and available for *BBS1-13*, but can only detect known point mutations (ASPER Biotech http://www.asperbio.com/ and CGC Genetics http://www.cgcgenetics.com/cgc/en/main-en.html). To examine copy number variations (coverage of whole exons to whole genes hence that are not detectable by sequencing or genotyping), deletion/duplication analysis is available for *BBS1-13* (Prevention Genetics http://www.preventiongenetics.com/) and *BBS14-15* (The Rare Disease Company Centogene http://www.centogene.com/) [44].

Recently, an *in-solution* targeted capture strategy based on next-generation sequencing was proposed as a high-throughput, cost-effective method [45] that detects novel and known point mutations, small insertions and deletions, large copy number variations [46], and some putative splicing mutations. However, the coverage of this new technique needs to be improved [47]. Methods that efficiently detect splicing mutations by examining DNA samples are still unavailable in part due to (1) large intron sizes, (2) high frequency of nonpathogenic intronic mutations, (3) poor reliability of splicing prediction tools, and (4) requirement of RNA samples to confirm splicing change.

Cloning of *BBS* Genes

BBS is a genetically heterogeneous disorder with 17 causal genes identified to date (Table 2.2). The contribution of each *BBS* gene to the mutational burden in BBS patients of European descent varies significantly, from 0.4% to 23.3% (Fig. 2.2) [65–68]. Collectively, the primary causal genetic lesion of ~80% of European BBS cases is accounted for by mutations in the 17 known *BBS* genes, suggesting that the remaining cases may be attributed to lesions in other genes and/or genomic structural variation. Here we present a summary of known *BBS* genes with the goal to provide insight into the isolation of unknown *BBS* genetic loci.

Positional Cloning

Historically, positional cloning in large BBS families led to the isolation of candidate genomic regions, which facilitated the discovery of causal genes. A prime example is the identification of *BBS6*. Katsanis et al. (2000) initially mapped a putative BBS locus to a 1.9 cM candidate region on 20p12 using genome-wide homozygosity mapping, linkage study, and haplotype analysis. The authors then sequenced the coding exons in this region for pathogenic mutations and identified loss of function mutations in *BBS6/MKKS* [69], aided by the recent, at that time, positional cloning of the phenotypically related MKKS gene for McKusick-Kaufman syndrome in the same genomic interval [70]. Similar studies led to the identification of five additional *BBS* genes: *BBS1* [71–74], *BBS2* [75–77], *BBS4* [78–80], *BBS10* [81–83], and *BBS16* [84]. In the case of *BBS16*, a candidate genomic region was defined by homozygosity mapping of large consanguineous BBS families, but sequencing the coding exons of five candidate genes in this region detected no mutations. However, a mutation was uncovered by RT-PCR analysis of mRNA from patient fibroblasts that identified a splicing variation in *SDCCAG8* (*BBS16*) caused by a homozygous intronic insertion [84].

Although positional cloning has contributed to the identification of six *BBS* genes (*BBS1*, *BBS2*, *BBS4*, *BBS6*, *BBS10*, *BBS16*), the application of this method is limited by the availability of large pedigrees. The identification of other BBS disease genes, as described below, has been expedited by the development of new techniques, combined with the improved knowledge about the cellular and molecular mechanisms underlying BBS.

Evolutionary Strategy

Evolutionary theory points to the possibility that the paralogs of known BBS proteins contribute to the etiopathology of BBS. Consistent with this notion, searching the database of expressed sequence tags (dbEST) and human genome translation with BBS2 peptide sequences led to the identification of *BBS7* [85]. Additionally, *BBS8* was identified because the BBS8 protein aligns partially with BBS4 and contains similar tetratricopeptide repeat domains [86].

Studies of the protein products of *BBS8* and *BBS4* point to their centrosome/basal body localization in ciliated tissues, which is consistent with cilium-related phenotypes in BBS patients, such as left-right axis defect, retinitis pigmentosa, polycystic kidney disease, and male infertility [86, 87], and suggests a role for the cilium in the pathology of BBS. On the basis of this

Table 2.2 Causative genes for Bardet-Biedl syndrome

Genes	Alternative names	Genomic position (human)	Genomic position (mouse)	Knockout mouse availability	Knockout mouse phenotypes
BBS1	BBS2L2	11q13	19	Yes	Stereociliary defect [41], anosmia [39], airway motile cilia defect [48], thermo- and mechanosensation defect [49], neuronal migration defect [50]
BBS2	BBS	16q21	8	Yes	Lack of sperm flagella, retinopathy, renal cysts, anosmia, defect in social dominance [51], obesity [52], cartilage abnormalities [53], vascular dysfunction [54], inflammatory filtration [55]
BBS3	ARL6, RP55	3p12-q13	16	Yes	Abnormal kidney and photoreceptor development [56], retinal degeneration, male infertility, obesity, severe hydrocephalus, elevated blood pressure [57]
BBS4	N/A	15q22.3-q23	9	Yes	Lack of sperm flagella [58], defect in social function [51], exencephaly, open eyelid, stereociliary defect [41], anosmia [39], liver dysfunction, hydrometrocolpos [59], airway motile cilia defect [48], retinal degeneration [60], thermo- and mechanosensation defect [49], obesity [52], inflammatory infiltration, renal cysts [55]
BBS5	N/A	2q31	2	No	N/A
BBS6	MKKS	20p12	2	Yes	Retinal degeneration, stereociliary defect [41], airway motile cilia defect [48], obesity [52], cartilage abnormalities [53], vascular dysfunction [54]
BBS7	BBS2L1	4q27	3	Yes	Retinal degeneration, hyperphagia, obesity, hydrocephalus, male infertility [57]
BBS8	TTC8, RP51	14q32.11	12	Yes	Anosmia, defects in axon targeting [61]
BBS9	PTHB1	7p14	9	No	N/A
BBS10	C12ORF58	12q21.2	10	No	N/A
BBS11	TRIM32, HT2A, LGMD2H, TATIP	9q33.1	4	Yes	Mild myopathic changes, motor axonal changes [62]
BBS12	C4ORF24	4q27	3	No	N/A
BBS13	MKS1	17q22	11	Yes	Structural abnormalities in the neural tube, biliary duct, limb patterning, bone development and the kidney [63]
BBS14	CEP290, MKS4, JBTS5, NPHP6, SLSN6, LCA10	12q21.32	10	Yes	Runting, retinal degeneration, midline fusion defect, mild foliation defect [64]
BBS15	Fritz, WDPCP, C2ORF86	2p15	11	No	N/A
BBS16	SDCCAG8, SLSN7, NPHP10	1q43	1	No	N/A
BBS17	LZTFL1	3p21.3	9	No	N/A

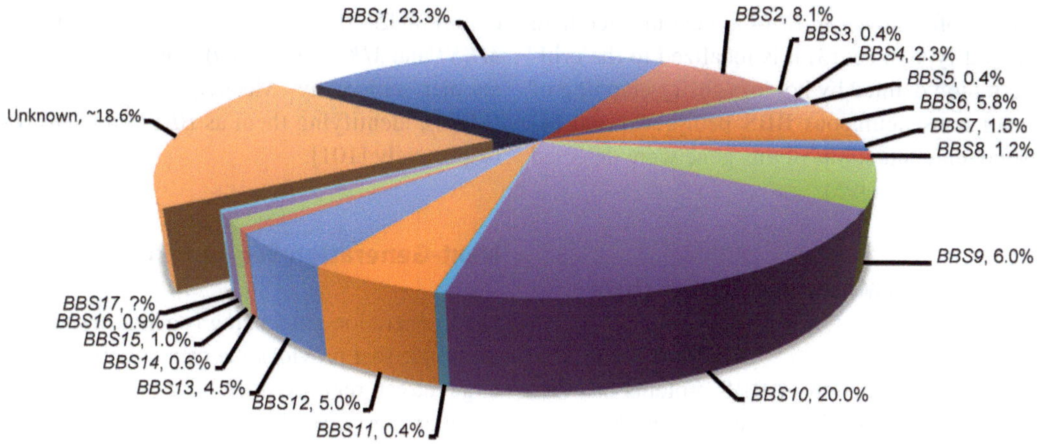

Fig. 2.2 The percentage contribution of *BBS* genes to the mutational burden of European patients with Bardet-Biedl syndrome

hypothesis, comparative genomics analyses of ciliated and non-ciliated species/tissues, coupled to evolutionary studies, led to the identification of new *BBS* genes. Li et al. (2004) studied the proteomes of humans, the ciliated green alga *Chlamydomonas*, and the non-ciliated plant *Arabidopsis*. Subtraction of the *Arabidopsis* proteome from the overlap of the human and *Chlamydomonas* proteomes defined a subset of proteins enriched for ciliary proteins. Two genes encoding proteins in this database were located in the candidate region for a putative *BBS* gene defined by positional cloning study of a Newfoundland family [88]. Sequencing identified pathogenic mutations in one of the genes, now called *BBS5* [89].

Chiang et al. (2004) and Fan et al. (2004) applied similar strategies to identify *BBS3*. Chiang et al. (2004) proposed that organisms expressing orthologs of the known *BBS* genes should also express orthologs of novel *BBS* genes. Based on this hypothesis, they selected several ciliated organisms (*H. sapiens*, *T. brucei*, *T. cruzi*, *C. reinhardtii*, and *C. intestinalis*) and non-ciliated organisms (*S. cerevisiae* and *A. thaliana*) and performed comparative genomic analysis to generate a database of candidate *BBS* genes. Sequencing of BBS patients identified pathogenic mutations in *ARL6* [90], one of the genes located in the 6 cM *BBS3* critical region on 3p12-13 [91–93]. Independently, Fan et al. (2004) searched the *Caenorhabditis elegans* genome for genes with an X-box domain, a promoter sequence that is bound by the transcription factor DAF-19 in ciliated sensory neurons [86]. The authors identified three putative *BBS* genes and showed subsequently that *ARL6* is *BBS3* by mutation screening in BBS patients [94].

Small Consanguineous Pedigrees

Large pedigrees are typically required for gene mapping. However, homozygosity mapping with small consanguineous BBS pedigrees can identify multiple candidate regions in single pedigrees. Genetic characterization of these regions, in combination with other techniques, such as an evolutionary approach, gene expression analysis, mutational screening, and functional studies, led to the identification of additional *BBS* genes, including *BBS9* [95], *BBS11* [66], and *BBS12* [96]. For example, to clone *BBS9*, Nishimura et al. (2005) combined comparative genomics, gene expression analysis, homozygosity mapping with small consanguineous pedigrees, and sequencing of candidate genes. The gene *PTHB1* was identified as *BBS9* because (1) it is expressed and conserved in organisms whose specific pathways containing all the known *BBS* genes are functional; (2) like other *BBS* genes, its expression level is more than twofold lower in *Bbs4* knockout mice than in wild-type mice; (3) it is localized to the critical region defined by homozygosity mapping of small consanguineous BBS pedigrees; and (4) pathogenic mutations of this gene were detected in BBS patients [95].

Cellular and Molecular Architecture of BBS

Studying the function of BBS proteins has first implicated dysfunction of cilium and/or basal body and the subsequent misregulation of cellular processes in the molecular pathology of the disease [86, 87]. These studies led to the hypothesis that additional genes encoding either ciliary proteins or components of cilium/basal body-related pathways could play roles in BBS. Wnt signaling is one of several well-characterized signal transduction pathways linked to the cilium/basal body. Sequencing of *FRITZ*, the coding gene of a protein that regulates both ciliogenesis and noncanonical Wnt signaling, led to the discovery of a homozygous splice mutation and two heterozygous missense mutations in BBS patients, defining *BBS15* [67].

Genetic Overlap with Other Ciliopathies

Ciliopathies are a group of diseases that are all attributed to the dysfunction of ciliary and/or basal body proteins and hence overlap in the clinical phenotypes [12, 97]. This disease category includes greater than 16 different disorders, such as nephronophthisis, Joubert syndrome, oral-facial-digital syndrome, and Meckel-Gruber syndrome. An overlap of disease genes between two or more conditions is observed [98]. Consistent with this rationale, Slavotinek et al. (2000) identified *BBS6* by sequencing BBS patients for mutations in *MKKS*, the causal gene of McKusick-Kaufman syndrome [99], a disease characterized with polydactyly, congenital heart disease, and genital abnormalities [100]. Similarly, Leitch et al. (2008) sequenced a BBS cohort of 155 families and detected mutations in *MKS1* and *MKS4* (*CEP290*), the causal genes of another ciliopathy Meckel-Gruber syndrome (MKS), identifying them as *BBS13* and *BBS14*, respectively [101].

Next-Generation Sequencing

Next-generation sequencing is a high-throughput technique that provides the capacity to sequence large target regions, including whole exomes, simultaneously, so that mutational screening of numerous genes in large candidate regions is possible. In a consanguineous BBS family with no mutation in *BBS1-16*, homozygosity mapping revealed nine large candidate regions. Without further narrowing down these regions for fewer candidate genes, whole exome sequencing was performed and identified a 5 bp deletion in *LZTFL1*/*BBS17* [102].

Inheritance of BBS

Pedigree analysis and sequencing of BBS patients suggests that two alleles of pathogenic mutations in one *BBS* gene are necessary for the pathology. However, some observations in these pedigrees, especially the non-penetrance and intrafamilial expressivity variation, cannot be explained by autosomal recessive inheritance. For example, with the possible exception of retinal degeneration, familial segregation of most BBS endophenotypes does not confine to Mendelian models. In turn, oligogenic models of inheritance have been proposed, highlighting the relationship between phenotypes and mutational load, which is the aggregate of deleterious mutations carried in multiple related genes of an individual.

Autosomal Recessive Inheritance and Its Limitations

In BBS pedigrees, the segregation of primary causal mutations suggests that BBS is an autosomal recessive disease. Mykytyn et al. (2003)

studied the role of *BBS1* in a cohort of 129 BBS probands, demonstrating a pattern of autosomal recessive inheritance [103]. Hichri et al. (2005) screened mutations in 6 *BBS* genes (*BBS1*, *BBS2*, *BBS4*, *BBS6*, *BBS7*, and *BBS8*) in 27 families with BBS and did not detect mutations in 2 *BBS* genes in a single patient, consistent with an autosomal recessive inheritance model. However, an excess of heterozygous single mutations in BBS patients left the possibility of both yet-identified *BBS* genes and complex inheritance [104].

An autosomal recessive model of inheritance cannot explain some observations in BBS pedigrees. These observations include (1) the incomplete or variable BBS phenotypes in family members other than the probands [19, 105, 106]; (2) decreased occurrence of consanguinity than expected in an autosomal recessive disease [19]; and (3) the presence of more affected males than affected females [19, 105, 107, 108], without linkage of BBS to the X chromosome to date. All these discrepancies suggest a more complex inheritance pattern, which was supported by later studies, partly due to an increased sample size of cohorts or the increased number of known BBS causal genes.

Phenotypic Effect of Heterozygous Mutations

In an autosomal recessive inheritance model, BBS heterozygous carriers should be phenotypically the same as the control population. However, mild BBS phenotypes are observed in carriers. Relative to family members with no known mutations in *BBS* genes, BBS heterozygous carriers have a higher frequency of obesity (especially in males), hypertension, diabetes mellitus, renal disease [109, 110], and retinal dysfunction [111]. On average, the parents of BBS patients are taller [110]. All these mild phenotypes in BBS carriers are attributed to the presence of one mutated copy of a *BBS* gene. These observations suggest that the presence of one mutant allele in *BBS* genes has a contributory effect for some BBS symptoms.

Oligogenic Inheritance

Penetrance and Expressivity Variation in BBS Homozygous Individuals

The autosomal recessive model is also challenged by the differences in penetrance and expressivity of BBS phenotypes observed between affected individuals within the same BBS family. The following are two examples of such pedigrees.

In the first example, BBS family AR259, each parent has a single copy of different nonsense mutations in *BBS2*, with the affected child (AR259-03) being a compound heterozygote for both alleles. Although an autosomal recessive model can explain the mode of inheritance in this trio, a sibling (AR259-05), who has the same *BBS2* genotype as the proband, is phenotypically normal, indicating that further explanation is required (Fig. 2.3a). Therefore, at least in family AR259, the presence of two nonsense *BBS2* alleles is insufficient to explain the spectrum of observed phenotypes [8].

In a second example, pedigree AR768, a range of phenotypes was observed in the probands and siblings. The father of this family bears a hypomorphic mutation in *BBS1*, and the mother has a frameshift mutation in the same gene. One of their two daughters (AR768-04) was diagnosed with BBS, presenting with obesity, severe mental retardation, delayed speech and development, and crowded teeth. Since AR768-04 is a compound heterozygote with respect to both mutant alleles in *BBS1*, this adheres to an autosomal recessive model. However, her sister (AR768-03) is also compound heterozygous for *BBS1* but did not meet the diagnostic criteria for BBS, given that she only presented with mild mental retardation, but her development, body weight, and teeth are all normal (Fig. 2.3b) [10].

Digenic and Triallelic Model

Such intrafamilial differences of penetrance and expressivity between individuals with the same mutations in one *BBS* gene require an expansion of the autosomal recessive model of inheritance. These models predate the molecular era. Bergsma and Brown (1975) proposed a hypothesis of polygenic inheritance, which suggests that multiple

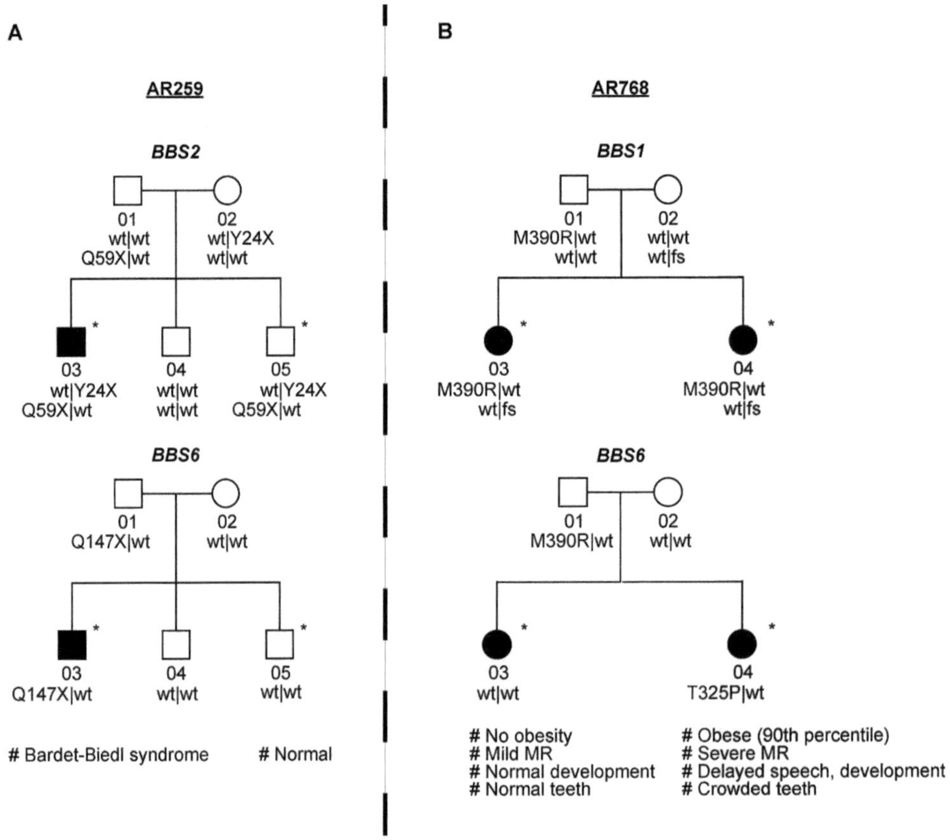

Fig. 2.3 Sample pedigrees demonstrate digenic and triallelic inheritance. (**a**) Pedigree AR259, in which two brothers both harbor compound heterozygous mutations in *BBS2*, but only the patient has the third mutant allele in *BBS6*. (**b**) Pedigree AR768, in which two sisters both harbor compound heterozygous mutations in *BBS1*, but only the one with a third mutant allele in *BBS6* manifests more severe phenotypes

genes exert a simultaneous effect in the inheritance of Bardet-Biedl syndrome, with the genetic interaction between genes determining phenotypes. Under this model, multiple genes could contribute to an outcome, or one gene could be the major causal locus with other genes acting as modifiers of penetrance and/or expressivity [112].

One example of a polygenic inheritance model is the digenic and triallelic model, which proposes that three mutant alleles in two *BBS* genes function together to give rise to the phenotypes in BBS patients [8, 113]. The contribution from the third allele is supported by the phenotypic effect of a single mutant *BBS* allele observed in the heterozygous carriers. Although other genetic and/or environmental factors may play a role in modulating penetrance and expressivity, such oligogenic models could explain the inheritance pattern observed in several BBS families.

As detailed above, the presence of two mutant alleles in *BBS2* is not sufficient to give rise to BBS phenotypes in pedigree AR259, so that AR259-05 is phenotypically normal. However, the affected individual (AR259-03) has a heterozygous nonsense mutant allele in a second *BBS* gene (*BBS6*), potentially acting as a modifier of penetrance (Fig. 2.3a) [8]. Similarly, the presence of a mutated allele in *BBS6* in addition to the two mutated alleles in *BBS1* could explain the phenotypic severity variation in the pedigree AR768. The sibling who does not harbor a *BBS6* mutation is mildly affected, whereas the sibling who is heterozygous for *BBS6* is severely affected (Fig. 2.3b) [10].

To date, *BBS1-10* and *BBS12* and *BBS13* are reported to participate in oligogenic inheritance [8–11, 101, 114, 115]. The frequency of triallelism varies between different *BBS* genes, from about 30% to almost 90% [113]. Oligogenic events were observed in 16% of BBS patients in a cohort from Denmark [116]. A survey based on systematic functional assays of all known BBS alleles showed that in addition to an enrichment of expected hypomorphic mutations, a significant fraction (33%) of *trans* modifying alleles in a second *BBS* gene are dominant-negative at the cellular level [117].

Modifying Genes

Genetic screening of BBS patients revealed modifying alleles in other loci, which cannot cause BBS independently even in homozygosity, but which likely interact with BBS causal genes to modify the penetrance and expressivity of the phenotype. The first reported BBS modifying gene was *MGC1203*, which is enriched in BBS patients, interacts genetically with *BBS* genes, modifies the severity of disease, and, at least in one family, acts as a likely modifier of penetrance. The protein product of *MGC1203* interacts biochemically and co-localizes with BBS proteins [118]. Some modifying alleles appear to have effects specific to a subset of organs and endophenotypes. For instance, the presence of the T allele at rs2435357 in the *RET* protooncogene is associated with Hirschsprung's disease in BBS patients [119]. Similarly, a common mutation A229T in *RPGRIP1L* is enriched in ciliopathy patients with retinitis pigmentosa, including BBS patients [120]. Screening of BBS cohorts detected the enrichment of some heterozygous mutations in *MKS3* [101], *KIF7* [121], and *TTC21B* [122]. Complementation assays utilizing a zebrafish modeling system were carried out to test the pathogenicity of mutations and demonstrated synergistic effects between these putative modifying genes and *BBS* genes [101, 121, 122]. However, the specific effect of these alleles on the human phenotype is not known.

Application of Oligogenic Models

Cumulatively, genetic and functional data suggest that BBS can be considered a quantitative trait, thus underlining the importance of mutational load in a pool of multiple relevant genes that encode proteins with convergent function. Oligogenic inheritance is not unique to BBS, but also observed in other disorders, such as cystic fibrosis [123], Huntington disease [124], and sensory neural deafness [125]. Notably, a survey of the literature about 10 years ago pointed to more than 50 examples of such phenomena [126], a catalog accelerating further with the advent of whole exome and whole genome sequencing.

Molecular Mechanisms of Bardet-Biedl Syndrome

Subcellular Localization of BBS Proteins

The first indication of the function of BBS proteins arose from studies on their subcellular localization. Most BBS proteins, under certain if not all conditions, have been shown to localize to or in proximity to the centrosome, to the basal body, and/or to the cilium [48, 84, 86, 87, 89, 96, 127–133], with three exceptions: (1) the E3 ubiquitin ligase TRIM32, encoded by *BBS11*, localizes throughout the cytoplasm as discrete speckles in mammalian cells [134]; (2) the planar cell polarity (PCP) effector FRITZ, encoded by *BBS15*, localizes to the proximal plasma membrane in the *Drosophila* pupal wing [135]; and (3) LZTFL1, encoded by *BBS17*, localizes to the cytoplasm in hTERT-RPE1 cells, although LZTFL1 regulates ciliary trafficking of proteins including the BBS family of proteins by inhibiting ciliary entry of these proteins [136].

The centrosome is the organization center for the microtubule network of the cell. This network provides mechanical power for cellular processes, such as vesicular transport, neuronal migration and axonal targeting, cytokinesis during mitosis or meiosis, and postmitotic cell polarity [137]. In postmitotic polarized cells, the mother centriole of the centrosome forms the basal body, a structure that nucleates the cilium [138], which plays major roles in development and homeostasis as described below. BBS proteins may participate in all these cilium-/basal body-/centrosome-related processes.

The relationship between the subcellular localization of BBS proteins and their function is exemplified by studies characterizing BBS6. BBS6 localizes to the pericentriolar material around the centrosome. During mitosis, BBS6 also resides at the midbody, an intercellular structure that forms during cytokinesis [129]. Some patient-derived mutations in BBS6 result in the mislocalization of BBS6, suggesting that BBS phenotypes might be linked to the mis-trafficking and dysfunction of proteins in cellular processes [129]. This notion is supported by in vitro and in vivo studies of cellular processes and development in the absence of BBS6. Knockdown of *BBS6* gives rise to multicentrosomal and multinucleated cells in cultured mammalian cell lines, suggesting defects in cytokinesis [129].

Cytoplasmic Functions of BBS Proteins

Based on their subcellular localization, BBS proteins can serve as both cytoplasmic and ciliary proteins either at the same time or at different stages of cell cycle. At the centrosome, BBS proteins may regulate the microtubule network or function as scaffold proteins, adaptors, substrates, or motors. Outlined below are some studies describing the role of BBS proteins in microtubule organization and intracellular transport.

Microtubule Network Organization

Pericentriolar material 1 (PCM1) is a component of the pericentriolar material at the centrosome and is important in the recruitment of centrosomal components such as centrin, kentrin, and pericentrin [139]. Kim et al. (2004) observed a random distribution of PCM1 and its cargo throughout the cytoplasm upon the depletion of BBS4 in cultured cells, suggesting that BBS4 is necessary for the organization of the centrosome and the assembly of the microtubule network. Furthermore, a truncated form of BBS4 colocalizes with PCM1 and associated cargo but cannot recruit them to the centrosome. These observations suggest that BBS4 may have multiple domains and be responsible for the association of PCM1 with the centriole [87]. The BBS4 protein has 13 tandem tetratricopeptide repeat (TPR) motifs, which are protein-protein interaction domains [140]. Yeast two-hybrid and Co-IP experiments provided evidence for the direct interaction between BBS4 and PCM1. In parallel, similar experiments resulted in the identification of the $p150^{glued}$ subunit of dynactin, an activator of the retrograde motor dynein [141], as another BBS4-interacting protein. BBS4 domain mapping experiments confirmed these interactions and identified the specific regions necessary for interaction of BBS4 with PCM1 and $p150^{glued}$, as well as the region required for the localization of BBS4 to the centrosome. These data led to a proposed mechanism for BBS4; by interacting with $p150^{glued}$, BBS4 moves PCM1 and associated cargo via retrograde transport by dynein, to the pericentriolar area to assemble the centrosome and organize the microtubule network [87].

Retrograde Intracellular Transport

The microtubule network at the centrosome plays a significant role in intracellular transport of vesicles and cellular organelles. A number of BBS proteins residing at the centrosome have been implicated in retrograde transport along the microtubule network [142].

Melanosomes are cellular organelles that provide pigment in the melanophores of skin cells. In response to visual and hormonal stimuli, melanosomes are transported along microtubules between the perinuclear region and the cell cortex of melanophores. The retraction of melanosomes to the perinuclear region is dependent on the retrograde motor dynein and its activator dynactin. As described above, based on an interaction with $p150^{glued}$, BBS4 participates in this process. Consistent with this idea, melanosome retraction delay was observed in zebrafish depleted of *bbs4*. Similarly, suppression of *bbs2*, *bbs5*, *bbs6*, *bbs7*, and *bbs8* in zebrafish also leads to melanosome retrograde transport defects [143]. In addition to the retrograde transport of melanosomes, BBS proteins have been suggested to participate in general organelle and vesicular transport along the microtubule network. For example, BBS3 belongs to the ARL-ARF family [94], of which several members are known to participate in vesicular transport from the endoplasmic reticulum to the Golgi [144–146].

Neuronal Development and Function

The microtubule network in neurons is essential for the transport of protein cargo throughout the axon and dendrites. Therefore, BBS proteins may play a role in neuronal function via retrograde transport along the microtubule network [147], which is consistent with behavioral defects observed in *Bbs2*, *Bbs4*, and *Bbs6* knockout mice [51, 148]. Loss of hearing is another symptom in both BBS patients and *Bbs* knockout mice [51, 148]. May-Simera et al. (2009) suggested that hearing defects in *Bbs4* knockout mice were the result of defective microtubule-dependent cytoplasmic transport [149]. BBS4 is expressed in the olfactory epithelium, and olfactory defects in *Bbs4* knockout mice can be explained by a disorganized microtubule network and trapping of olfactory receptor proteins in dendrites and cell bodies in olfactory sensory neurons [87].

A caveat to the prediction that neuronal phenotypes in *Bbs* knockout mice are driven by defects in microtubule transport is that BBS proteins are also required for ciliary function. For example, a reduced ciliated border was observed in the olfactory sensory neurons of *Bbs4* knockout mice [39]. Similarly, a critical role for BBS proteins in the sensory cilia of *C. elegans* was also established in paradigms that model behavioral plasticity and associative learning in humans [150].

BBS proteins may also be required for neuronal development. *Bbs8* is expressed in the neural plate of 8.5 dpc mice [151], and loss of *Bbs8* in mice leads to reduction of cilia and aberrant axonal targeting from olfactory sensory neuron to the olfactory bulb [61].

Ciliary Functions of BBS Proteins

Given the localization of BBS proteins to the basal body and cilium, it is not surprising that BBS proteins can regulate the assembly of the cilium, participate in the transport of cargo along the ciliary axoneme, and modulate signal transduction pathways.

Ciliogenesis

The role of BBS proteins in ciliogenesis was first observed by examining cilia formation in *Bbs2*, *Bbs4*, and *Bbs6* knockout mice. Although no major structural defects were discovered in nonmotile cilia, spermatozoa flagella (motile cilia) were absent in mutant mice [51, 58, 148]. Interestingly, not all motile cilia were absent, as motile cilia in the airway of these mice were present, although morphologically abnormal [48]. In *Xenopus*, when *bbs15* (*fritz*) is knocked down, multiciliated epidermis cells display fewer and shorter cilia [67]. These findings indicate that the depletion of BBS proteins may cause aberrant ciliogenesis rather than complete loss of cilia.

Work described by Nachury et al. (2007) provided an alternative hypothesis to the molecular mechanism of BBS proteins in ciliogenesis. Seven highly conserved BBS proteins (BBS1, BBS2, BBS4, BBS5, BBS7, BBS8, and BBS9) can form a stable complex called the BBSome, which was shown to localize to the ciliary membrane as well as to the centriolar satellites in the cytoplasm of cultured cells. Perturbation of the BBSome leads to defects in ciliogenesis, which is partially mediated by Rab8 GDP/GTP exchange factor. Based on the role of $Rab8^{GTP}$ in vesicle trafficking to the primary cilium, the BBSome was proposed to contribute to the same process [133]. Another complex consisting of three BBS proteins that form the type II chaperonin subfamily (BBS6, BBS10, and BBS12) has been identified. This complex participates in ciliogenesis by mediating the assembly of the BBSome complex [152]. Finally, BBS14 (CEP290) is necessary for the ciliary localization of the GTPase Rab8 in cultured hTERT-RPE cells and hence for ciliogenesis in vitro [153].

Intraflagellar Transport

Intraflagellar transport (IFT) is a process by which protein cargo is trafficked along the ciliary axoneme. IFT utilizes motor proteins to shuttle cargo from the basal body to the tip of cilium (anterograde transport) and from the tip of cilium back to the basal body (retrograde transport) [154]. BBS7 and BBS8 were the first BBS proteins described to regulate intraflagellar transport. Blacque et al. (2004) demonstrated that mutations in *bbs7* and *bbs8* in *C. elegans* led to the mislocalization of IFT components and ciliary defects [128]. Ou et al. (2005) showed that IFT components form a functional particle containing two subunits. These two subunits are driven by two different motors to sequentially build distinct parts of the cilium. BBS7 and BBS8 stabilize the IFT particle by keeping the two subunits in a complex [155]. Pan et al. (2006) further explored the mechanistic details of the two IFT subunits and proposed a mechanical competition model, in which BBS7 and BBS8 provide tension on the IFT particle to stabilize the complex [156]. Further studies have suggested that other BBS proteins contribute to intraflagellar transport [94, 157] and proposed that these BBS proteins form an IFT-BBS complex to facilitate IFT [157]. The relationship between an IFT-BBS complex and the BBSome is unclear and has led to additional studies suggesting that the BBSome and IFT-BBS complexes are not the same and that the BBSome is the cargo but not an integral component of the IFT system [158].

Given that IFT is necessary for the assembly, maintenance, and function of the cilium, dysfunction of the IFT system leads to defects in ciliogenesis and cellular processes in which the cilium participates. The fact that BBS proteins are necessary for IFT can explain some BBS phenotypes, such as retinal degeneration associated with mislocalization of phototransduction proteins in photoreceptors, which is IFT dependent [51, 60].

Signaling Pathways

Initial interest in the cilium was centered on motile cilia and a role in fluid propulsion along the cell surface and locomotion of cells (such as sperm motility) [159]. Non-motile cilia were thought to be vestigial organelles, and their importance was underappreciated until about 10 years ago. The sensory role of non-motile cilia first came to light through work conducted on the ciliary disorder polycystic kidney disease (PKD). The two causal genes of autosomal dominant PKD encode calcium channel proteins PC1 and PC2, which localize to the cilium [160]. The calcium channel opens in response to ciliary bending under pressure from extracellular fluid flow [161]. Besides mechanosensation in the kidney and cochlea, chemosensation in the olfactory epithelium, and photosensation in the retina, the detection of morphogens is an emerging function of the primary cilium [162]. Morphogenetic signaling pathways play vital roles in development; it is now known that phenotypes of BBS can be attributed to morphogenetic signaling defects brought about by a malfunctioning cilium.

Sonic Hedgehog Signaling

Sonic Hedgehog (Shh) signaling was first linked to the cilium by the observation of Shh signaling phenotypes in mice with mutations of IFT subunits [163]. Several components of the Shh signaling pathway, including the receptor Patched1 (PTC) [164], the effectors Smoothened (SMO) [165] and GLI2 and GLI3, and the negative regulator SUFU [166], localize to cilium. Localization of Patched1 at the cilium appears to be involved in the inhibition of Smoothened accumulation. When Shh ligand binds to Patched1, Patched1 is transported from the cilium, which allows Smoothened to be transported into the cilium [164]. Localization of Smoothened to the cilium is required for Shh signaling [165], possibly through the activation of the proteolytic processing of GLI3 from the repressor form to the activator form [167]. The IFT subunit IFT88 is required for the processing of GLI3 and thus the activation of Shh signaling [166] (Fig. 2.4a).

As BBS proteins are known to function in ciliogenesis and intraflagellar transport, defects in either the localization or processing of Shh signaling components were predicted in BBS mutants.

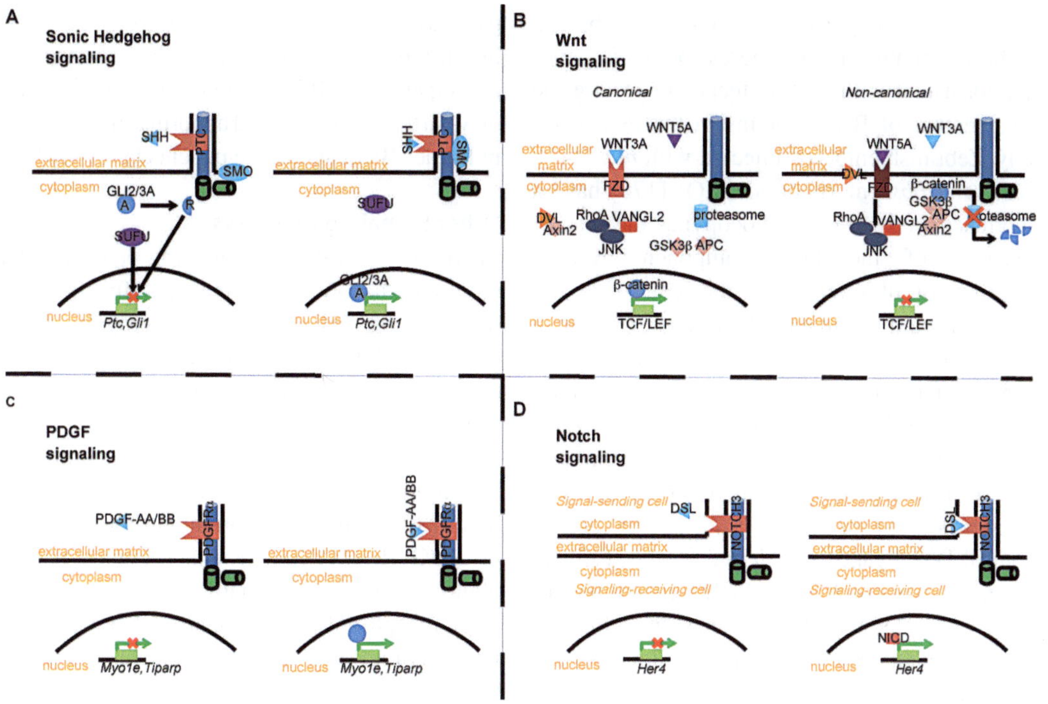

Fig. 2.4 The components of selected signaling pathways and the subcellular localization of some components to the cilium or the basal body. (**a**) In the Sonic Hedgehog signaling pathway, the receptor PTC, the effectors SMO and GLI2/3, and the negative regulator SUFU localize to the cilium. (**b**) In Wnt signaling pathways, the effector VANGL2 localizes to the cilium and the basal body, and the effector APC localizes to the basal body. (**c**) In the PDGF signaling pathway, the receptor PDGFRα localizes to the cilium. (**d**) In the Notch signaling pathway, the receptor NOTCH3 localizes to the cilium

BBS1, BBS3, BBS5, and BBS17 (LZTFL1) are required for localization of Smoothened to the cilium [136]. *Kif7*, a putative modifier of BBS, has dual functions in the regulation of Shh signaling via SUFU-dependent positive regulation and SUFU-independent negative regulation, probably by regulating the localization of SUFU-GLI complex along the cilium [168]. The expression pattern of *shh* is altered in zebrafish *bbs1* and *bbs7* morphants, leading to abnormal fin skeletal structure [169]. In *bbs4*, *bbs6*, and *bbs8* zebrafish morphants, the expression level of *patched1* decreases, suggesting perturbation of Shh signaling. This disruption of Shh signaling may explain craniofacial dysmorphology and Hirschsprung's disease in Bardet-Biedl syndrome patients [31]. Zebrafish morphants of *bbs15* (*fritz*) also display craniofacial dysmorphology and defective Shh signaling [67]. Taken together, these studies support the idea that BBS proteins participate in Shh signaling. Defective Shh signaling explains, at least in part, polydactyly, craniofacial dysmorphology, and the central nervous system and peripheral nervous system symptoms in individuals affected with BBS.

Wnt Signaling

The Wnt signaling pathway is broadly conceptualized as canonical and noncanonical branches. Canonical Wnt signaling regulates cell proliferation and differentiation [170], through the mediator β-catenin [171], while noncanonical Wnt signaling controls polarized convergent extension movements during gastrulation and neurulation in vertebrates, through the planar cell polarity (PCP) pathway [172]. Abnormal convergent extension movements affect early development and result in a shortened body axis in zebrafish [173] and neural tube closure defects in mice [173, 174].

Some phenotypes observed in zebrafish embryos and mice upon suppression of *bbs* genes are consistent with PCP defects, suggesting the involvement of BBS proteins in the PCP pathway. Zebrafish embryos injected with *bbs4* [41], *bbs1*, and *bbs6* morpholino (MO) [175] have a shortened body axis, phenocopying the loss of function of the PCP component *vangl2*. Localization of VANGL2 to the basal body and cilium in cultured mammalian cells and human respiratory epithelial cells (Fig. 2.4b), plus a genetic interaction between *bbs4* and *vangl2*, indicates that Bbs4 participates in the PCP pathway as a basal body/ciliary protein [41]. Similarly, genetic interaction was also observed between *bbs* genes (*bbs1*, *bbs4*, and *bbs6*) and the noncanonical Wnt ligands *wnt5b* and *wnt11* [175]. In mice, knockout of *Bbs4* and *Bbs6* causes phenotypes associated with PCP defects, including the presence of an open eyelid, open neural tube, and disrupted cochlear stereociliary bundles [41].

Involvement of BBS proteins in canonical Wnt signaling pathway was also reported. Suppression of *bbs1*, *bbs4*, and *bbs6* results in upregulation of TCF-/LEF-dependent transcription in both zebrafish embryos and mammalian ciliated cells, which was phenocopied by depletion of axonemal protein KIF3A but not by chemical disruption of the cytoplasmic microtubule network, suggesting that regulation of canonical Wnt signaling by BBS proteins is cilium-related. Given the observation of proteasome dysfunction and concomitant β-catenin accumulation when *BBS4* is suppressed, part of the molecular mechanism underlying canonical Wnt regulation by BBS proteins is attributable to defective proteasomal degradation of β-catenin [175]. The same work also dissected the relationship between the two branches of Wnt signaling pathway and demonstrated that the noncanonical branch inhibits the canonical branch in a *BBS4*-dependnet manner [175]. However, another study demonstrated overexpression of another BBS gene, *BBS3*, lead to hyperactivation of canonical Wnt signaling [132].

Despite the debate about which branch and which direction of Wnt signaling is regulated by BBS proteins, accumulating evidence supports the participation of BBS proteins in Wnt signaling pathways. Based on the known role of Wnt signaling in kidney development and homeostasis, the participation of BBS proteins in Wnt signaling may partially explain renal abnormalities observed in Bardet-Biedl syndrome patients [176, 177].

Other Signaling Pathways

There are several other signaling pathways that require normal ciliary structure and function. The receptor of platelet-derived growth factor (PDGF), PDGFRα, localizes to the cilium (Fig. 2.4c), can be activated by serum starvation or the ligands PDGF-AA and PDGF-BB, and is then phosphorylated to activate signaling. A hypomorphic mutation of the IFT subunit IFT88 perturbs both the localization and the activation of PDGFRα [178]. An intact cilium is also required for Notch signaling in the epidermis, and a receptor of Notch signaling, Notch3, localizes to cilium (Fig. 2.4d) [179]. Given the role of BBS proteins in ciliogenesis, these proteins are likely to participate in the regulation of PDGF and Notch signaling pathways in addition to Wnt and Shh signaling pathways.

Nuclear Functions of BBS7

Although most BBS proteins mainly localize to the centrosome/basal body and/or cilium [48, 84, 86, 87, 89, 96, 127–133] and play a role in the cilium/basal body or cytoplasmic microtubule network as described above, temporary localization of BBS7 to the nucleus and involvement of BBS7 in transcription regulation were reported. In silico analysis of the BBS7 amino acid sequence predicted a nuclear export signal, and chemical inhibition of nuclear export resulted in increased BBS7 protein levels in the nucleus. Interaction between BBS7 and the transcription repressor RNF2 was observed by yeast two-hybrid and co-immunoprecipitation. Suppression of *BBS7* leads to accumulation of RNF2 in vitro, possibly due to defective proteasomal degradation of RNF2, and concomitant decreased expression levels of RNF2 target genes in both cells and zebrafish embryos [180]. This work provided the first piece of evidence about the nuclear role of

BBS proteins. The possible nuclear role of other BBS proteins was also discussed, based on the presence of nuclear export signals in other BBS proteins and the interaction between RNF2 and other BBS proteins [180].

Summary

The study of BBS has provided insights from a genetic standpoint as a model of oligogenic inheritance and from a cell biology perspective to help understand the functions of the centrosome, basal body, and cilium. The study of diseases inherited in an oligogenic manner is vitally important as it provides a link between Mendelian inheritance (a single gene defect) and complex inheritance (due to defects in multiple genes). The digenic and triallelic model of inheritance in BBS is a modified autosomal recessive model and also the simplest form of complex inheritance. Interaction between the casual gene and additional alleles affecting components of the same ciliary module expands the standard autosomal recessive model that has limited application to the majority of human genetic diseases and sheds a light on the mechanism by which multiple genes interact in complex diseases.

The study of BBS also informs how cilia regulate many aspects of development and homeostasis. Different symptoms observed in BBS are due to deficiencies in different tissues and organs that initiate at different stages of life. These data point to the ubiquity of the cilium and its fine-tuned functions in multiple processes of development and homeostasis. As the causal genes and clinical presentation of the ciliopathies overlap, understanding of the pathogenesis of BBS and the associated ciliary biology may be applied to other ciliopathies as well.

Acknowledgments We thank Edwin Oh for critical reading and editorship of this chapter. This work was supported by a grant from the National Institute of Child Health and Human Development (HD042601) and grants from the National Institute of Diabetes and Digestive and Kidney Disorders (DK072301 and DK075972). NK is a distinguished Brumley Professor.

References

1. Klein D, Ammann F. The syndrome of Laurence-Moon-Bardet-Biedl and allied diseases in Switzerland. Clinical, genetic and epidemiological studies. J Neurol Sci. 1969;9(3):479–513.
2. Beales PL, et al. Bardet-Biedl syndrome: a molecular and phenotypic study of 18 families. J Med Genet. 1997;34(2):92–8.
3. Farag TI, Teebi AS. Bardet-Biedl and Laurence-Moon syndromes in a mixed Arab population. Clin Genet. 1988;33(2):78–82.
4. Farag TI, Teebi AS. High incidence of Bardet Biedl syndrome among the Bedouin. Clin Genet. 1989;36(6):463–4.
5. Green JS, et al. The cardinal manifestations of Bardet-Biedl syndrome, a form of Laurence-Moon-Biedl syndrome. N Engl J Med. 1989;321(15):1002–9.
6. Bardet G. Sur un syndrome d'obesite infantile avec polydactylie et retinite pigmentaire (contribution a l'etude des formes cliniques de l'obesite hypophysaire). Paris: Universite de Paris; 1920.
7. Biedl A. Ein Geschwisterpaar mit adiposo-genitaler Dystrophie. Dtsch Med Wschr. 1922;48:1630.
8. Katsanis N, et al. Triallelic inheritance in Bardet-Biedl syndrome, a Mendelian recessive disorder. Science. 2001;293(5538):2256–9.
9. Katsanis N, et al. BBS4 is a minor contributor to Bardet-Biedl syndrome and may also participate in triallelic inheritance. Am J Hum Genet. 2002;71(1):22–9.
10. Badano JL, et al. Heterozygous mutations in BBS1, BBS2 and BBS6 have a potential epistatic effect on Bardet-Biedl patients with two mutations at a second BBS locus. Hum Mol Genet. 2003; 12(14):1651–9.
11. Beales PL, et al. Genetic interaction of BBS1 mutations with alleles at other BBS loci can result in non-Mendelian Bardet-Biedl syndrome. Am J Hum Genet. 2003;72(5):1187–99.
12. Badano JL, et al. The ciliopathies: an emerging class of human genetic disorders. Annu Rev Genomics Hum Genet. 2006;7(author):125–48.
13. Beales PL, et al. New criteria for improved diagnosis of Bardet-Biedl syndrome: results of a population survey. J Med Genet. 1999;36(6):437–46.
14. Al-Adsani A, Gader FA. Combined occurrence of diabetes mellitus and retinitis pigmentosa. Ann Saudi Med. 2010;30(1):70–5.
15. Pasinska M, et al. Prenatal and postnatal diagnostics of a child with Bardet-Biedl syndrome: case study. J Mol Genet Med. 2015;9(4):189.
16. Chakravarti HN, et al. Bardet–Biedl syndrome in two siblings: a rare entity revisited. QJM. 2016;109(2):123–4.
17. Karmous-Benailly H, et al. Antenatal presentation of Bardet-Biedl syndrome may mimic Meckel syndrome. Am J Hum Genet. 2005;76(3):493–504.

18. Baker K, et al. Neocortical and hippocampal volume loss in a human ciliopathy: a quantitative MRI study in Bardet-Biedl syndrome. Am J Med Genet A. 2011;155A(1):1–8.
19. Beales PL, P.P.a.K.N. The Bardet-Biedl and Alstrom syndromes. In: Flinter F, Maher ER, Saggar-Malik A, editors. Genetics of renal disease. London: Oxford University Press; 2004. p. 361–98.
20. Heon E, et al. Ocular phenotypes of three genetic variants of Bardet-Biedl syndrome. Am J Med Genet A. 2005;132A(3):283–7.
21. Azari AA, et al. Retinal disease expression in Bardet-Biedl syndrome-1 (BBS1) is a spectrum from maculopathy to retina-wide degeneration. Invest Ophthalmol Vis Sci. 2006;47(11):5004–10.
22. Moore SJ, et al. Clinical and genetic epidemiology of Bardet-Biedl syndrome in Newfoundland: a 22-year prospective, population-based, cohort study. Am J Med Genet A. 2005;132(4):352–60.
23. Ramirez N, et al. Orthopaedic manifestations of Bardet-Biedl syndrome. J Pediatr Orthop. 2004;24(1):92–6.
24. Barnett S, et al. Behavioural phenotype of Bardet-Biedl syndrome. J Med Genet. 2002;39(12):e76.
25. Mehrotra N, Taub S, Covert RF. Hydrometrocolpos as a neonatal manifestation of the Bardet-Biedl syndrome. Am J Med Genet. 1997;69(2):220.
26. Uguralp S, et al. Bardet-Biedl syndrome associated with vaginal atresia: a case report. Turk J Pediatr. 2003;45(3):273–5.
27. Stoler JM, Herrin JT, Holmes LB. Genital abnormalities in females with Bardet-Biedl syndrome. Am J Med Genet. 1995;55(3):276–8.
28. Friedman NJ, Kaiser PK. Essentials of ophthalmology. Philadelphia: Saunders Elsevier; 2007.
29. Parfrey PS, Davidson WS, Green JS. Clinical and genetic epidemiology of inherited renal disease in Newfoundland. Kidney Int. 2002;61(6):1925–34.
30. O'Dea D, et al. The importance of renal impairment in the natural history of Bardet-Biedl syndrome. Am J Kidney Dis. 1996;27(6):776–83.
31. Tobin JL, et al. Inhibition of neural crest migration underlies craniofacial dysmorphology and Hirschsprung's disease in Bardet-Biedl syndrome. Proc Natl Acad Sci U S A. 2008;105(18):6714–9.
32. Lorda-Sanchez I, et al. Does Bardet-Biedl syndrome have a characteristic face? J Med Genet. 2001;38(5):E14.
33. Rooryck C, et al. Bardet-biedl syndrome and brain abnormalities. Neuropediatrics. 2007;38(1):5–9.
34. Cherian MP, Al-Sanna'a NA. Clinical spectrum of Bardet-Biedl syndrome among four Saudi Arabian families. Clin Dysmorphol. 2009;18(4):188–94.
35. Lorda-Sanchez I, Ayuso C, Ibanez A. Situs inversus and hirschsprung disease: two uncommon manifestations in Bardet-Biedl syndrome. Am J Med Genet. 2000;90(1):80–1.
36. Elbedour K, et al. Cardiac abnormalities in the Bardet-Biedl syndrome: echocardiographic studies of 22 patients. Am J Med Genet. 1994;52(2):164–9.
37. Pagon RA, et al. Hepatic involvement in the Bardet-Biedl syndrome. Am J Med Genet. 1982;13(4):373–81.
38. Cramer B, et al. Sonographic and urographic correlation in Bardet-Biedl syndrome (formerly Laurence-Moon-Biedl syndrome). Urol Radiol. 1988;10(4):176–80.
39. Kulaga HM, et al. Loss of BBS proteins causes anosmia in humans and defects in olfactory cilia structure and function in the mouse. Nat Genet. 2004;36(9):994–8.
40. Iannaccone A, et al. Clinical evidence of decreased olfaction in Bardet-Biedl syndrome caused by a deletion in the BBS4 gene. Am J Med Genet A. 2005;132(4):343–6.
41. Ross AJ, et al. Disruption of Bardet-Biedl syndrome ciliary proteins perturbs planar cell polarity in vertebrates. Nat Genet. 2005;37.(author(10):1135–40.
42. Deffert C, et al. Recurrent insertional polydactyly and situs inversus in a Bardet-Biedl syndrome family. Am J Med Genet A. 2007;143(2):208–13.
43. Schachat AP, Maumenee IH. Bardet-Biedl syndrome and related disorders. Arch Ophthalmol. 1982;100(2):285–8.
44. Forsythe E, Beales PL Bardet-Biedl syndrome. In: Adam MP, Ardinger HH, Pagon RA, Wallace SE, et al., editors. GeneReviews. Seattle: University of Washington; 2017.
45. Schuster SC. Next-generation sequencing transforms today's biology. Nat Methods. 2008;5(1):16–8.
46. Medvedev P, Stanciu M, Brudno M. Computational methods for discovering structural variation with next-generation sequencing. Nat Methods. 2009;6(11 Suppl):S13–20.
47. Redin C, et al. Targeted high-throughput sequencing for diagnosis of genetically heterogeneous diseases: efficient mutation detection in Bardet-Biedl and Alstrom syndromes. J Med Genet. 2012;49(8):502–12.
48. Shah AS, et al. Loss of Bardet-Biedl syndrome proteins alters the morphology and function of motile cilia in airway epithelia. Proc Natl Acad Sci U S A. 2008;105(9):3380–5.
49. Tan PL, et al. Loss of Bardet Biedl syndrome proteins causes defects in peripheral sensory innervation and function. Proc Natl Acad Sci U S A. 2007;104(44):17524–9.
50. Ishizuka K, et al. DISC1-dependent switch from progenitor proliferation to migration in the developing cortex. Nature. 2011;473(7345):92–6.
51. Nishimura DY, et al. Bbs2-null mice have neurosensory deficits, a defect in social dominance, and retinopathy associated with mislocalization of rhodopsin. Proc Natl Acad Sci U S A. 2004;101(47):16588–93.
52. Rahmouni K, et al. Leptin resistance contributes to obesity and hypertension in mouse models of Bardet-Biedl syndrome. J Clin Invest. 2008; 118(4):1458–67.
53. Kaushik AP, et al. Cartilage abnormalities associated with defects of chondrocytic primary cilia in

Bardet-Biedl syndrome mutant mice. J Orthop Res. 2009;27(8):1093–9.
54. Beyer AM, et al. Contrasting vascular effects caused by loss of Bardet-Biedl syndrome genes. Am J Physiol Heart Circ Physiol. 2010;299(6):H1902–7.
55. Guo DF, et al. Inactivation of Bardet-Biedl syndrome genes causes kidney defects. Am J Physiol Ren Physiol. 2011;300(2):F574–80.
56. Schrick JJ, et al. ADP-ribosylation factor-like 3 is involved in kidney and photoreceptor development. Am J Pathol. 2006;168(4):1288–98.
57. Zhang Q, et al. Bardet-Biedl syndrome 3 (Bbs3) knockout mouse model reveals common BBS-associated phenotypes and Bbs3 unique phenotypes. Proc Natl Acad Sci U S A. 2011;108(51):20678–83.
58. Mykytyn K, et al. Bardet-Biedl syndrome type 4 (BBS4)-null mice implicate Bbs4 in flagella formation but not global cilia assembly. Proc Natl Acad Sci U S A. 2004;101(23):8664–9.
59. Eichers ER, et al. Phenotypic characterization of Bbs4 null mice reveals age-dependent penetrance and variable expressivity. Hum Genet. 2006;120(2):211–26.
60. Abd-El-Barr MM, et al. Impaired photoreceptor protein transport and synaptic transmission in a mouse model of Bardet-Biedl syndrome. Vis Res. 2007;47(27):3394–407.
61. Tadenev AL, et al. Loss of Bardet-Biedl syndrome protein-8 (BBS8) perturbs olfactory function, protein localization, and axon targeting. Proc Natl Acad Sci U S A. 2011;108(25):10320–5.
62. Kudryashova E, et al. Deficiency of the E3 ubiquitin ligase TRIM32 in mice leads to a myopathy with a neurogenic component. Hum Mol Genet. 2009;18(7):1353–67.
63. Weatherbee SD, Niswander LA, Anderson KV. A mouse model for Meckel syndrome reveals Mks1 is required for ciliogenesis and Hedgehog signaling. Hum Mol Genet. 2009;18(23):4565–75.
64. Lancaster MA, et al. Defective Wnt-dependent cerebellar midline fusion in a mouse model of Joubert syndrome. Nat Med. 2011;17(6):726–31.
65. Zaghloul NA, Katsanis N. Mechanistic insights into Bardet-Biedl syndrome, a model ciliopathy. J Clin Invest. 2009;119(3):428–37.
66. Chiang AP, et al. Homozygosity mapping with SNP arrays identifies TRIM32, an E3 ubiquitin ligase, as a Bardet-Biedl syndrome gene (BBS11). Proc Natl Acad Sci U S A. 2006;103(16):6287–92.
67. Kim SK, et al. Planar cell polarity acts through septins to control collective cell movement and ciliogenesis. Science. 2010;329(5997):1337–40.
68. Schaefer E, et al. Mutations in SDCCAG8/NPHP10 cause Bardet-Biedl syndrome and are associated with penetrant renal disease and absent polydactyly. Mol Syndromol. 2011;1(6):273–81.
69. Katsanis N, et al. Mutations in MKKS cause obesity, retinal dystrophy and renal malformations associated with Bardet-Biedl syndrome. Nat Genet. 2000;26(1):67–70.
70. Stone DL, et al. Genetic and physical mapping of the McKusick-Kaufman syndrome. Hum Mol Genet. 1998;7(3):475–81.
71. Leppert M, et al. Bardet-Biedl syndrome is linked to DNA markers on chromosome 11q and is genetically heterogeneous. Nat Genet. 1994;7(1):108–12.
72. Katsanis N, et al. Delineation of the critical interval of Bardet-Biedl syndrome 1 (BBS1) to a small region of 11q13, through linkage and haplotype analysis of 91 pedigrees. Am J Hum Genet. 1999;65(6):1672–9.
73. Young TL, et al. A founder effect in the newfoundland population reduces the Bardet-Biedl syndrome I (BBS1) interval to 1 cM. Am J Hum Genet. 1999;65(6):1680–7.
74. Mykytyn K, et al. Identification of the gene (BBS1) most commonly involved in Bardet-Biedl syndrome, a complex human obesity syndrome. Nat Genet. 2002;31(4):435–8.
75. Kwitek-Black AE, et al. Linkage of Bardet-Biedl syndrome to chromosome 16q and evidence for non-allelic genetic heterogeneity. Nat Genet. 1993;5(4):392–6.
76. Beales PL, et al. Genetic and mutational analyses of a large multiethnic Bardet-Biedl cohort reveal a minor involvement of BBS6 and delineate the critical intervals of other loci. Am J Hum Genet. 2001;68(3):606–16.
77. Nishimura DY, et al. Positional cloning of a novel gene on chromosome 16q causing Bardet-Biedl syndrome (BBS2). Hum Mol Genet. 2001;10(8):865–74.
78. Bruford EA, et al. Linkage mapping in 29 Bardet-Biedl syndrome families confirms loci in chromosomal regions 11q13, 15q22.3-q23, and 16q21. Genomics. 1997;41(1):93–9.
79. Carmi R, et al. Phenotypic differences among patients with Bardet-Biedl syndrome linked to three different chromosome loci. Am J Med Genet. 1995;59(2):199–203.
80. Mykytyn K, et al. Identification of the gene that, when mutated, causes the human obesity syndrome BBS4. Nat Genet. 2001;28(2):188–91.
81. Laurier V, et al. Pitfalls of homozygosity mapping: an extended consanguineous Bardet-Biedl syndrome family with two mutant genes (BBS2, BBS10), three mutations, but no triallelism. Eur J Hum Genet. 2006;14(11):1195–203.
82. Stoetzel C, et al. BBS10 encodes a vertebrate-specific chaperonin-like protein and is a major BBS locus. Nat Genet. 2006;38(5):521–4.
83. White DR, et al. Autozygosity mapping of Bardet-Biedl syndrome to 12q21.2 and confirmation of FLJ23560 as BBS10. Eur J Hum Genet. 2007;15(2):173–8.
84. Otto EA, et al. Candidate exome capture identifies mutation of SDCCAG8 as the cause of a retinal-renal ciliopathy. Nat Genet. 2010;42(10):840–50.
85. Badano JL, et al. Identification of a novel Bardet-Biedl syndrome protein, BBS7, that shares structural

features with BBS1 and BBS2. Am J Hum Genet. 2003;72(3):650–8.
86. Ansley SJ, et al. Basal body dysfunction is a likely cause of pleiotropic Bardet-Biedl syndrome. Nature. 2003;425(6958):628–33.
87. Kim JC, et al. The Bardet-Biedl protein BBS4 targets cargo to the pericentriolar region and is required for microtubule anchoring and cell cycle progression. Nat Genet. 2004;36(5):462–70.
88. Young TL, et al. A fifth locus for Bardet-Biedl syndrome maps to chromosome 2q31. Am J Hum Genet. 1999;64(3):900–4.
89. Li JB, et al. Comparative genomics identifies a flagellar and basal body proteome that includes the BBS5 human disease gene. Cell. 2004;117(4):541–52.
90. Chiang AP, et al. Comparative genomic analysis identifies an ADP-ribosylation factor-like gene as the cause of Bardet-Biedl syndrome (BBS3). Am J Hum Genet. 2004;75(3):475–84.
91. Sheffield VC, et al. Identification of a Bardet-Biedl syndrome locus on chromosome 3 and evaluation of an efficient approach to homozygosity mapping. Hum Mol Genet. 1994;3(8):1331–5.
92. Young TL, et al. Canadian Bardet-Biedl syndrome family reduces the critical region of BBS3 (3p) and presents with a variable phenotype. Am J Med Genet. 1998;78(5):461–7.
93. Ghadami M, et al. Bardet-Biedl syndrome type 3 in an Iranian family: clinical study and confirmation of disease localization. Am J Med Genet. 2000;94(5):433–7.
94. Fan Y, et al. Mutations in a member of the Ras superfamily of small GTP-binding proteins causes Bardet-Biedl syndrome. Nat Genet. 2004;36(9):989–93.
95. Nishimura DY, et al. Comparative genomics and gene expression analysis identifies BBS9, a new Bardet-Biedl syndrome gene. Am J Hum Genet. 2005;77(6):1021–33.
96. Stoetzel C, et al. Identification of a novel BBS gene (BBS12) highlights the major role of a vertebrate-specific branch of chaperonin-related proteins in Bardet-Biedl syndrome. Am J Hum Genet. 2007;80(1):1–11.
97. Hildebrandt F, Benzing T, Katsanis N. Ciliopathies. N Engl J Med. 2011;364(16):1533–43.
98. Zaghloul NA, Katsanis N. Functional modules, mutational load and human genetic disease. Trends Genet. 2010;26(4):168–76.
99. Slavotinek AM, et al. Mutations in MKKS cause Bardet-Biedl syndrome. Nat Genet. 2000;26(1): 15–6.
100. Robinow M, Shaw A. The McKusick-Kaufman syndrome: recessively inherited vaginal atresia, hydrometrocolpos, uterovaginal duplications, anorectal anomalies, postaxial polydactyly, and congenital heart disease. J Pediatr. 1979;94(5):776–8.
101. Leitch CC, et al. Hypomorphic mutations in syndromic encephalocele genes are associated with Bardet-Biedl syndrome. Nat Genet. 2008;40(4): 443–8.
102. Marion V, et al. Exome sequencing identifies mutations in LZTFL1, a BBSome and smoothened trafficking regulator, in a family with Bardet – Biedl syndrome with situs inversus and insertional polydactyly. J Med Genet. 2012;49(5):317–21.
103. Mykytyn K, et al. Evaluation of complex inheritance involving the most common Bardet-Biedl syndrome locus (BBS1). Am J Hum Genet. 2003;72(2):429–37.
104. Hichri H, et al. Testing for triallelism: analysis of six BBS genes in a Bardet-Biedl syndrome family cohort. Eur J Hum Genet. 2005;13(5):607–16.
105. Polychronakos D, Tsipas D, Leanis D. Laurence-Moon-Bardet-Biedl syndrome. Acta Ophthal Hetair Borei Hellad. 1963;12:45–54.
106. Klein D. Genetic approach to the nosology of retinal disorders. Birth Defects Orig Artic Ser. 1971;7(3):52–82.
107. Macklin MT. The Laurence-Moon Biedl syndrome: a genetic study. J Hered. 1936;27:97–104.
108. Stern C. Principles of human genetics. San Francisco: W.H. Freeman and Co; 1960. p. 240–375.
109. Croft JB, Swift M. Obesity, hypertension, and renal disease in relatives of Bardet-Biedl syndrome sibs. Am J Med Genet. 1990;36(1):37–42.
110. Croft JB, et al. Obesity in heterozygous carriers of the gene for the Bardet-Biedl syndrome. Am J Med Genet. 1995;55(1):12–5.
111. Cox GF, et al. Retinal function in carriers of Bardet-Biedl syndrome. Arch Ophthalmol. 2003;121(6):804–10.
112. Bergsma DR, Brown KS. Assessment of ophthalmologic, endocrinologic and genetic findings in the Bardet-Biedl syndrome. Birth Defects Orig Artic Ser. 1975;11(2):132–6.
113. Katsanis N. The oligogenic properties of Bardet-Biedl syndrome. Hum Mol Genet. 2004;13 Spec No 1:R65–R71.
114. Slavotinek AM, et al. Mutation analysis of the MKKS gene in McKusick-Kaufman syndrome and selected Bardet-Biedl syndrome patients. Hum Genet. 2002;110(6):561–7.
115. Chen J, et al. Molecular analysis of Bardet-Biedl syndrome families: report of 21 novel mutations in 10 genes. Invest Ophthalmol Vis Sci. 2011;52(8):5317–24.
116. Hjortshoj TD, et al. Bardet-Biedl syndrome in Denmark – report of 13 novel sequence variations in six genes. Hum Mutat. 2010;31(4):429–36.
117. Zaghloul NA, et al. Functional analyses of variants reveal a significant role for dominant negative and common alleles in oligogenic Bardet-Biedl syndrome. Proc Natl Acad Sci U S A. 2010;107(23):10602–7.
118. Badano JL, et al. Dissection of epistasis in oligogenic Bardet-Biedl syndrome. Nature. 2006;439(7074):326–30.
119. de Pontual L, et al. Epistatic interactions with a common hypomorphic RET allele in syndromic Hirschsprung disease. Hum Mutat. 2007;28(8):790–6.

120. Khanna H, et al. A common allele in RPGRIP1L is a modifier of retinal degeneration in ciliopathies. Nat Genet. 2009;41(6):739–45.
121. Putoux A, et al. KIF7 mutations cause fetal hydrolethalus and acrocallosal syndromes. Nat Genet. 2011;43(6):601–6.
122. Davis EE, et al. TTC21B contributes both causal and modifying alleles across the ciliopathy spectrum. Nat Genet. 2011;43(3):189–96.
123. Pirzada O, Taylor C. Modifier genes and cystic fibrosis liver disease. Hepatology. 2003;37(3):714. author reply 714
124. Li JL, et al. A genome scan for modifiers of age at onset in Huntington disease: the HD MAPS study. Am J Hum Genet. 2003;73(3):682–7.
125. Pandya A, et al. Frequency and distribution of GJB2 (connexin 26) and GJB6 (connexin 30) mutations in a large North American repository of deaf probands. Genet Med. 2003;5(4):295–303.
126. Badano JL, Katsanis N. Beyond Mendel: an evolving view of human genetic disease transmission. Nat Rev Genet. 2002;3(10):779–89.
127. Bialas NJ, et al. Functional interactions between the ciliopathy-associated Meckel syndrome 1 (MKS1) protein and two novel MKS1-related (MKSR) proteins. J Cell Sci. 2009;122(Pt 5):611–24.
128. Blacque OE, et al. Loss of C. elegans BBS-7 and BBS-8 protein function results in cilia defects and compromised intraflagellar transport. Genes Dev. 2004;18(13):1630–42.
129. Kim JC, et al. MKKS/BBS6, a divergent chaperonin-like protein linked to the obesity disorder Bardet-Biedl syndrome, is a novel centrosomal component required for cytokinesis. J Cell Sci. 2005;118(Pt 5):1007–20.
130. Marion V, et al. Transient ciliogenesis involving Bardet-Biedl syndrome proteins is a fundamental characteristic of adipogenic differentiation. Proc Natl Acad Sci U S A. 2009;106(6):1820–5.
131. Sayer JA, et al. The centrosomal protein nephrocystin-6 is mutated in Joubert syndrome and activates transcription factor ATF4. Nat Genet. 2006;38(6):674–81.
132. Wiens CJ, et al. Bardet-Biedl syndrome-associated small GTPase ARL6 (BBS3) functions at or near the ciliary gate and modulates Wnt signaling. J Biol Chem. 2010;285(21):16218–30.
133. Nachury MV, et al. A core complex of BBS proteins cooperates with the GTPase Rab8 to promote ciliary membrane biogenesis. Cell. 2007;129(6):1201–13.
134. Locke M, et al. TRIM32 is an E3 ubiquitin ligase for dysbindin. Hum Mol Genet. 2009;18(13):2344–58.
135. Strutt D, Warrington SJ. Planar polarity genes in the Drosophila wing regulate the localisation of the FH3-domain protein multiple wing hairs to control the site of hair production. Development. 2008;135(18):3103–11.
136. Seo S, et al. A novel protein LZTFL1 regulates ciliary trafficking of the BBSome and smoothened. PLoS Genet. 2011;7(11):e1002358.
137. Badano JL, Teslovich TM, Katsanis N. The centrosome in human genetic disease. Nat Rev Genet. 2005;6(3):194–205.
138. Beisson J, Wright M. Basal body/centriole assembly and continuity. Curr Opin Cell Biol. 2003;15(1):96–104.
139. Dammermann A, Merdes A. Assembly of centrosomal proteins and microtubule organization depends on PCM-1. J Cell Biol. 2002;159(2):255–66.
140. Blatch GL, Lassle M. The tetratricopeptide repeat: a structural motif mediating protein-protein interactions. BioEssays. 1999;21(11):932–9.
141. Gill SR, et al. Dynactin, a conserved, ubiquitously expressed component of an activator of vesicle motility mediated by cytoplasmic dynein. J Cell Biol. 1991;115(6):1639–50.
142. Blacque OE, Leroux MR. Bardet-Biedl syndrome: an emerging pathomechanism of intracellular transport. Cell Mol Life Sci. 2006;63(18):2145–61.
143. Yen HJ, et al. Bardet-Biedl syndrome genes are important in retrograde intracellular trafficking and Kupffer's vesicle cilia function. Hum Mol Genet. 2006;15(5):667–77.
144. Stearns T, et al. ADP-ribosylation factor is functionally and physically associated with the Golgi complex. Proc Natl Acad Sci U S A. 1990;87(3):1238–42.
145. Dascher C, Balch WE. Dominant inhibitory mutants of ARF1 block endoplasmic reticulum to Golgi transport and trigger disassembly of the Golgi apparatus. J Biol Chem. 1994;269(2):1437–48.
146. Lowe SL, Wong SH, Hong W. The mammalian ARF-like protein 1 (Arl1) is associated with the Golgi complex. J Cell Sci. 1996;109(Pt 1):209–20.
147. Gerdes JM, Katsanis N. Small molecule intervention in microtubule-associated human disease. Hum Mol Genet. 2005;14 Spec No. 2:R291–R300.
148. Fath MA, et al. Mkks-null mice have a phenotype resembling Bardet-Biedl syndrome. Hum Mol Genet. 2005;14(9):1109–18.
149. May-Simera HL, et al. Patterns of expression of Bardet-Biedl syndrome proteins in the mammalian cochlea suggest noncentrosomal functions. J Comp Neurol. 2009;514(2):174–88.
150. Torayama I, Ishihara T, Katsura I. Caenorhabditis elegans integrates the signals of butanone and food to enhance chemotaxis to butanone. J Neurosci. 2007;27(4):741–50.
151. Takada T, et al. Expression of ADP-ribosylation factor (ARF)-like protein 6 during mouse embryonic development. Int J Dev Biol. 2005;49(7):891–4.
152. Seo S, et al. BBS6, BBS10, and BBS12 form a complex with CCT/TRiC family chaperonins and mediate BBSome assembly. Proc Natl Acad Sci U S A. 2010;107(4):1488–93.
153. Kim J, Krishnaswami SR, Gleeson JG. CEP290 interacts with the centriolar satellite component PCM-1 and is required for Rab8 localization to the primary cilium. Hum Mol Genet. 2008;17(23):3796–805.
154. Rosenbaum JL, Witman GB. Intraflagellar transport. Nat Rev Mol Cell Biol. 2002;3(11):813–25.

155. Ou G, et al. Functional coordination of intraflagellar transport motors. Nature. 2005;436(7050):583–7.
156. Pan X, et al. Mechanism of transport of IFT particles in C. elegans cilia by the concerted action of kinesin-II and OSM-3 motors. J Cell Biol. 2006;174(7):1035–45.
157. Ou G, et al. Sensory ciliogenesis in Caenorhabditis elegans: assignment of IFT components into distinct modules based on transport and phenotypic profiles. Mol Biol Cell. 2007;18(5):1554–69.
158. Lechtreck KF, et al. The Chlamydomonas reinhardtii BBSome is an IFT cargo required for export of specific signaling proteins from flagella. J Cell Biol. 2009;187(7):1117–32.
159. Afzelius BA. The immotile-cilia syndrome: a microtubule-associated defect. CRC Crit Rev Biochem. 1985;19(1):63–87.
160. Yoder BK, Hou X, Guay-Woodford LM. The polycystic kidney disease proteins, polycystin-1, polycystin-2, polaris, and cystin, are co-localized in renal cilia. J Am Soc Nephrol. 2002;13(10):2508–16.
161. Nauli SM, et al. Polycystins 1 and 2 mediate mechanosensation in the primary cilium of kidney cells. Nat Genet. 2003;33(2):129–37.
162. Davis EE, Brueckner M, Katsanis N. The emerging complexity of the vertebrate cilium: new functional roles for an ancient organelle. Dev Cell. 2006;11(1):9–19.
163. Huangfu D, et al. Hedgehog signalling in the mouse requires intraflagellar transport proteins. Nature. 2003;426(6962):83–7.
164. Rohatgi R, Milenkovic L, Scott MP. Patched1 regulates hedgehog signaling at the primary cilium. Science. 2007;317(5836):372–6.
165. Corbit KC, et al. Vertebrate smoothened functions at the primary cilium. Nature. 2005;437(7061):1018–21.
166. Haycraft CJ, et al. Gli2 and Gli3 localize to cilia and require the intraflagellar transport protein polaris for processing and function. PLoS Genet. 2005;1(4):e53.
167. Dai P, et al. Sonic Hedgehog-induced activation of the Gli1 promoter is mediated by GLI3. J Biol Chem. 1999;274(12):8143–52.
168. Hsu SH, et al. Kif7 promotes hedgehog signaling in growth plate chondrocytes by restricting the inhibitory function of Sufu. Development. 2011;138(17):3791–801.
169. Tayeh MK, et al. Genetic interaction between Bardet-Biedl syndrome genes and implications for limb patterning. Hum Mol Genet. 2008;17(13):1956–67.
170. Logan CY, Nusse R. The Wnt signaling pathway in development and disease. Annu Rev Cell Dev Biol. 2004;20:781–810.
171. Willert K, Nusse R. Beta-catenin: a key mediator of Wnt signaling. Curr Opin Genet Dev. 1998;8(1):95–102.
172. De Marco P, et al. Human neural tube defects: genetic causes and prevention. Biofactors. 2011;37(4):261–8.
173. Tada M, Concha ML, Heisenberg CP. Non-canonical Wnt signalling and regulation of gastrulation movements. Semin Cell Dev Biol. 2002;13(3):251–60.
174. Torban E, et al. Independent mutations in mouse Vangl2 that cause neural tube defects in looptail mice impair interaction with members of the Dishevelled family. J Biol Chem. 2004;279(50):52703–13.
175. Gerdes JM, et al. Disruption of the basal body compromises proteasomal function and perturbs intracellular Wnt response. Nat Genet. 2007;39.(author(11):1350–60.
176. Benzing T, Simons M, Walz G. Wnt signaling in polycystic kidney disease. J Am Soc Nephrol. 2007;18(5):1389–98.
177. Lancaster MA, Gleeson JG. Cystic kidney disease: the role of Wnt signaling. Trends Mol Med. 2010;16(8):349–60.
178. Schneider L, et al. PDGFRalphaalpha signaling is regulated through the primary cilium in fibroblasts. Curr Biol. 2005;15(20):1861–6.
179. Ezratty EJ, et al. A role for the primary cilium in notch signaling and epidermal differentiation during skin development. Cell. 2011;145(7):1129–41.
180. Gascue C, et al. Direct role of Bardet-Biedl syndrome proteins in transcriptional regulation. J Cell Sci. 2012;125(Pt 2):362–75.

Cystic Kidney Diseases Associated with Increased Cancer Risk: Tuberous Sclerosis Complex, Von Hippel-Lindau, and Birt-Hogg-Dubé

3

John J. Bissler

Introduction

In a commentary about the use of a tyrosine kinase inhibitor in polycystic kidney disease, Grantham used a title that is timeless, "Time to treat polycystic kidney diseases like the neoplastic disorders that they are" [1]. Decades of literature have tried to definitively resolve any relationship between autosomal dominant polycystic kidney disease and malignancy. While this risk, if any, seems to be very small, there are malignancy predisposition syndromes in which renal cystic disease can be an impressive phenotype. Tuberous sclerosis complex (TSC), von Hippel-Lindau (VHL) disease and Birt-Hogg-Dubé (BHD) disease are autosomal dominant tumor suppressor-associated syndromes that are characterized by solid and cystic renal lesions. These diseases can also have a purely renal cystic disease phenotype. Phenotypic expression of these diseases also occurs through a somatic mutation mechanism, specifically the combination of an acquired somatic mutation occurring in a patient with an inherited inactivating mutation in the TSC gene loci (*TSC1* gene on chromosome 9q34 or the *TSC2* gene on chromosome 16p13.32), the *VHL* gene locus (on chromosome 3p25.3), or the *FLCN* gene (on chromosome 17p11.2), respectively. The second somatic mutation results in complete cellular deficiency of the protein products hamartin (TSC1), tuberin (TSC2), von Hippel-Lindau tumor suppressor protein (pVHL), or folliculin (FLCN). These proteins have a pivotal role in normal gene expression and are linked in an intricate pathway that regulates cell growth, proliferation, vascular supply, and renal cilia [2].

TSC Renal Disease

Genetics of Tuberous Sclerosis Complex Renal Cystic Disease

Tuberous sclerosis complex (TSC) is an autosomal dominant genetic disorder affecting every organ system and exhibits a birth incidence of ~1:5800, thus affecting approximately *one million patients worldwide* [3, 4]. Proper diagnosis can be missed if one relies on the outdated Vogt's triad for TSC (facial angiofibromas, developmental delay, and intractable epilepsy) because less than 40% of affected patients exhibit these classical features [5]. In fact, only about half of patients demonstrate cognitive impairment, autism, or

J. J. Bissler, MD, FAAP, FASN (✉)
Chief, Division of Nephrology, Department of Pediatrics, Director, Tuberous Sclerosis Center of Excellence at Le Bonheur Children's Hospital, Medical Director, Nephrology, St. Jude Children's Research Hospital, University of Tennessee Health Science Center, Children's Foundation Research Center, Memphis, TN, USA
e-mail: jbissler@UTHSC.edu

B. D. Cowley, Jr., J. J. Bissler (eds.), *Polycystic Kidney Disease*,
https://doi.org/10.1007/978-1-4939-7784-0_3

other behavioral disorders [6]. There are two loci associated with TSC: the *TSC1* gene, located on chromosome 9, and the *TSC2* gene, located on chromosome 16. The identification of the *TSC2* gene location was assisted because of an astute genetic observation in a family with autosomal dominant polycystic kidney disease. The family members who manifested polycystic disease did so because they suffered from a balanced translocation involving the *PKD1* gene. A child in this family not only had autosomal dominant polycystic kidney disease but also had tuberous sclerosis complex. The cause of simultaneous ADPKD and TSC in this child was an unbalanced translocation, while the family members with only autosomal dominant polycystic disease had balanced translocations, and this fact aided in the positional cloning of the *TSC2* gene [7].

Tuberous sclerosis complex is phenotypically expressed by a somatic silencing event of the nonmutant allele, either through a second somatic mutation or other possible silencing mechanisms. Both TSC and autosomal dominant polycystic kidney disease are phenotypically expressed due to a second hit or somatic mutation mechanism [8–10]. The kidney disease associated with the *PKD1* and the *TSC2* loci accounts for a majority of their respective diseases, and both exhibit a more severe phenotype compared to the disease associated with the *PKD2* and *TSC1* loci. The association of these genes with more severe disease appears to have a molecular underpinning. Both the *PKD1* and *TSC2* loci are immediately adjacent, in a tail-to-tail orientation, on chromosome 16p. The proximity of the genes is important because the *PKD1* gene contains an intronic sequence with unique structural properties [11] that can predispose to mutation because this tract interferes with DNA replication and leads to double-strand breaks and thus an array of somatic mutational effects [12, 13]. Synergizing this predisposition to DNA double-strand breaks, the renal microenvironment also inhibits DNA damage recognition [14–16]. This renal microenvironmental predisposition to disease may also help explain the multifocal and bilateral nature of the TSC cystic disease as well as the angiomyolipomata.

TSC and Renal Function

Premature impairment of glomerular filtration rate (GFR) has been reported in up to 40% of patients with TSC [17]. Practically speaking, the reduction of renal function is similar to that expected if the TSC patient population were 30 years older. This reduction in function occurs in the absence of overt bleeding from angiomyolipomata or interventions [18]. This underscores the need to use methods that preserve kidney function when treating angiomyolipomata preemptively to prevent bleeding and for hypertension control. To assess renal function at the time of diagnosis, as well as on an annual basis, blood tests need to be done to estimate glomerular filtration rate (GFR) using creatinine [19, 20] or cystatin C equations [21]. Renal function in patients with TSC is of critical importance because many of the drugs commonly used to treat patients are renally cleared (Table 3.1).

Intersection of Cilial Cystogenic and Oncogenic Signaling Pathways in TSC Renal Cystic Disease

Tuberous sclerosis complex proteins regulate cell growth and proliferation, crucial features of organogenesis, organ maintenance, and malignancy. As reviewed in Chap. 5, the mammalian target of rapamycin complex 1 (mTORC1) signaling pathway integrates intra- and extracellular environmental information in order to regulate metabolism, protein translation, growth, proliferation, autophagy, and survival (Fig. 3.1). The TSC2 protein interacts with polycystin-1 to control the mTORC1 pathway by way of the cleaved C-terminal tail of polycystin-1 [22]. AKT phosphorylation of TSC2 causes its retention at the cell membrane in order to regulate mTOR. This phosphorylation step is inhibited by the uncleaved membrane-bound C-terminal tail of polycystin-1. Without this phosphorylation, TSC2 complexes with TSC1 to inhibit mTORC1.

The integrated role of the primary cilium and the mTORC1 pathway in cystogenesis is

Table 3.1 Renal clearance of commonly used medications in TSC

Generic (brand)	Metabolism/elimination	Renal dosing
Carbamazepine (Tegretol)	Hepatic	Cl_{cr} <10 mL/min: administer 75% of recommended dose; monitor serum levels
Clobazam (Onfi)	Hepatic	Cl_{cr} ≥30 mL/min: no dosage adjustment required
		Cl_{cr} <30 mL/min: use with caution, has not been studied
Clonazepam (Klonopin)	Hepatic	No dosage adjustment provided in manufacturer's labeling; use with caution. Clonazepam metabolites may accumulate in patients with renal impairment Hemodialysis: supplemental dose not necessary
Divalproex (Depakote)	Extensive in the liver via glucuronide conjugation and oxidation	Cl_{cr} <10 mL/min: no dosage adjustment is needed for patients on hemodialysis
Everolimus (Afinitor)	Hepatic	No dosage adjustment necessary
Lamotrigine (Lamictal)	>75% metabolized in the liver via glucuronidation	Use with caution; has not been adequately studied; base initial dose on patient's Anti-epileptic drug regimen; decreased maintenance dosage may be effective in patients with significant renal impairment
Metyrosine (Demser)	Primarily in the urine (53–88% as unchanged drug)	No dosage adjustment provided in manufacturer's labeling
Oxcarbazepine (Trileptal)	Hepatic	Cl_{cr} <30 mL/min: initial dose—administer 50% of the normal starting dose; slowly increase the dose if needed, using a slower dosage titration than normal
Phenytoin (Dilantin)	Metabolized in the liver; major metabolite (via oxidation) HPPA undergoes enterohepatic recycling and elimination in urine as glucuronides	Phenytoin serum concentrations may be difficult to interpret in renal failure. Monitoring of free (unbound) concentrations or adjustment to allow interpretation is recommended
Quetiapine (Seroquel)	Hepatic	No dosage adjustment required
Risperidone (Risperdal)	Hepatic	Cl_{cr} <30 mL/min: starting dose of 0.5 mg twice daily; titration should progress slowly in increments of no more than 0.5 mg twice daily; increases to dosages >1.5 mg twice daily should occur at intervals of ≥1 week. Clearance of the active moiety is decreased by 60% in patients with moderate-to-severe renal disease (Cl_{cr} <60 mL/min) compared to healthy subjects
Sirolimus (Rapamune)	In the intestinal wall via P-glycoprotein and hepatic via CYP3A4	No dosage adjustment (in loading or maintenance dose) is necessary in renal impairment. However, adjustment of regimen (including discontinuation of therapy) should be considered when used concurrently with cyclosporine and elevated or increasing serum creatinine is noted
Topiramate (Topamax)	70% excreted unchanged in the urine	Cl_{cr} <70 mL/min/1.73 m^2: administer 50% of the usual dose; titrate more slowly due to prolonged half-life. Significantly hemodialyzed; dialysis clearance: 120 mL/min (4–6 times higher than in adults with normal renal function); supplemental doses may be required
Trazodone	Hepatic	No dosage adjustment required
Vigabatrin (Sabril)	Eliminated via urine	Cl_{cr} >50–80 mL/min: decrease dose by 25%
		Cl_{cr} >30–50 mL/min: decrease dose by 50%
		Cl_{cr} >10–30 mL/min: decrease dose by 75%

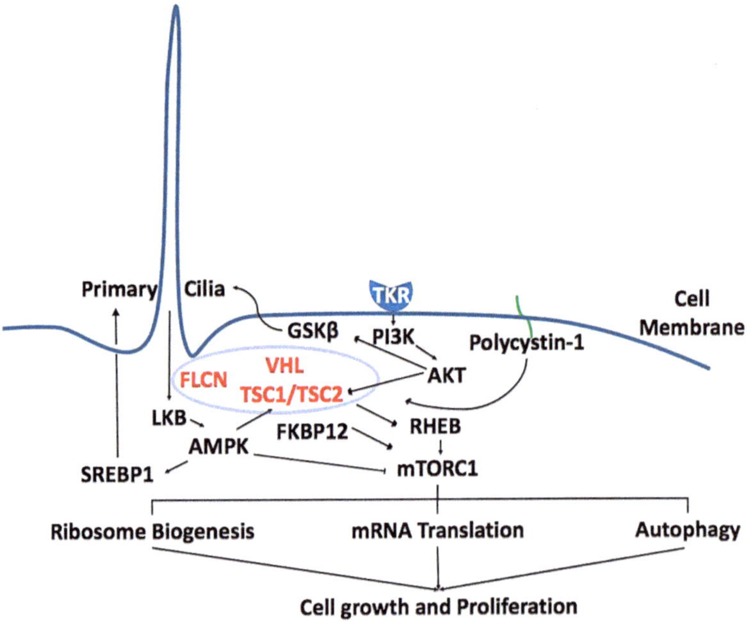

Fig. 3.1 Diagram to help depict the relationship between primary cilia and the mTORC1 pathway. TSC, VHL, and BHP proteins are larger and in red. Blue oval contains cilia mTORC1 facilitating proteins. Cilia deflection signals through the BHD-associated protein called folliculin (FLCN). Cilia hoisting and maintenance are functions of pVHL and GSKβ, while SREBP1 inhibits cilia formation

supported by experiments using unilateral nephrectomy. Transgenic mice that underwent adult-induced cilia loss and subsequent unilateral nephrectomy showed an increase in cyst severity, and the cilia mutants showed significantly higher levels of mTORC1 activity in the remaining kidney compared to controls [23].

mTORC1 activity is also modulated by cilia deflection or mechanosensation. Specifically, cilia-mediated detection of fluid flow modulated cell volume by inhibiting the mTORC1 signaling cascade. When adult cells that had cilia expression disrupted were cultured in the presence of flow, they did not adjust cell volume and were significantly larger than the same cells that continued to express cilia. The size phenotype in the mutant cells could be normalized using mTORC1 inhibitors [24]. Although there is an interaction between polcystin-1 and TSC2 protein as discussed above, this effect of cilia transduction through mTORC1 was mediated through LKB1. LKB1, a cilium-localized kinase, phosphorylates AMP-activated protein kinase (AMPK). AMPK inhibits mTOR activity but is upregulated as a consequence of cilia sensing flow under normal conditions [24].

Activation of AMPK by LKB1 is required for cell polarization and essential for formation of epithelial tight junctions [25]. A curious potential mechanism linking LKB1 signaling to AMPK is through the activity of sterol response element-binding proteins (SREBPs), which regulate cell metabolic processes. Increased SREPB1 activity may be, at least in part, involved in lipid synthesis in the angiomyolipomata. In addition, increased expression of SREBP1 causes loss of cilia and fatty acid synthesis. Remarkably, inhibition of fatty acid synthesis is sufficient to restore cilia [26]. An additional association with cystogenic pathways includes the relationship between SREPB1 and Wnt signaling. SREBP1, signaling through downstream fatty acid synthase (FASN), promotes palmitoylation of a group of protein targets including Wnt. This protein is a key regulator of planar cell polarity (PCP) [27]. Specifically, palmitoylated Wnt is stabilized at the cell and ciliary membrane, stabilizing cytoplasmic expression of its major canonical effector β-catenin [27]. Stabilization of β-catenin in the cytoplasm contributes to cell cycle entry and limits the cilial hedgehog/sonic hedgehog (Hh/Shh) signaling that supports differentiation rather than proliferation. β-Catenin also increases expression of NEDD9 which also may play a role in the SREBP1-associated loss of cilia [28].

Perturbations in the TSC proteins can also affect the physical cilial structure. Mutations disrupting the activity of TSC2 and its heterodimerizing partner TSC1 de-suppress mTOR signaling, and this activity has been associated with lengthened cilia [29, 30]. Mechanistically, TSC negatively regulates PLK1 [31], and LKB1 negatively regulates NEDD9 [32, 33], suggesting mechanisms for dialogue between regulation of the mTOR pathway and the presence of cilia.

Practical Clinical Considerations of TSC Renal Cystic Disease

Renal cystic disease is much more common than once appreciated in the TSC population and increases the patient's risk for hypertension. Most patients with TSC exhibit at least stage I chronic kidney disease (CKD), and blood pressure control is important to slow progression of CKD. Hypertension in TSC is thought to be renin-mediated and responds very well to angiotensin-converting enzyme inhibitors or angiotensin receptor blockers. There is evidence that the TSC-associated renal angiomyolipomata express the angiotensin II receptor type 1 [34], and early reduction of the renin-angiotensin-aldosterone system in autosomal dominant polycystic kidney disease slows cystic disease progression [35]. Despite a significant burden of renal parenchymal abnormalities observed by imaging, renal function often is preserved.

Nephrolithiasis is not infrequent in patients with TSC because of their renal disease manifestations as well as side effects of some anticonvulsant therapies. For example, topiramate is an effective anticonvulsant for some forms of TSC-associated epilepsy. The drug enhances GABA-activated chloride channels and inhibits excitatory neurotransmission, thereby reducing seizure activity. Topiramate also inhibits carbonic anhydrase, particularly subtypes II and IV, leading to reduced renal citrate excretion and subsequently increased risk of nephrolithiasis. While a ketogenic diet can significantly improve seizure control for some patients with TSC, it is also associated with hypercalciuria, hypocitraturia, and decreased uric acid solubility caused by the low urine pH. These three factors synergize to increase the risk of nephrolithiasis in patients treated with a ketogenic diet. Significant renal cystic disease also increases the risk of nephrolithiasis because of altered distal tubular function and subsequent hypocitraturia. Diagnosing nephrolithiasis in a developmentally delayed patient can be difficult because they may not be able to articulate their symptoms well. Understanding the risk factors can help guide imaging and diagnosis. Successful medical therapy for nephrolithiasis in this patient population is relatively simple, involving adequate hydration and citrate supplementation when required. Minimally invasive treatment of nephrolithiasis includes extracorporeal shock wave lithotripsy (ESWL), percutaneous nephrolithotomy (PCNL), and ureteroscopic stone removal (URS). ESWL may result in renal subcapsular hematoma formation, and PCNL involves accessing by puncture and dilation of the renal collecting system via the renal parenchyma. Because patients with TSC renal disease have a well-known potential for renal hemorrhage, such approaches may pose an unacceptable risk. Ureteroscopic stone removal by stone baskets to remove small stones and a laser fiber to direct pulsed laser energy that will fragment stones are better options.

Some patients also experience nocturnal enuresis. This can be part of a normal development and can be prolonged in part because of developmental delay, as well as renal cystic disease-induced urinary concentration defect. This can be quite trying for patients and families, and the topic belongs in a chapter about renal cystic disease because families will seek help wherever they can. Well-meaning practitioners may use desmopressin (ddAVP), a synthetic replacement for vasopressin, to reduce the nocturnal urine volume. This approach is contraindicated in patients with cystic disease given the role of vasopressin/cyclic adenosine monophosphate in cyst enlargement [36].

Because about a third of TSC-associated angiomyolipomata can have fat-poor components, and because at least half of the patients affected with TSC will have cystic disease, it is not uncommon that some patients will have a solid mass, which may even enhance, associated with their cystic components. This basic finding should raise concern for renal cell carcinoma in the general population but should not raise the same level of concern in the population with TSC because renal cell carcinoma is actually very rare in the population of TSC patients. Such lesions can be serially measured and assessed for grow characteristics that can help sort the fat-poor angiomyolipoma from the malignancy [37]. Current research focuses on noninvasive approaches to help better delineate malignancy from fat-poor angiomyolipoma [38].

Recognizable Patterns of TSC-Associated Renal Cystic Disease

TSC renal cystic disease can be detected by conventional MRI in approximately 50% of patients with TSC and is associated with mutations in either the *TSC1* or *TSC2* genes [39–41]. The size of the renal cysts in TSC renal disease ranges from the microscopic glomerulocystic disease [42] to a polycystic renal phenotype associated with the TSC2/PKD1 contiguous gene syndrome [43]. To better understand the natural history and communicate about TSC renal cystic disease, the five basic patterns of cystic disease are described below.

TSC Polycystic Kidney Disease

This syndrome usually involves deletions that encompass a portion of the adjacent *TSC2* and *PKD1* genes on chromosome 16p13 and accounts for about 2% of TSC patients [44]. However, there are cases that appear identical to this contiguous gene syndrome that are linked to *TSC1*. Renal cysts in TSC can arise from all nephron segments [42]. There is a high number of mosaic cases [45], and often these children have some cystic disease in utero or shortly after birth but develop very significant disease by 2 months of age (Fig. 3.2). Hypertension usually develops by the first 2 weeks of life but can take up to several months and is best treated with angiotensin-converting enzyme inhibitors or angiotensin receptor blockers. Because of the severity of renal parenchyma disruption, these children develop a urinary concentrating defect very early, and this may further drive cystogenesis by increasing antidiuretic hormone secretion [46]. There are also practical considerations. Because the kidney mass can be so large, balance can be affected, so the ambulation developmental

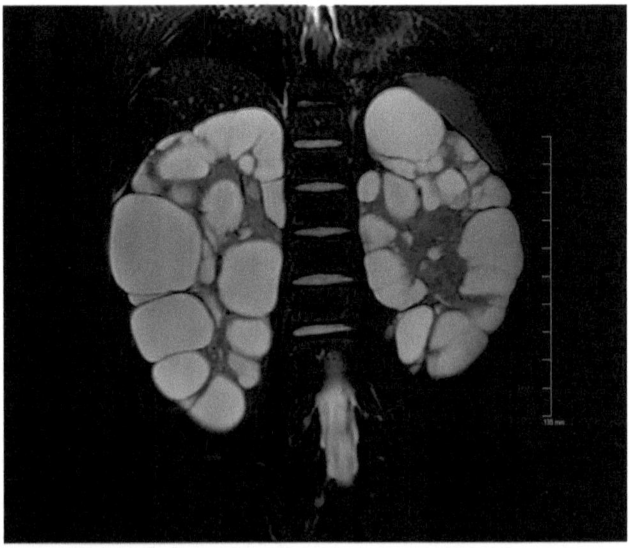

Fig. 3.2 Polycystic variant of TSC renal disease. Coronal MRI of a preteen boy with the polycystic variety of TSC

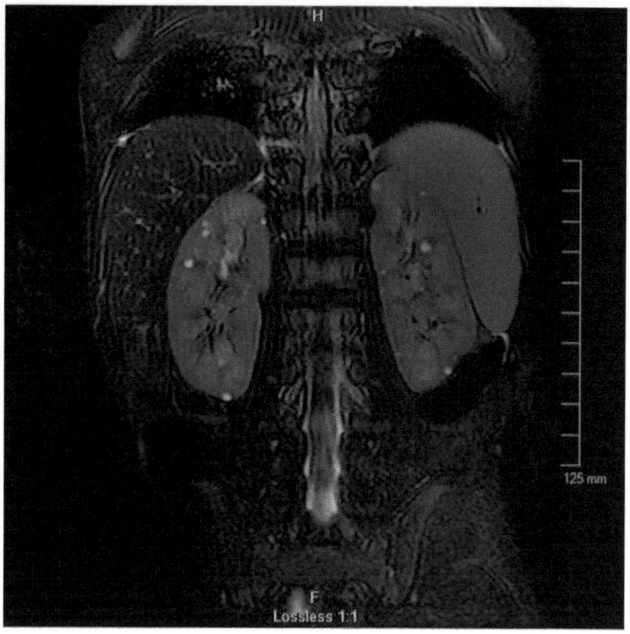

Fig. 3.3 Cortical TSC cystic kidney disease. TSC cystic renal disease is limited to the cortex and columns of Bertin

milestone can be delayed. Likewise, nocturnal enuresis can be prolonged because of the concentration defect and *must not* be treated with ddAVP given the cyst-promoting potential. Even clothing options for the child can be a source of frustration for the family as the protuberant abdomen often can be an impediment for proper-fitting trousers; fortunately, bib overalls are still in style for infants and toddlers.

TSC Cortical Cystic Kidney Disease

Another recognizable pattern of TSC cystic renal disease is that it is limited to the cortex and columns of Bertin (Fig. 3.3). This cystic disease occurs early on, and the cysts are remarkably uniform in size. This imaging pattern may suggest glomerulocystic disease or even dilatation of other tubular segments. There are usually a number of cysts but often less than two dozen or so.

TSC Multicystic Kidney Disease

Cysts can also be distributed throughout the cortical and medullary tissue and exhibit variable sizes (Fig. 3.4). This pattern is also associated with either *TSC1* or *TSC2* mutations and with significant chronic kidney disease. It can also resemble the polycystic variety but genetically is different than TSC2/PKD1 contiguous gene syndrome.

TSC Cortical Microcystic Kidney Disease

Initially the findings of cortical microcystic disease are subtle and detected by careful inspection of the abdominal MRI (Fig. 3.5). The renal cortex will exhibit an increased water signal of fast spin echo T2 or similar sequences before overt discrete cortical cysts can be identified. Eventually, the cortex may exhibit an increased echotexture similar to that seen in the medullary pyramids in autosomal recessive polycystic renal disease. Identification of this pattern is important because it is also associated with a more rapid decline in renal function, not uncommonly developing chronic kidney disease stage II or III in the late teens or early 20s. The renal pyramids are spared, the urinary concentration capacity is preserved, sometimes there is evidence of tubular proteinuria with the creatinine increase, and hypertension is not common until significant chronic kidney disease develops.

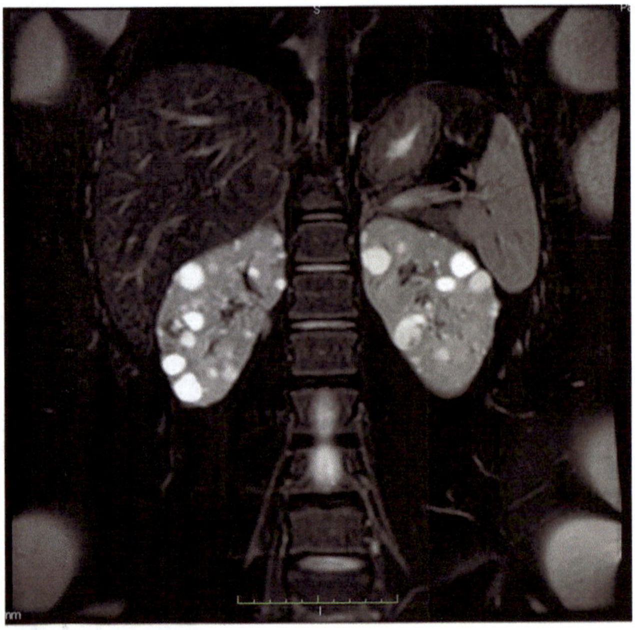

Fig. 3.4 TSC multicystic kidney disease. Cysts are distributed throughout the cortical and medullary tissue and exhibit variable sizes

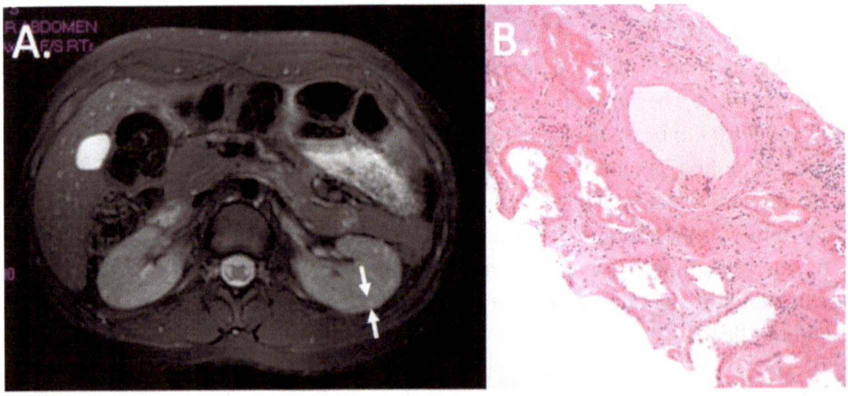

Fig. 3.5 TSC cortical microcystic kidney disease. (**a**) MRI imaging. Note cortical cysts and increased water signal (white) in the cortex (between white arrows). (**b**) Note microcystic disease on hematoxylin and eosin staining

TSC Focal Cystic Kidney Disease

Focal cystic disease appears to result in a somatic mutation during branching of the ureteric bud such that there is significant cystogenesis in a localized renal pyramid (Fig. 3.6). The developmental timing can be such that a small child can have an isolated renal pyramid with profound cystic disease, while the other pyramids are structurally normal. I posit that the mutation can occur *after* a critical time period during induction and only be phenotypically expressed after acute kidney injury. Following renal injury, TSC patients develop cystic disease in an isolated renal pyramid. This renal injury has been postulated to constitute a "third hit" in autosomal dominant polycystic kidney disease and results in rapid cyst formation in adult research animals [47]. TSC focal cystic kidney disease appears to follow the same sort of temporal sequence. Risk factors for acute kidney injury in TSC patients include certain anticonvulsant and nonsteroidal anti-inflammatory medications, as well as rhabdomyolysis and hypoxia induced by status epilepticus [48].

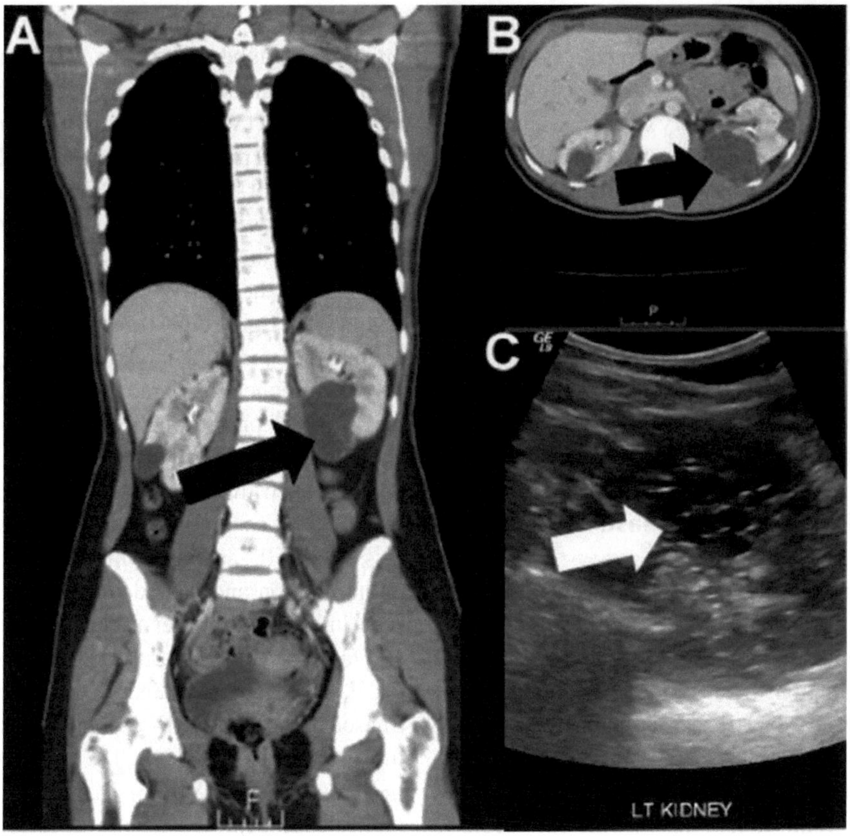

Fig. 3.6 TSC focal cystic kidney disease. (**a**) Coronal CT scan showing focal cystic disease (black arrow), corresponding to (**b**). Axial CT showing cystic disease. (**c**) Ultrasound showing individual cysts

Von Hippel-Lindau Renal Disease

Genetics of Von Hippel-Lindau Renal Disease

The birth incidence of VHL disease is approximately 1 in 36,000, and roughly 20% are new mutations [49, 50]. The disease most often presents with retinal or cerebellar hemangioblastomas, clear cell renal cell carcinoma (RCC), pheochromocytomas, and pancreatic endocrine tumors (reviewed in [51]). The mean age of onset is 35–40 years [51], and patients have an ~70% lifetime risk of developing RCC.

VHL phenotypic expression is divided into four different patterns. Type 1 is characterized by the absence of pheochromocytoma and associated with large mutations deleting or truncating fragments of the *VHL* gene causing the complete inactivation of the gene and high HIF activity. Type 2 is characterized by the presence of pheochromocytomas and more moderate changes in the *VHL* gene, including those preserving some pVHL activity toward HIF-αs. Type 2 VHL disease is subdivided into type 2A which is characterized by a low incidence of renal lesions, type 2B characterized by a high risk of RCC, and type 2C that is characterized by the development of only pheochromocytoma.

Like TSC, VHL is typically phenotypically expressed following a second somatic mutation in a patient who already has a mutant allele. This loss of VHL expression in the cell predisposes to the development of cysts, which occur in the kidney, pancreas, epididymis, and broad ligament. The renal cystic disease can initially be diagnosed as atypical autosomal dominant polycystic kidney disease until other manifestations are identified [52, 53]. In such cases of renal cystic disease and a family history of VHL, a single retinal or cerebellar hemangioblastoma, renal cell carcinoma, or pheochromocytoma is sufficient to make the diagnosis of VHL. If there is no family history, two or more retinal or cerebellar hemangioblastomas or a single hemangioblastoma and a related visceral tumor are required to make the diagnosis.

Intersection of Cilial Cystogenic and Oncogenic Signaling Pathways in VHL Renal Cystic Disease

Although many pVHL functions would appear to confer tumor suppressor capabilities, the loss of pVHL function alone is insufficient for renal tumor initiation. The kidneys of patients with familial VHL disease can contain thousands of sites which have lost pVHL function, but most are single cells [54]. Murine experimental data also support this mutational insufficiency because the loss of VHL alone does not lead to significant cystic disease or conventional renal cell carcinoma [55, 56], though some models can eventually develop cysts [57]. These observations indicate that additional factors, including possible additional mutations, are required for the phenotypic expression. Although the loss of the VHL gene is insufficient to lead to renal cell carcinoma, this loss appears to be associated with and perhaps required for VHL-associated renal cell carcinoma. For example, approximately 38,000 new cases of sporadic renal cell carcinoma occur per year, and the majority are the clear cell variety, of which 50–80% of cases are associated with mutations in the VHL locus [58].

pVHL occupies a central regulatory position in several different signaling pathways, including those directly modulating cellular transcription as well as those controlling the activity of cytoskeletal proteins. The most well-established role of pVHL is its E3 ubiquitin ligase function as part of a multiprotein complex containing elongins C and B, Cullin2, and the RING-H2 finger protein Rbx-1. This multiprotein complex ubiquitinates a number of proteins, including HIF-αs, atypical protein kinase C (aPKC), deubiquitinating enzyme-1 (VDU-1), and two subunits, Rpb1 and Rpb7, of the RNA polymerase II complex (RNAPII) (for review see [59]). During normoxia, HIF-αs are hydroxylated on proline 564 and 402 residues located within L(XY)LAP motifs, by the O2, Fe(II), and oxoglutarate-regulated Egl-9-type proline hydroxylases (Eglns1–3), resulting in HIF-α's ubiquitination and subsequent degradation [60]. During hypoxia, the proline hydroxylation is inhibited, and ubiquitination and degradation of HIF-αs are reduced such that HIF-α accumulates. A gratuitous HIF-α accumulation also occurs with the loss of pVHL activity, which prevents normal ubiquitination and degradation of HIF-α, and is seen in the sporadic renal clear cell carcinomas and familial VHL disease [61]. As a downstream event, HIF activity is increased and stimulates transcription of the HIF-responsive genes including angiogenic factors, such as vascular endothelial growth factor (VEGF), that contribute to the highly angiogenic phenotype of RCC and other tumors associated with the loss of pVHL activity. The glucose transporter Glut1 and several glycolytic enzymes are also HIF responsive, and this helps to explain the Warburg effect, i.e., a metabolic switch in the source of ATP generation toward anaerobic glycolysis and away from mitochondrial oxidative phosphorylation in RCC cells. HIF-2α also stimulates expression of transforming growth factor-α (TGF-α), a potent renal cell mitogen [62]. TGF-α is released from RCC cells and interacts with EGFR on the cell surface, activating it and driving proliferation [62]. This pathway is considered to be primarily responsible for HIF-2α-induced cell proliferation, because knockdown of EGFR inhibits formation of tumors by VHL(-) cells in nude mouse xenograft assays [63]. This HIF-2-/TGF-α-dependent activation of EGFR also leads to increased activity of PI3K/AKT/NF-kappaB cascade and induction of NF-kappaB anti-apoptotic gene targets [64, 65]. Understanding the activation of EGFR through TGF-α or in any other VHL-dependent mechanism is likely critical because 85% of human

RCC exhibit overexpression or inappropriate activation of EGFR [66, 67]. pVHL also has multiple activities unrelated or indirectly related to HIF activity and has also been implicated in cystogenesis.

Beyond its oxygen-sensing capacity, pVHL controls microtubule dynamics [68, 69] and is necessary for the formation of primary cilia in cultured cancer cell lines and immortalized cells [70–72]. Cell culture experiments suggest a cooperative interaction between pVHL, PI3K, and GSK3β in primary cilium maintenance [73, 74]. Under normal conditions, serum starvation induces primary cilium formation regardless of VHL status, but cells devoid of pVHL lose their primary cilia with GSK3β inhibition or PI3K signaling activation [73, 74]. Dysregulation of β-catenin is also associated with both TSC and VHL disease, and disturbances in this pathway have likewise been linked to renal cystic disease [75, 76]. Taken together, these data indicate that pVHL is active in the regulation of multiple HIF-dependent and HIF-independent pathways, and the loss of pVHL contributes to renal oncogenesis and cystogenesis at multiple levels including those that converge at the primary cilia.

Birt-Hogg-Dubé Renal Disease

Genetics of Birt-Hogg-Dubé

Birt-Hogg-Dubé syndrome is caused by germline mutations in the *BHD* gene found at chromosome 17p11.2, encoding folliculin(FLCN), a 64-kDa polypeptide that shares little sequence similarity with any other known proteins [77]. Like TSC, patients with BHD also exhibit pulmonary cysts, although it is more common and there is no gender bias as seen in TSC [78]. About 90% of BHD patients have pulmonary cysts, and 24–29% develop recurrent pneumothorax at the average age of 36 years [79–84]. The cysts predominantly are seen in lower and/or peripheral regions of the lungs [84]. Histologically, BHD-associated lung cysts exhibit cuboidal cells resembling type 2 pneumocytes in the innermost layers that show the activation of mTORC1 and hypoxia-inducible factor-vascular endothelial growth factor pathways [85–88].

Between 16% and 34% of BHD patients develop bilateral, multifocal renal tumors at the average age of 50 years [81, 89–91]. Histologically these tumors include hybrid oncocytic/chromophobe tumors (50%), chromophobe renal cell carcinoma (34%), clear cell renal cell carcinoma (9%), oncocytoma (5%), and papillary renal cell carcinoma (2%) [92]. Multifocal renal oncocytosis, composed of cells filled with mitochondria and observed in the surrounding normal kidney of BHD-associated renal tumors in 50–58% of patients, is possibly a precancerous lesion [92–94]. Small papillary tufts are often observed in the periphery of the tumor and are helpful for diagnosing BHD-associated renal tumors [95–97]. Usually, the progression of these tumors is slow, and nephron-sparing surgery is indicated for these types of tumor, although there is one case report of metastasis [81]. Renal cystic disease also has been reported and recapitulated in the mouse model [98].

Intersection of Cilial Cystogenic and MTORC1 Signaling Pathways in BHD Renal Cystic Disease

Folliculin complexes with AMPK and folliculin-interacting protein 1 (FNIP1), although what this association does for folliculin function is unclear [99]. Folliculin-deficient mouse models develop polycystic kidneys and renal cell carcinoma that are similar to those found in patients with BHD [98, 100]. Likewise, the inactivation of FNIP1, together with its homolog FNIP2, in mice produces similar phenotypes, suggesting that FNIP1 may be required for folliculin function [101]. Analyses of tumor cells from BHD patients as well as folliculin-deficient animals reveal a consistent relationship with the activity of mammalian target of rapamycin complex 1 (mTORC1) [85, 99, 102–105].

This abnormality in mTORC1 signaling is thought to contribute to the pathobiology of BHD, as inhibition of mTORC1 reduces BHD tumor growth in animal models [98, 100], although exactly how folliculin regulates mTORC1 is not understood. At G_0, most eukaryotic cells possess a primary cilium [106]. As discussed above, this structure plays a critical role in maintaining tissue homeostasis and functioning as an environmental sensor for extracellular fluidic shear stress and chemicals [107, 108]. Many of the cell growth and proliferation signaling pathways are regulated by the primary cilia, including the mTORC1 pathway [109–111]. Several upstream regulators of mTORC1, such as TSC1 and TSC2, LKB1, and AMPK, localize to primary cilia [22, 24, 29]. Primary cilia can modulate mTORC1 signaling through an LKB1- and AMPK-dependent mechanism to effect cell size in response to flow stress [24, 112]. FLCN is a critical element of a flow sensory mechanism that regulates mTORC1 through the primary cilia [113].

Commonalities of Biology and Approach to Tuberous Sclerosis Complex, Von Hippel-Lindau, and Birt-Hogg-Dubé

All three diseases, TSC, VHL, and BHD, can present with renal cystic disease and of course have an association with renal malignancy. All three diseases are associated with the primary cilia signaling and abnormal mTORC1 axis. These commonalities have practical, patient-care implications.

The cornerstone of reducing patient chronic kidney disease and malignancy risk is surveillance. For TSC renal disease, including cystic disease, the recommended screening for disease discovery is to use MRI every 1–3 years [114]. Because renal disease progresses for the vast majority of patients throughout life, this means lifelong monitoring. Likewise for VHL renal disease, abdominal MRI is also recommended every 2–3 years after the age of 16 years. For BHD, kidney surveillance is recommended to commence after the age of 20 years [115]. As recommended for TSC and VHL disease, computed tomography or magnetic resonance imaging is far more appropriate than ultrasonography, because computed tomography and magnetic resonance imaging detect renal masses of 15–20 mm with 100% detection rates, whereas ultrasonography can detect those masses with 58% detection rates [116]. mTORC1 inhibitors are Food and Drug Administration approved for TSC-associated renal angiomyolipomata and renal cell carcinoma and are being studied for renal tumors in BHD (NCT02504892). There is preclinical evidence, and research just starting, to examine the possible role of mTORC1 inhibitors in the treatment or prevention of the renal cystic disease in TSC and soon possibly VHL and BHD.

References

1. Grantham JJ. Time to treat polycystic kidney diseases like the neoplastic disorders that they are. Kidney Int. 2000;57:339–40.
2. Siroky BJ, Czyzyk-Krzeska MF, Bissler JJ. Renal involvement in tuberous sclerosis complex and von Hippel-Lindau disease: shared disease mechanisms? Nat Clin Pr Nephrol. 2009;5:143–56.
3. Crino PB, Nathanson KL, Henske EP. The tuberous sclerosis complex. N Engl J Med. 2006;355:1345–56.
4. Yates JR. Tuberous sclerosis. Eur J Hum Genet. 2006;14:1065–73.
5. Curatolo P. The International Child Neurology Association: personal view. J Child Neurol. 2003;18:786–94.
6. Franz DN, Bissler JJ, McCormack FX. Tuberous sclerosis complex: neurological, renal and pulmonary manifestations. Neuropediatrics. 2010;41:199–208.
7. European Chromosome 16 Tuberous Sclerosis Consortium. Identification and characterization of the tuberous sclerosis gene on chromosome 16. Cell. 1993;75:1305–15.
8. Henske EP, et al. Allelic loss is frequent in tuberous sclerosis kidney lesions but rare in brain lesions. Am J Hum Genet. 1996;59:400–6.
9. Brasier JL, Henske EP. Loss of the polycystic kidney disease (PKD1) region of chromosome 16p13 in renal cyst cells supports a loss-of-function model for cyst pathogenesis. J Clin Invest. 1997;99:194–9.
10. Giannikou K, et al. Whole exome sequencing identifies TSC1/TSC2 Biallelic loss as the primary and sufficient driver event for renal angiomyolipoma development. PLoS Genet. 2016;12:e1006242.
11. Blaszak RT, Potaman V, Sinden RR, Bissler JJ. DNA structural transitions within the PKD1 gene. Nucleic Acids Res. 1999;27:2610–7.

12. Patel HP, Lu L, Blaszak RT, Bissler JJ. PKD1 intron 21: triplex DNA formation and effect on replication. Nucleic Acids Res. 2004;32:1460–8.
13. Liu G, et al. Replication fork stalling and checkpoint activation by a PKD1 locus mirror repeat Polypurine-Polypyrimidine (Pu-Py) tract. J Biol Chem. 2012;287:33412–23.
14. Dixon BP, Lu L, Chu A, Bissler JJ. RecQ and RecG helicases have distinct roles in maintaining the stability of polypurine.polypyrimidine sequences. Mutat Res. 2008;643:20–8.
15. Dixon BP, Chu A, Henry J, Kim R, Bissler JJ. Increased cancer risk of augmentation cystoplasty: possible role for hyperosmolal microenvironment on DNA damage recognition. Mutat Res. 2009;670:88–95.
16. Dixon BP, et al. Cell cycle control and DNA damage response of conditionally immortalized urothelial cells. PLoS One. 2011;6:e16595.
17. Bissler JJ, Kingswood JC. Optimal treatment of tuberous sclerosis complex associated renal angiomyolipomata: a systematic review. Ther Adv Urol. 2016:1–12. https://doi.org/10.1177/1756287216641353.
18. Nikolskaya N, Cox JA, Kingswood JC. TSC patients with different renal phenotypes. In: Nephrology dialysis transplantation. ERA-EDTA Congress, Amsterdam, Netherlands. 2014.
19. Levey AS, et al. A new equation to estimate glomerular filtration rate. Ann Intern Med. 2009; 150:604–12.
20. Schwartz GJ, et al. New equations to estimate GFR in children with CKD. J Am Soc Nephrol. 2009;20:629–37.
21. Nehus EJ, Laskin BL, Kathman TI, Bissler JJ. Performance of cystatin C-based equations in a pediatric cohort at high risk of kidney injury. Pediatr Nephrol. 2013;28:453–61.
22. Dere R, Wilson PD, Sandford RN, Walker CL. Carboxy terminal tail of polycystin-1 regulates localization of TSC2 to repress mTOR. PLoS One. 2010;5:e9239.
23. Bell PD, et al. Loss of primary cilia upregulates renal hypertrophic signaling and promotes cystogenesis. J Am Soc Nephrol. 2011;22:839–48.
24. Boehlke C, et al. Primary cilia regulate mTORC1 activity and cell size through Lkb1. Nat Cell Biol. 2010;12:1115–22.
25. Zheng B, Cantley LC. Regulation of epithelial tight junction assembly and disassembly by AMP-activated protein kinase. Proc Natl Acad Sci U S A. 2007;104:819–22.
26. Willemarck N, et al. Aberrant activation of fatty acid synthesis suppresses primary cilium formation and distorts tissue development. Cancer Res. 2010;70:9453–62.
27. Fiorentino M, et al. Overexpression of fatty acid synthase is associated with palmitoylation of Wnt1 and cytoplasmic stabilization of beta-catenin in prostate cancer. Lab Investig. 2008;88:1340–8.
28. Li Y, et al. HEF1, a novel target of Wnt signaling, promotes colonic cell migration and cancer progression. Oncogene. 2011;30:2633–43.
29. Hartman TR, et al. The tuberous sclerosis proteins regulate formation of the primary cilium via a rapamycin-insensitive and polycystin 1-independent pathway. Hum Mol Genet. 2009;18:151–63.
30. Dibella LM, Park A, Sun Z. Zebrafish Tsc1 reveals functional interactions between the cilium and the TOR pathway. Hum Mol Genet. 2008;18:595–606.
31. Astrinidis A, Senapedis W, Henske EP. Hamartin, the tuberous sclerosis complex 1 gene product, interacts with polo-like kinase 1 in a phosphorylation-dependent manner. Hum Mol Genet. 2006;15:287–97.
32. Ji H, et al. LKB1 modulates lung cancer differentiation and metastasis. Nature. 2007;448:807–10.
33. Tikhmyanova N, Little JL, Golemis EA. CAS proteins in normal and pathological cell growth control. Cell Mol Life Sci. 2010;67:1025–48.
34. Siroky BJ, et al. Evidence for pericyte origin of TSC-associated renal angiomyolipomas and implications for angiotensin receptor inhibition therapy. Am J Physiol Ren Physiol. 2014;307:F560–70.
35. Schrier RW, et al. Blood pressure in early autosomal dominant polycystic kidney disease. N Engl J Med. 2014;371:2255–66.
36. Ong ACM, Devuyst O, Knebelmann B, Walz G. Autosomal dominant polycystic kidney disease: the changing face of clinical management. Lancet. 2015;385:1993–2002.
37. Patel U, Simpson E, Kingswood JC, Saggar-Malik AK. Tuberose sclerosis complex: analysis of growth rates aids differentiation of renal cell carcinoma from atypical or minimal-fat-containing angiomyolipoma. Clin Radiol. 2005;60:664–5.
38. Ho C-L, et al. Dual-tracer PET/CT in renal angiomyolipoma and subtypes of renal cell carcinoma. Clin Nucl Med. 2012;37:1075–82.
39. Dabora SL, et al. Mutational analysis in a cohort of 224 tuberous sclerosis patients indicates increased severity of TSC2, compared with TSC1, disease in multiple organs. Am J Hum Genet. 2001;68:64–80.
40. Ewalt DH, Sheffield E, Sparagana SP, Delgado MR, Roach ES. Renal lesion growth in children with tuberous sclerosis complex. J Urol. 1998;160: 141–5.
41. Rakowski SK, et al. Renal manifestations of tuberous sclerosis complex: incidence, prognosis, and predictive factors. Kidney Int. 2006;70:1777–82.
42. Bissler JJ, Siroky BJ, Yin H. Glomerulocystic kidney disease. Pediatr Nephrol. 2010;25:2049.
43. Dixon BP, Hulbert JC, Bissler JJ. Tuberous sclerosis complex renal disease. Nephron Exp Nephrol. 2011;118:e15–20.
44. Sampson JR, et al. Renal cystic disease in tuberous sclerosis: role of the polycystic kidney disease 1 gene. Am J Hum Genet. 1997;61:843–51.
45. Brook-Carter PT, et al. Deletion of the TSC2 and PKD1 genes associated with severe infantile poly-

cystic kidney disease – a contiguous gene syndrome. Nat Genet. 1994;8:328–32.
46. Terryn S, Ho A, Beauwens R, Devuyst O. Fluid transport and cystogenesis in autosomal dominant polycystic kidney disease. Biochim Biophys Acta. 2011;1812:1314–21.
47. Patel V, et al. Acute kidney injury and aberrant planar cell polarity induce cyst formation in mice lacking renal cilia. Hum Mol Genet. 2008;17:1578–90.
48. de Chadarevian JP, Legido A, Miles DK, Katsetos CD. Epilepsy, atherosclerosis, myocardial infarction, and carbamazepine. J Child Neurol. 2003;18:150–1.
49. Maher ER, et al. Von Hippel-Lindau disease: a genetic study. J Med Genet. 1991;28:443–7.
50. Richards FM, et al. Molecular analysis of de novo germline mutations in the von Hippel-Lindau disease gene. Hum Mol Genet. 1995;4:2139–43.
51. Von Maher ER. Hippel-Lindau disease. Curr Mol Med. 2004;4:833–42.
52. Clifford SC, et al. Contrasting effects on HIF-1alpha regulation by disease-causing pVHL mutations correlate with patterns of tumourigenesis in von Hippel-Lindau disease. Hum Mol Genet. 2001;10:1029–38.
53. Choyke PL, et al. von Hippel-Lindau disease: genetic, clinical, and imaging features. Radiology. 1995;194:629–42.
54. Mandriota SJ, et al. HIF activation identifies early lesions in VHL kidneys: evidence for site-specific tumor suppressor function in the nephron. Cancer Cell. 2002;1:459–68.
55. Ma W, et al. Hepatic vascular tumors, angiectasis in multiple organs, and impaired spermatogenesis in mice with conditional inactivation of the VHL gene. Cancer Res. 2003;63:5320–8.
56. Haase VH, Glickman JN, Socolovsky M, Jaenisch R. Vascular tumors in livers with targeted inactivation of the von Hippel-Lindau tumor suppressor. Proc Natl Acad Sci U S A. 2001;98:1583–8.
57. Rankin EB, Tomaszewski JE, Haase VH. Renal cyst development in mice with conditional inactivation of the von Hippel-Lindau tumor suppressor. Cancer Res. 2006;66:2576–83.
58. Jemal A, et al. Cancer statistics, 2006. CA Cancer J Clin. 2006;56:106–30.
59. Czyzyk-Krzeska MF, von Meller J. Hippel-Lindau tumor suppressor: not only HIF's executioner. Trends Mol Med. 2004;10:146–9.
60. Kaelin WG. Proline hydroxylation and gene expression. Annu Rev Biochem. 2005;74:115–28.
61. Kaelin WGJ. Molecular basis of the VHL hereditary cancer syndrome. Nat Rev Cancer. 2002;2:673–82.
62. Gunaratnam L, et al. Hypoxia inducible factor activates the transforming growth factor-alpha/epidermal growth factor receptor growth stimulatory pathway in VHL(-/-) renal cell carcinoma cells. J Biol Chem. 2003;278:44966–74.
63. Smith K, et al. Silencing of epidermal growth factor receptor suppresses hypoxia-inducible factor-2-driven VHL-/- renal cancer. Cancer Res. 2005;65:5221–30.
64. An J, Rettig MB. Mechanism of von Hippel-Lindau protein-mediated suppression of nuclear factor kappa B activity. Mol Cell Biol. 2005;25:7546–56.
65. Qi H, Ohh M. The von Hippel-Lindau tumor suppressor protein sensitizes renal cell carcinoma cells to tumor necrosis factor-induced cytotoxicity by suppressing the nuclear factor-kappaB-dependent antiapoptotic pathway. Cancer Res. 2003;63:7076–80.
66. Jermann M, et al. A phase II, open-label study of gefitinib (IRESSA) in patients with locally advanced, metastatic, or relapsed renal-cell carcinoma. Cancer Chemother Pharmacol. 2006;57:533–9.
67. Perera AD, Kleymenova EV, Walker CL. Requirement for the von Hippel-Lindau tumor suppressor gene for functional epidermal growth factor receptor blockade by monoclonal antibody C225 in renal cell carcinoma. Clin Cancer Res. 2000;6:1518–23.
68. Lolkema MP, et al. The von Hippel-Lindau tumor suppressor protein influences microtubule dynamics at the cell periphery. Exp Cell Res. 2004;301: 139–46.
69. Hergovich A, Lisztwan J, Barry R, Ballschmieter P, Krek W. Regulation of microtubule stability by the von Hippel-Lindau tumour suppressor protein pVHL. Nat Cell Biol. 2003;5:64–70.
70. Schermer B, et al. The von Hippel-Lindau tumor suppressor protein controls ciliogenesis by orienting microtubule growth. J Cell Biol. 2006;175:547–54.
71. Lutz MS, Burk RD. Primary cilium formation requires von hippel-lindau gene function in renal-derived cells. Cancer Res. 2006;66:6903–7.
72. Esteban MA, Harten SK, Tran MG, Maxwell PH. Formation of primary cilia in the renal epithelium is regulated by the von Hippel-Lindau tumor suppressor protein. J Am Soc Nephrol. 2006;17:1801–6.
73. Thoma CR, Frew IJ, Krek W. The VHL tumor suppressor: riding tandem with GSK3beta in primary cilium maintenance. Cell Cycle. 2007;6:1809–13.
74. Frew IJ, et al. Combined Vhlh and Pten mutation causes genital tract cystadenoma and squamous metaplasia. Mol Cell Biol. 2008;28:4536–48.
75. Kugoh H, Kleymenova E, Walker CL. Retention of membrane-localized beta-catenin in cells lacking functional polycystin-1 and tuberin. Mol Carcinog. 2002;33:131–6.
76. Huan Y, van Adelsberg J. Polycystin-1, the PKD1 gene product, is in a complex containing E-cadherin and the catenins. J Clin Invest. 1999;104:1459–68.
77. Nickerson ML, et al. Mutations in a novel gene lead to kidney tumors, lung wall defects, and benign tumors of the hair follicle in patients with the Birt-Hogg-Dubé syndrome. Cancer Cell. 2002;2:157–64.
78. Hasumi H, Baba M, Hasumi Y, Furuya M, Yao M. Birt-Hogg-Dubé syndrome: clinical and molecular aspects of recently identified kidney cancer syndrome. Int J Urol. 2015;23:11–3.
79. Tobino K, et al. Differentiation between Birt-Hogg-Dube syndrome and lymphangioleiomyomatosis:

quantitative analysis of pulmonary cysts on computed tomography of the chest in 66 females. Eur J Radiol. 2012;81:1340–6.
80. Predina JD, Kotloff RM, Miller WT, Singhal S. Recurrent spontaneous pneumothorax in a patient with Birt-Hogg-Dube syndrome. Eur J Cardiothorac Surg. 2011;39:404–6.
81. Houweling AC, et al. Renal cancer and pneumothorax risk in Birt-Hogg-Dubé syndrome; an analysis of 115 FLCN mutation carriers from 35 BHD families. Br J Cancer. 2011;105:1912–9.
82. Toro JR, et al. Lung cysts, spontaneous pneumothorax, and genetic associations in 89 families with birt-Hogg-Dubé syndrome. Am J Respir Crit Care Med. 2007;175:1044–53.
83. Zbar B, et al. Risk of renal and colonic neoplasms and spontaneous pneumothorax in the Birt-Hogg-Dube syndrome. Cancer Epidemiol Biomark Prev. 2002;11:393–400.
84. Kumasaka T, et al. Characterization of pulmonary cysts in Birt-Hogg-Dube syndrome: histopathological and morphometric analysis of 229 pulmonary cysts from 50 unrelated patients. Histopathology. 2014;65:100–10.
85. Furuya M, et al. Pulmonary cysts of Birt-Hogg-Dube syndrome: a clinicopathologic and immunohistochemical study of 9 families. Am J Surg Pathol. 2012;36:589–600.
86. Furuya M, Nakatani Y. Birt-Hogg-Dube syndrome: clinicopathological features of the lung. J Clin Pathol. 2013;66:178–86.
87. Nishii T, et al. Unique mutation, accelerated mTOR signaling and angiogenesis in the pulmonary cysts of Birt-Hogg-Dubé syndrome. Pathol Int. 2013;63:45–55.
88. Koga S, et al. Lung cysts in Birt-Hogg-Dubé syndrome: histopathological characteristics and aberrant sequence repeats: original article. Pathol Int. 2009;59:720–8.
89. Pavlovich CP, et al. Evaluation and management of renal tumors in the Birt-Hogg-Dubé syndrome. J Urol. 2005;173:1482–6.
90. Toro JR, et al. BHD mutations, clinical and molecular genetic investigations of Birt-Hogg-Dube syndrome: a new series of 50 families and a review of published reports. J Med Genet. 2008;45:321–31.
91. Benusiglio PR, et al. Renal cell tumour characteristics in patients with the Birt-Hogg-Dubé cancer susceptibility syndrome: a retrospective, multicentre study. Orphanet J Rare Dis. 2014;9:163.
92. Pavlovich CP, et al. Renal tumors in the Birt-Hogg-Dubé syndrome. Am J Surg Pathol. 2002;26:1542–52.
93. Hasumi H, et al. Regulation of mitochondrial oxidative metabolism by tumor suppressor FLCN. J Natl Cancer Inst. 2012;104:1750–64.
94. Nagashima Y, et al. Renal oncocytosis. Pathol Int. 2005;55:210–5.
95. Kuroda N, et al. Review of renal tumors associated with Birt-Hogg-Dube syndrome with focus on clinical and pathobiological aspects. Pol J Pathol. 2014;65:93–9.
96. Kuroda N, et al. Review of renal oncocytosis (multiple oncocytic lesions) with focus on clinical and pathobiological aspects. Histol Histopathol. 2012;27:1407–12.
97. Kuroda N, et al. Intratumoral peripheral small papillary tufts: a diagnostic clue of renal tumors associated with Birt-Hogg-Dub?? syndrome. Ann Diagn Pathol. 2014;18:171–6.
98. Chen J, et al. Deficiency of FLCN in mouse kidney led to development of polycystic kidneys and renal neoplasia. PLoS One. 2008;3:e3581.
99. Baba M, et al. Folliculin encoded by the BHD gene interacts with a binding protein, FNIP1, and AMPK, and is involved in AMPK and mTOR signaling. Proc Natl Acad Sci U S A. 2006;103:15552–7.
100. Baba M, et al. Kidney-targeted Birt-Hogg-Dube gene inactivation in a mouse model: Erk1/2 and Akt-mTOR activation, cell hyperproliferation, and polycystic kidneys. J Natl Cancer Inst. 2008;100: 140–54.
101. Hasumi H, et al. Folliculin-interacting proteins Fnip1 and Fnip2 play critical roles in kidney tumor suppression in cooperation with Flcn. Proc Natl Acad Sci U S A. 2015;112:E1624–31.
102. Baba M, et al. The folliculin-FNIP1 pathway deleted in human Birt-Hogg-Dubé syndrome is required for murine B-cell development. Blood. 2012;120:1254–61.
103. Hasumi Y, et al. Homozygous loss of BHD causes early embryonic lethality and kidney tumor development with activation of mTORC1 and mTORC2. Proc Natl Acad Sci U S A. 2009;106:18722–7.
104. Hartman TR, et al. The role of the Birt-Hogg-Dubé protein in mTOR activation and renal tumorigenesis. Oncogene. 2009;28:1594–604.
105. Hudon V, et al. Renal tumour suppressor function of the Birt-Hogg-Dubé syndrome gene product folliculin. J Med Genet. 2010;47:182–9.
106. Satir P, Pedersen LB, Christensen ST. The primary cilium at a glance. J Cell Sci. 2010;123:499–503.
107. Singla V, Reiter JF. The primary cilium as the cell's antenna: signaling at a sensory organelle. Science. (80). 2006;313:629–33.
108. Pazour GJ, Witman GB. The vertebrate primary cilium is a sensory organelle. Curr Opin Cell Biol. 2003;15:105–10.
109. Goetz SC, Anderson KV. The primary cilium: a signalling centre during vertebrate development. Nat Rev Genet. 2010;11:331–44.
110. Berbari NF, Connor AKO, Haycraft CJ, Yoder BK. The primary cilium as a complex signaling center. Curr Biol. 2009;19:R526–35.
111. Huber TB, Walz G, Kuehn EW. mTOR and rapamycin in the kidney: signaling and therapeutic implications beyond immunosuppression. Kidney Int. 2011;79:502–11.
112. Aznar N, Billaud M. Primary cilia bend LKB1 and mTOR to their will. Dev Cell. 2010;19:792–4.

113. Zhong M, et al. Tumor suppressor folliculin regulates mTORC1 through Primary Cilia. J Biol Chem. 2016;291:11689–97. https://doi.org/10.1074/jbc.M116.719997.
114. Krueger DA, et al. Tuberous sclerosis complex surveillance and management: recommendations of the 2012 international tuberous sclerosis complex consensus conference. Pediatr Neurol. 2013;49:255–65.
115. Khoo SK, et al. Clinical and genetic studies of Birt-Hogg-Dube syndrome. J Med Genet. 2002;39:906–12.
116. Jamis-Dow CA, et al. Small (< or = 3-cm) renal masses: detection with CT versus US and pathologic correlation. Radiology. 1996;198:785–8.

Part II

PKD: Mechanisms of Disease

Aberrant Cellular Pathways in PKD

4

Alison Grazioli, Patricia Outeda, and Terry Watnick

Introduction

Cystic kidney diseases are a heterogeneous group of genetic, developmental, and acquired disorders characterized by dilated or cystic tubular segments caused by dysregulation of tubular morphology. Very often, these diseases are associated with a wide spectrum of extrarenal abnormalities with bilateral renal cysts being just one feature of a systemic disorder. Cystic kidney diseases fall into two broad categories: (1) polycystic kidney disease which has two prevalent subtypes, autosomal dominant polycystic kidney disease (ADPKD) and autosomal recessive polycystic kidney disease (ARPKD), characterized by renal enlargement due to cyst burden and (2) hereditary diseases such as Bardet-Biedl syndrome and nephronophthisis which feature small kidneys, significant interstitial fibrosis, and tubular atrophy [1–4]. Of these, ADPKD is the most prevalent and extensively studied cystic kidney disease and the most common cause of genetic renal disease [5].

A. Grazioli, MD · P. Outeda, PhD
T. Watnick, MD (✉)
Department of Medicine, Division of Nephrology, University of Maryland School of Medicine, Baltimore, MD, USA
e-mail: twatnick@som.umaryland.edu

The overarching question for these diseases is how does the normal tubular epithelium give way to cyst formation? In broadest terms, renal cyst development involves dilatation of the renal tubule, with formation of a saccular cyst filled with fluid derived from glomerular filtrate. Progressive expansion eventually leads to separation of cysts from the tubule of origin. Subsequent enlargement of the newly independent cyst is driven by transepithelial fluid secretion and cyst epithelial cell proliferation. Expanding cysts cause parenchymal changes such as macrophage infiltration, fibrosis, and neovascularization, ultimately resulting in renal failure. Several pathologic hallmarks have been identified to explain the abnormal cellular phenotype of cystic epithelium. Though not without some controversy, these include enhanced proliferation, increased apoptosis, remodeling of the extracellular matrix, a secretory phenotype, dysregulated metabolism, and an inability to maintain planar cell polarity [6].

Extensive work over the last few decades has identified many of the genes responsible for inherited forms of cystic kidney disease. This has provided an entry into the identification of cystogenic pathways that result in the pathologic hallmarks described above. In this review, we discuss our current understanding of some of the key signaling pathways that are disrupted in the most common form of renal cystic disease, autosomal dominant polycystic kidney disease (ADPKD).

B. D. Cowley, Jr., J. J. Bissler (eds.), *Polycystic Kidney Disease*,
https://doi.org/10.1007/978-1-4939-7784-0_4

Genetic Mechanisms of Cystogenesis in ADPKD

ADPKD arises when there is an inherited or sporadic mutation in one copy of either *PKD1*, encoding polycystin 1 (PC1), or *PKD2*, encoding polycystin 2 (PC2) [7, 8]. Most cases of ADPKD have a delayed clinical onset and are identified in adulthood between the ages of 30 and 50 [9]. Early microdissection studies performed on kidneys retrieved from patients with ADPKD revealed that cysts are focal lesions capable of affecting any segment of an otherwise normal-appearing renal tubule [10]. Surprisingly, no more than 1–5% of nephrons develop cysts despite each renal tubular cell harboring a germ line mutation of a polycystin gene.

The earliest proposed mechanism for explaining this phenomenon, along with the adult onset of disease, was a "two-hit hypothesis" not unlike that proposed to explain the origin of cancer [11]. Under this premise, a somatic mutation or "second hit" of the remaining wild-type allele is acquired in a tubular cell already containing an inherited germ line PKD mutation (Fig. 4.1). Somatic mutation is followed by clonal expansion of the now PKD-deficient cell, thereby setting the stage for cyst formation and enlargement [11, 12]. Genetic analysis of cyst lining epithelium in both *PKD1* and *PKD2* kidneys ultimately confirmed that independent somatic mutations could be identified in a large fraction of renal cysts [13–17]. The same mechanism was also shown to be operative in ADPKD-associated liver cysts [18].

Studies in mouse models support the two-hit hypothesis. Wu et al. described a *Pkd2* mouse model with an unstable allele that undergoes random somatic mutation to produce a functionally null allele [19]. Mice that are heterozygous for this allele in combination with a germ line null develop polycystic kidney and liver disease that mimics human disease [19]. In addition, mice bearing floxed alleles of *Pkd1* or *Pkd2* that allow regulated deletion of these genes also develop human-like ADPKD [20–22]. However, the data generated in murine models do not exclude the possibility that there may be other mechanisms that lower polycystin signaling in human ADPKD.

The two-hit hypothesis has been refined based on evidence supporting the idea that a reduction in polycystin signaling below a critical threshold

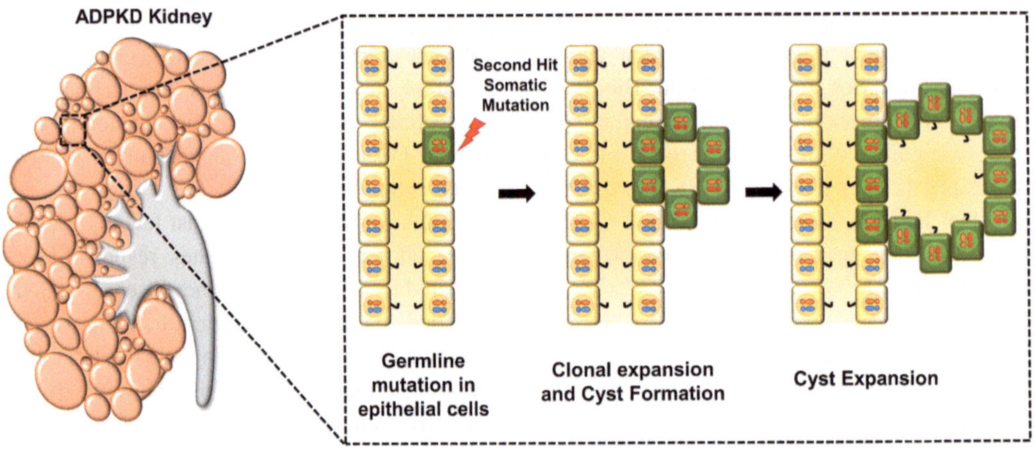

Fig. 4.1 The two-hit model of focal cyst formation in ADPKD. Cyst formation in ADPKD is a focal process that affects a small fraction of nephrons. Each epithelial cell in a renal tubule from an ADPKD kidney harbors the same germ line *PKD* mutation. When a cell acquires a mutation in the *PKD* allele inherited from the unaffected parent, the level of polycystin signaling falls below a critical threshold and that cell undergoes clonal expansion eventually forming a cyst. Cyst expansion is accompanied by increased cell proliferation and fluid secretion through aberrant regulation of a variety of signaling pathways discussed in the text

level is the most significant factor for cyst formation [23–26]. This was initially suggested by a mouse model with a cystic phenotype carrying an aberrantly spliced variant of the *Pkd1* gene, lowering its expression to 13–20% normal levels [25]. Further evidence that gene dosage is important came with the identification of ADPKD families with individuals carrying homozygous, hypomorphic *Pkd1* mutations [23]. Another corollary of this model is that the threshold of polycystin signaling that is required to maintain tubular architecture may vary depending on the renal milieu. Therefore cyst formation may occur when there is an imbalance in the supply and demand of polycystin signaling based on environmental factors, genetic modifiers, physiologic demands particularly in response to injury, and temporality of a second hit [26]. In fact, the timing of polycystin loss appears to be a major determinant of the rapidity of cyst formation [27–29]. In conditional mouse models, inactivation of *Pkd1* before about postnatal day 13 results in severely cystic kidneys within 3 weeks [27, 28]. In contrast, inactivation of *Pkd1* at about postnatal day 14 or later resulted in cysts after a delay of ~5 months and mimiced adult onset ADPKD. Developmentally regulated gene expression profiles within the kidney are thought to underlie the differential effect of *Pkd1* loss on rapidity of cyst formation. Thus, the pathologic consequences of inactivation are seemingly defined by cellular developmental status [27].

The discordance between rapid cyst growth in neonates with germ line deletion of *Pkd1* and slower cyst growth in mouse models with adult *Pkd1* inactivation prompted the hypothesis that there might be a "third hit" required for rapid cyst development [30, 31]. It has since been shown that in an adult onset mouse model, ischemia reperfusion injury significantly accelerates cyst growth [30]. Dysregulated apoptosis, increased cell proliferation, disruption of planar cell polarity, and disoriented mitotic spindle formation, almost all seen following renal injury, are thought to contribute to cyst formation in current prevailing models [6, 32].

The Role of the Cilium in Cyst Formation

Over the past 15 years or so, there has been intense focus on the role of the primary cilium in the maintenance of renal tubular architecture. Mutations in many genes associated with PKD are involved in the assembly or function of the cilium and their protein products, including PC1 and PC2, localize to the cilia-basal body complex [33–37]. The primary cilium is a structure that protrudes from the surface of most cells and acts as a sensor for a variety of chemical and mechanical stimuli with subsequent transmission of these environmental signals to the interior of the cell. Specialized translocation machinery, referred to as intraflagellar transport (IFT), is required to develop, maintain, and traffic both structural and signaling proteins into and out of cilia [38, 39]. Cilia are critical for the integrity of an ever-growing list of signaling pathways including sonic Hedgehog and Wnt (reviewed in [40, 41]). Kidney cysts arise following inactivation of genes that disrupt either the structure or function of the primary cilium, including the IFT genes [37].

Since both polycystins localize to the primary cilium and the primary cilium remains intact in both *Pkd1* and *Pkd2* mutant cells, it has been speculated that the polycystin complex is not required for ciliary assembly but rather for detecting external stimuli that results in altered regulation of downstream signaling pathways [22, 35, 36]. Some of the major implicated effector pathways of abnormal ciliary signaling include the Wnt signaling-planar cell polarity pathway, mTOR, cAMP, intracellular calcium, CFTR, and MAPK/ERK [5, 26, 42, 43]. Until recently, it was assumed that the cellular pathway alterations caused by loss of PC1 or PC2 were due to the disruption in normal ciliary function when these cystoproteins were eliminated. In this paradigm, the cellular defects resulting from polycystin loss would likely parallel the effects of loss of structurally intact cilia (independent of PC1 and PC2 knockout). However, recent experimental data suggests that it is much more complicated than previously thought (Fig. 4.2). Ablation of cilia

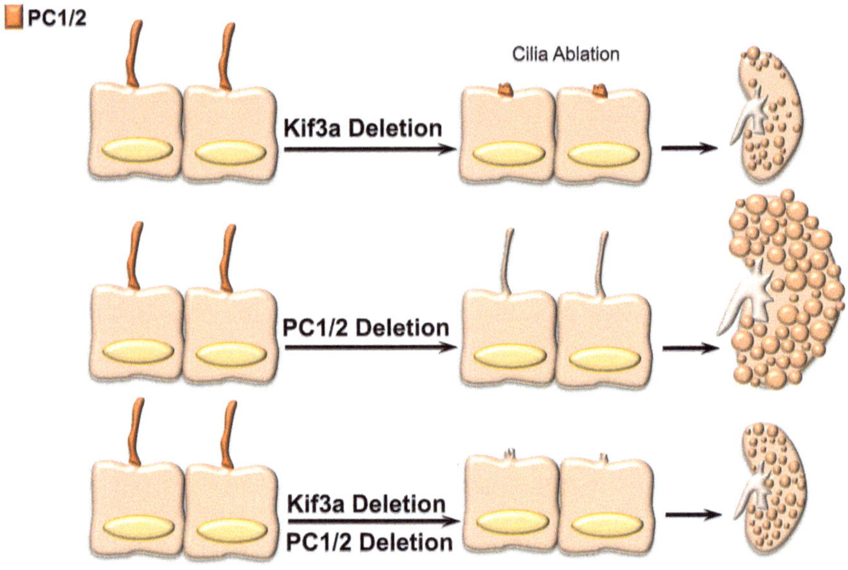

Fig. 4.2 Schematic illustration showing that loss of cilia slows cystogenesis in *Pkd* mutant mice (see reference [22]). Polycystin 1 and polycystin 2 are found in the cilia of renal epithelial cells. When cilia are ablated in renal epithelial cells by conditional inactivation of Kif3a (a gene required for ciliogenesis), slowly progressive cystic kidney disease ensues (top panel). When a *Pkd* gene is deleted by conditional inactivation in renal epithelial cells, cilia remain intact but cyst formation with massive renal enlargement occurs (middle panel). When both cilia and a *Pkd* gene are lost, cystogenesis is reduced and the kidney does not exhibit massive enlargement (bottom panel). This interaction occurs regardless of whether deletion occurs early or late

(via knockout of IFT proteins: Kif3a or IFT20) reduces cyst growth in *Pkd1* or *Pkd2* mutant kidneys irrespective of the timing of polycystin gene inactivation [22]. Additionally, loss of cilia alone also resulted in slow cyst growth with neither reduction or overexpression of PC1 impacting the phenotype in vivo. In essence, structurally intact cilia are stimulators of cyst growth in *Pkd1* or *Pkd2* mutant kidneys. This work brings to light the existence of distinct signaling pathways that promote cystogenesis via (1) cilia-dependent (polycystin-independent) activation or (2) the loss of polycystin-dependent inhibition of ciliary pathways which promote cyst growth [22, 44]. The identity of the so named "cilia-dependent cyst activation" signal remains elusive [44].

Calcium Signaling in PKD

PC2 is a member of the transient receptor potential (TRP) family of ion channels, and many groups using a variety of experimental systems have reported that it is a nonselective, calcium-permeable cation channel [45–52]. Recent cryo-EM studies have solved the three-dimensional structure of PC2 in lipid bilayers and have provided new insights into its novel structural features [53–55]. PC1 is the main binding partner of PC2, and together these proteins are speculated to form a receptor-channel complex that is a hub for signaling pathways utilizing Ca^{2+} as a second messenger [46, 49, 52, 56]. This is an attractive hypothesis since calcium is a highly versatile intracellular signaling molecule that regulates numerous cellular processes implicated in PKD including secretion, proliferation, and apoptosis [57]. The precise alterations in intracellular calcium homeostasis that occur in ADPKD, however, remain controversial [58]. This is in part because the PC1/PC2 complex is found in multiple cellular compartments including the cilium, the plasma membrane, and the endoplasmic reticulum (ER) [49, 59–62]. In addition, heterologously expressed PC2 is retained in the ER, making direct electrophysiologic characterization of the channel properties at the plasma membrane challenging [58].

Because the cilium is thought to be of prime importance in the development of polycystic kidney disease, intense effort has been devoted toward defining the link between the polycystins, cilia, and calcium signaling. The idea that the primary cilium might function as a mechanosensor was first suggested by the seminal studies of Praetorius and Spring who showed that bending the cilium by a variety of methods, including laminar flow, resulted in an increase in cytosolic calcium concentration $[Ca^{2+}]$ [63, 64]. Since PC1 and PC2 were detected in the cilium and PC2 was presumed to be a Ca^{2+} channel, it seemed logical that the polycystin complex might contribute to ciliary mechanosensation. In order to test this hypothesis, Nauli et al. isolated renal epithelial cells from *Pkd1*$^{-/-}$ embryos and showed that unlike wild-type cells, they failed to increase intracellular Ca^{2+} in response to fluid flow [65]. Wild-type cells treated with blocking antibodies to PC2 as well as human ADPKD cyst lining epithelia were similarly defective [65, 66]. These findings led to the theory that PC1 induces ciliary Ca^{2+} influx via PC2 in response to flow triggered ciliary bending and that this calcium signal is presumably propagated to the cell body. Loss of this PC1-/PC2-dependent calcium signal was thought to ultimately result in cystogenesis [67, 68].

Over the past several years, however, challenges to this model have been accumulating from a variety of directions. Knockdown of the calcium channel TRPV4, which complexes with PC2, abrogates the intracellular calcium response to sheer stress or flow in cultured renal epithelial cells, but TRPV4 knockout in mice or zebrafish doesn't result in a cystic phenotype [69]. In addition, a series of technical advances have yielded more precise characterization of ciliary calcium dynamics, casting doubt on a simple flow model [70–72]. Delling et al. generated transgenic mice with a genetically encoded, ratiometric calcium indicator targeted to primary cilia that allowed for control of motion artifacts and yielded more accurate Ca^{2+} measurements [72]. These investigators measured responses to flow in the primary cilia of kidney epithelial cells, in the cilia of the embryonic node, and in intact kidney thick ascending tubules and failed to show ciliary calcium influx in response to fluid flow.

Delling et al. also used these tools to demonstrate that the resting ciliary calcium concentration, $[Ca^{2+}]$, is approximately 600 nM, which is ~sixfold higher than the normal resting cytoplasmic $[Ca^{2+}]$ of ~100 nM [71]. The cilia's resting membrane potential is also ~30 mV more positive in comparison with the cytoplasm [71]. The combination of a high ciliary $[Ca^{2+}]$ and the more positive resting potential promotes calcium efflux from cilia to cytoplasm. However, because the volume of the cytoplasm is large in comparison to the cilium, cytoplasmic $[Ca^{2+}]$ appears to be unaffected by variations in ciliary $[Ca^{2+}]$ which makes direct propagation of ciliary Ca^{2+} signal to the cell body seem unlikely [71].

There has also been disagreement as to whether PC2 is indeed a ciliary calcium channel at all. Several labs have developed methods that allowed sensitive and direct recording of ciliary currents using patch clamp methods [70, 73]. Knockdown of either *PKD1* or *PKD2* in retinal pigment epithelial (RPE) cells with short interfering RNAs did not reduce ciliary calcium current, whereas knockdown of *PKD1L1* or *PKD2L1* did [70]. *PKD1L1* and *PKD2L1* are members of the PC1 and PC2 family, respectively, and similarly interact to form a receptor-channel complex [70, 71]. Ciliary currents were also much reduced in *Pkd2L1* homozygous knockout mouse embryonic fibroblasts (MEFs) [70]. These results suggest that PKD2L1 is the primary ciliary calcium channel, at least in the cell types tested. On the other hand, direct ciliary patch clamp recordings from wild-type and *Pkd2* knockout murine IMCD-3 cells did in fact detect a ciliary current that is dependent on *Pkd2* [73]. Characterization of this channel suggests that it has high conductance with permeability to $K^+ > Ca^{2+} > Na^+$ [73]. Similar biophysical properties were reported when a chimeric protein containing only the PC2 pore in a PKD2L1 backbone (thus allowing PC2 to reach the plasma membrane) was heterologously expressed in HEK293T cells [53]. The inconsistent results in RPE cells versus IMCD cells could be due to context-dependent differences in ciliary signaling or other differences in experimental protocols. More work will be required to resolve these contradictory findings.

Since PC2 is abundant in the ER, another line of inquiry has focused on the role of the polycystin complex in regulating intracellular calcium stores [45, 74]. In a variety of overexpression studies, PC1 and PC2 have each been shown to interact with various ER calcium channels and proteins including the inositol 1,4,5-trisphosphate (IP3) receptor (PC1 and PC2), the ryanodine receptor (PC2), and STIM1 (PC1) [75–79]. The IP3 receptor and the ryanodine receptor are the two major Ca^{2+} channels localized in the ER and sarcoplasmic reticulum (SR) that initiate calcium release from internal stores (ER/SR) (reviewed in [80, 81]). STIM1 is an ER protein that senses ER [Ca^{2+}] and stimulates store-operated Ca^{2+} entry via plasma membrane ORAI1 calcium channels when ER calcium is depleted [81]. Taken together the data suggest that the polycystin complex interacts with these proteins to modulate ER calcium levels, but whether the result is an increased, decreased, or unchanged ER [Ca^{2+}] remains controversial. Most groups have concluded that the polycystins prevent depletion of calcium stores by inhibiting leakage of calcium out of the SR/ER and thereby preserving the integrity of intracellular Ca^{2+} flux [45, 78, 82–85]. However, in other studies overexpression of PC2 has been reported to increase ER Ca^{2+} leak resulting in decreased ER Ca^{2+} concentration and decreased release of ER Ca^{2+} upon stimulation [86]. In these studies, *PKD2* knockdown causes the reverse and augments the amount of releasable ER Ca^{2+}. Whether alterations in ER calcium levels result in a lower resting cytosolic calcium concentration remains controversial, but several studies have reported a reduction in some cell types [87].

There are many additional unanswered questions related to the role of polycystins in Ca^{2+} signaling. The final six transmembrane spanning segments of PC1 bear sequence homology to PC2, raising the question of whether PC1 is itself a channel [88, 89]. Several studies have shown that binding between PC1 and PC2 is required for the polycystin complex to reach the cilium/cell membrane, but whether PC1 forms an integral part of the channel pore versus serving as a chaperone remains unclear [46, 90–92]. Modeling of the PC1 channel-like domain based on the cryo-EM structure of PC2, however, led Grieben et al. to conclude that there are differences in key amino acid residues that make it less likely that PC1 is an ion channel [54]. Finally, if flow doesn't activate the polycystin complex, then what does? Kim et al. reported that a variety of Wnts bind to the extracellular domain of PC1, which activates PC2-dependent (whole cell) calcium influx [93]. However, these findings could not be reproduced by another group [53, 72].

In summary, there is agreement that PC2 is likely to function as a calcium channel, but an integrated understanding of the function of PC2 in the various cellular compartments where it is found remains elusive. The consequence of polycystin loss on downstream calcium signaling will continue to be a subject of intense investigation.

cAMP, an Essential Second Messenger in PKD

Cyclic 3′,5′ adenosine monophosphate (cAMP) is an important second messenger that is synthesized from adenosine triphosphate (ATP) by adenylate cyclase (AC), which is activated by adenylate cyclase stimulatory G (Gs)-protein-coupled receptors (GsPCRs) such as vasopressin (AVP) receptors and inhibited by inhibitory G (Gi)-protein-coupled receptors (GiPCRs) [87, 94, 95]. The degradation of cAMP via hydrolysis is mediated by the activity of phosphodiesterases [96]. cAMP activates protein kinase A (PKA) which in turn targets and phosphorylates many substrates including aquaporin 2, CFTR, ROMK, and ENaC [95, 97–100]. cAMP has been reported to be elevated in almost all PKD models studied to date [101–106] and as described in more detail below has been implicated in driving the secretion of luminal fluid and cell proliferation, thus, propagating cyst enlargement [101–103, 107, 108].

The mechanisms underlying elevations in cytosolic cAMP in PKD remain incompletely understood but are thought to involve an imbalance in the production and breakdown of cAMP. It has been hypothesized that perturbations in cytosolic Ca^{2+} flux underlie changes in cAMP concentration through effects on both cAMP synthesis (via adenylate cyclase) and hydrolysis (via phosphodiesterase) (reviewed in [109]). If cell calcium is indeed reduced in ADPKD cells, this might result in the stimulation of calcium inhibitable ACs, notably, AC6 (*Adcy6*), and an inhibition of calcium-dependent cAMP phosphodiesterases like PDE1. Consistent with this model, introduction of an *Adcy6* mutant allele ameliorates cystic disease in mice with collecting duct deletion of *Pkd1* [110]. In addition, knockdown of *Pde1a* by morpholino or gene targeting exacerbates cystic disease in *Pkd2* zebrafish morphants and in *Pkd2* mutant mice, respectively [111, 112]. There are several other factors that have been proposed to contribute to elevations in cAMP levels, for example, disruption of PC1 binding to the heterotrimeric G-proteins, which inhibit AC activity and accumulation of other agonists of AC activity in cyst fluid such as endogenous forskolin [95, 113, 114].

The most important contributor to elevated renal cAMP levels in ADPKD, however, is the vasopressin pathway. Vasopressin, acting on the Gs-coupled V2 receptor, is the major agonist of adenylate cyclase in the renal collecting duct. A large body of data indicates that upregulation of this pathway is significant in the progression of polycystic kidney disease [87, 95]. Impaired urinary concentrating capacity is one of the earliest manifestations of ADPKD, and this presumably is the basis for increased activity of the vasopressin pathway [115, 116]. Copeptin, a vasopressin surrogate which is produced when AVP is processed to its active form, is elevated in ADPKD and has been correlated with disease severity in several studies [117–119]. In addition, expression of other vasopressin pathway members, such as the V2 receptor and aquaporin 2, is increased in cystic kidneys from multiple rodent models including *Pkd2* mutant mice [102, 103]. Perhaps the most compelling piece of data comes from experiments in an ARPKD rat model (PCK) showing that introduction of a vasopressin null allele nearly abolishes cystic disease in these animals, while treatment with DDAVP causes cystic disease to re-emerge [120]. As further proof of the importance of the vasopressin pathway, V2 receptor antagonists have been shown to improve cystic disease in all rodent models where they have been tested, and these finding have formed the basis for human clinical trials that are discussed elsewhere [102, 103, 121–123].

So why are elevated levels of cAMP detrimental in ADPKD? cAMP has been implicated in differential modulation of cell proliferation, which is an important feature of cyst expansion (reviewed in [95]). cAMP has a pro-proliferative effect on cultured cells derived from human ADPKD cysts, whereas an inhibitory effect is observed in normal renal epithelial cells (NHK) [107, 124]. The effect of cAMP and its agonists on proliferation in PKD cells is mediated by PKA stimulation of the mitogen-activated protein kinase kinase/extracellular-regulated kinase (MEK/ERK) pathway [124–126]. This pathway is activated in many malignancies and promotes cell proliferation (reviewed in [127]). Yamaguchi et al. showed that treatment of ADPKD cells with 8-Br-cAMP stimulated ERK phosphorylation, and this could be prevented by treatment with either PKA or MEK inhibitors [124]. In contrast 8-Br-cAMP had no effect on P-ERK levels in normal human kidney cells. The activation of MEK/ERK in ADPKD cells appears to occur at the level of B-Raf, a kinase upstream of the Ras/Raf/MEK/ERK pathway. cAMP treatment of ADPKD cells (but not normal human kidney cells) resulted in augmented B-Raf kinase activity, an effect that could be abrogated by pretreatment with a PKA inhibitor [95, 124].

The relationship between calcium homeostasis and cAMP signaling in ADPKD cells has been further studied in vitro. Yamaguchi et al. treated M1 collecting duct cells and normal human kidney cells with calcium channel blockers (nifedipine and verapamil) and found that this maneuver converted these cells to an ADPKD, cAMP growth-stimulated phenotype [128].

Under calcium-restricted conditions, cAMP was able to stimulate ERK and B-Raf activity. Conversely increasing intracellular calcium in ADPKD cyst cells, by either activating L-type Ca^{2+} channels or by treating the cells with a calcium ionophore, inhibited cAMP-dependent proliferation, ERK phosphorylation, as well as activation of B-Raf [129]. In aggregate these data have been interpreted to link the differential response to cAMP in ADPKD cells versus normal human kidney cells to a reduction in intracellular Ca^{2+} associated with mutations in *PKD1*/*PKD2* [87, 95, 109]. However, whether pharmacologic maneuvers in cell culture, which presumably cause dramatic alterations in calcium homeostasis, mimic in vivo conditions in ADPKD remains uncertain. A more detailed and integrated understanding of the role that the polycystin complex plays in regulating cell calcium is needed to draw a more definitive conclusion.

In addition to cell proliferation, cAMP is also an important mediator of chloride-driven transepithelial fluid secretion, which is responsible for cyst enlargement in polycystic kidney disease [130–132]. In the absence of fluid secretion, it is believed that the relatively small degree of increased cell proliferation would not be sufficient to cause the parenchymal distortion that occurs secondary to the large cyst burden that is characteristic of the ADPKD kidney [133]. Early studies using intact cysts dissected from ADPKD kidneys showed that they secrete fluid and enlarge when treated with forskolin, thereby linking fluid secretion to elevated cAMP [130, 132, 134]. Like other secretory epithelia, fluid flux is driven by active chloride secretion [130, 132].

Much attention has been focused on the role of the cystic fibrosis transmembrane conductance regulator (CFTR) in this process. CFTR is an ABC transporter-class ion channel activated by cAMP/protein kinase A that allows flow of chloride ions down an electrochemical gradient and plays an important role in chloride-driven fluid flux by other secretory epithelia [135, 136]. Immunolocalization studies in ADPKD kidneys showed that CFTR is located in the apical membrane of cyst epithelium [137–139]. Moreover, inhibitors of CFTR or genetic introduction of a CFTR mutation were able to block cAMP-induced cyst formation in *Pkd1* null murine kidneys grown in metanephric organ culture [140–142]. There are several reports describing a small number of families harboring both CFTR and ADPKD mutations with some investigators concluding that a CFTR mutation may be protective in the context of ADPKD and others finding no effect [143–145]. It is difficult, however, to establish a definitive correlation from these anecdotal reports since the numbers of individuals with both *PKD* and *CFTR* mutations are small. There are no published reports describing whether a *CFTR* null allele is protective in an orthologous adult ADPKD mouse model. In any case, CFTR is unlikely to be the sole channel responsible for chloride secretion in ADPKD given the heterogeneity of its expression in cyst epithelium [137, 146]. In addition to CFTR-mediated chloride secretion, apical calcium-activated chloride channels have also been implicated in luminal Cl^- secretion in in vitro and ex vivo PKD models [147, 148].

Taken together many lines of evidence support the idea that cAMP levels are associated with ADPKD progression and that cAMP is a "bad actor" in the context of cyst progression. The vasopressin pathway is an important player in upregulating cAMP levels presumably in those cysts arising from renal tubular segments where vasopressin is active. The cAMP-vasopressin axis continues to be an important therapeutic target in clinical trials.

The Role of mTOR in ADPKD Pathogenesis

A spotlight on mTOR's involvement in PKD dates back over two decades when it was discovered that many individuals afflicted with infantile onset ADPKD had large deletions of chromosome 16 affecting *PKD1* and the adjacent *TSC2* gene [149]. *TSC1* and *TSC2* mutations give rise to tuberous sclerosis, a rare multi-system genetic disease with renal cysts as one of its features [150]. Given the increased severity and infantile onset of renal cystogenesis in individuals with mutations in *PKD1* and *TSC2*, a regulator of the mammalian target of rapamycin (mTOR) pathway, it seemed plausible that *PKD1* might also have a role in mTOR signaling.

The mammalian target of rapamycin (mTOR) is a conserved serine/threonine kinase that senses cellular states of energy, stress, nutrition, and oxygenation and integrates this information to regulate complex cellular pathways that control growth and survival (reviewed in [151–154]). In general, when nutrients are plentiful and specific growth stimuli are present, mTOR signaling is turned on to coordinate anabolic processes such as nutrient import and macromolecular synthesis all of which increase cell size and mass [154].

mTOR exits in two distinct large multiprotein complexes, mTOR complex 1 (mTORC1) and mTOR complex 2 (mTORC2). Both complexes share core components including the kinase mTOR, GβL/mLST8, and DEPTOR, but each also contains unique proteins [151]. mTORC1 is in a complex with raptor and PRAS40 and is inhibited by the rapamycin-FKB12 (FK506 binding protein) complex, while mTORC2 is distinguished by interaction with Rictor, mSin1, and Protor [151, 153, 154]. A large body of work has focused on regulators of mTORC1, which to date is much better characterized than mTORC2. The best-known regulator of mTORC1 is the TSC1-TSC2 complex, which is a heterodimer composed of TSC1 (known as hamartin) and TSC2 (known as tuberin) [155]. This complex acts as a GTPase-activating protein (GAP) for the Rheb GTPase. When in its GTP-bound form, Rheb stimulates mTORC1 kinase activity through direct interaction. TSC1/TSC2 converts Rheb to its inactive, GDP-bound form, thereby inhibiting mTORC1 [156]. The TSC1/TSC2 complex is a target for several kinases. Phosphorylation events can either inhibit TSC1/TSC2 (thereby increasing mTOR signaling) or the reverse [153, 155, 157]. Negative regulators of TSC1/TSC2 include PI3K/Akt and ERK1/2, while positive regulators include AMPK and GSk3β (reviewed in [155, 157]).

There is also a body of data suggesting that there is cross talk between polycystin pathways and TSC1/TSC2. Distefano et al. noted that MDCK cells stably overexpressing PC1 were smaller than controls, whereas *Pkd1* null mouse embryonic fibroblasts (*Pkd1*$^{-/-}$ MEFS) were larger than their wild-type counterparts [158]. This "large cell" phenotype in *Pkd1*$^{-/-}$ MEFs was associated with upregulation of mTOR signaling (as measured by levels of phosphorylated 70S6K and 4EBP1) along with activation of MEK/ERK. Inhibition of mTOR with rapamycin, as well as application of MEK/ERK inhibitors, was able to return cell size to normal. These authors proposed that loss of polycystins activate the MEK/ERK pathway, which in turn phosphorylates tuberin and relieves its repression of mTOR. It should be noted that other investigators failed to show constitutive upregulation of mTOR signaling in *Pkd1*$^{-/-}$ MEFs, which may be due to variation in clonal cell isolates or to differences in experimental protocol [159].

The cell-based studies described above were complemented by findings that mTOR signaling is upregulated in cyst lining epithelial cells from rodent models of PKD [160–163] as well as in human ADPKD [159, 160]. Consistent with this, blocking mTOR activity with sirolimus (formerly rapamycin) or everolimus had a beneficial effect in numerous rodent models of PKD including ORPK-rescue (*Tg737*$^{orpk/orpk}$;*TgRsq*), *bpk*, HanSPRD, *Pkd1*$^{cond/cond}$;*Nestin-Cre*, and *Pkd2*$^{WS25/-}$ [160–168]. These preclinical data formed the basis for clinical trials of mTOR inhibitors in human ADPKD that are discussed elsewhere in this monograph [169, 170]. Unfortunately, the results of these studies were disappointing for a variety of reasons. One possibility is that the mTOR pathway may not be the most proximate upstream initiator of cyst formation given the existence of subsets of ADPKD cysts that are found which lack mTORC1 upregulation [22, 159]. Another proposed explanation is that the standard doses of mTOR inhibitors used to achieve immunosuppression in the transplant setting may not be sufficient to inhibit mTOR in the kidney [171, 172]. One approach that has been tried to circumvent this problem is to target rapamycin to the kidney by targeting it to the folate receptor, which is expressed in both normal and cystic kidney at high levels [173].

This approach has been successful in a non-orthologous *bpk* mouse model of PKD [173]. There is also complex cross talk between the mTORC1 and mTORC2 complexes [151, 157]. Whether inhibitors of both complexes would be more effective remains to be formally tested [168]. Additional strategies aimed at metabolic reprogramming are also being pursued as discussed below.

Metabolism in PKD

The link between ADPKD and increased cell proliferation and growth has led to comparisons between the processes of cystogenesis and neoplasia [6, 174]. Therefore, it is no surprise that metabolic reprogramming of pathways involved in energy production and biosynthesis has been discovered in PKD, a phenomenon that has been long associated with cancer (Fig. 4.3). Evidence of metabolic alterations in ADPKD was shown through transcriptomic and urine metabolomic analysis in mice with inducible inactivation of *Pkd1* [175, 176]. These analyses showed an enrichment for genes linked to metabolic pathways in mutant signature sets, notably HNF4α [175]. HNF4α is a transcription factor downstream of mTOR that is involved in regulation of development and metabolism and, notably, has been implicated as a regulator of glucose homeostasis [177].

Further evidence that cystic epithelia have metabolic alterations came from reports that *Pkd1*$^{-/-}$ MEFs, *Pkd1* mutant mouse kidneys and human cyst lining epithelial cells all have high levels of glycolysis [178, 179]. This finding is akin to the Warburg effect found in many malignancies that harbor a preference for aerobic glycolysis [180, 181]. The rewiring of metabolism in these neoplasms causes an addiction to glucose rendering them susceptible to agents that inhibit glucose utilization. Cancer cells that rely on aerobic glycolysis are glucose dependent largely because the PI3K/Akt/mTOR pathway directs metabolic substrates into lipid and protein synthesis and away from catabolism [181]. It is conceivable that the same may be true in ADPKD. Treatment of *Pkd1* mutant mice with the glucose analog 2-deoxyglucose (2-DG) which inhibits glycolysis was effective in reducing the cystic phenotype [178, 179, 182]. This benefit was observed regardless of whether the *Pkd1* gene was inactivated early (aggressive early onset model) or late after renal development is complete.

Follow-up studies by other groups have added weight to the general principle of metabolic reprogramming in ADPKD but failed to confirm that cystic disease or *Pkd1* mutation in MEFs is associated with the Warburg effect [183, 184]. A study describing transcriptional and metabolomic profiling in a large data set of more than 30 control and 30 cystic *Pkd1* murine kidney samples failed to detect differences in lactic acid levels or glycolytic activity and instead found defects in fatty acid oxidation which was confirmed by seahorse analysis of *Pkd1* mutant cell lines [183]. Interestingly, in this study male mice had more severe cystic kidney disease than females, and it was speculated that differences in lipid metabolic pathways might account for the protection seen in females [183]. In several studies calorie restriction and fat restriction appear to have salutatory effect on cyst progression in various mouse models [183–185].

The mechanistic link between *Pkd1/Pkd2* mutation, cystogenesis, and metabolic reprogramming, however, has yet to be defined. Rowe et al. suggested that activation of glycolytic genes in *Pkd1* mutant cells and mice is being driven by the transcription factor HIF1α which can be stabilized in cystic epithelia by either hypoxia or mTOR [178]. As noted above, the ERK pathway, which is upregulated in ADPKD, is implicated as an upstream mediator of metabolic alterations through its activation of the mTORC1 complex and its inhibition of the LKB1-AMPK axis [157, 158, 178]. LKB1-AMPK signaling serves as a key nutrient sensor, which is critical for maintenance of cellular metabolic homeostasis [186]. LKB1 phosphorylates and activates AMPK in response to an increase in the intracellular AMP to ATP ratio. AMPK, in turn, phosphorylates numerous substrates controlling processes that contribute to a shift from anabolism to catabolism

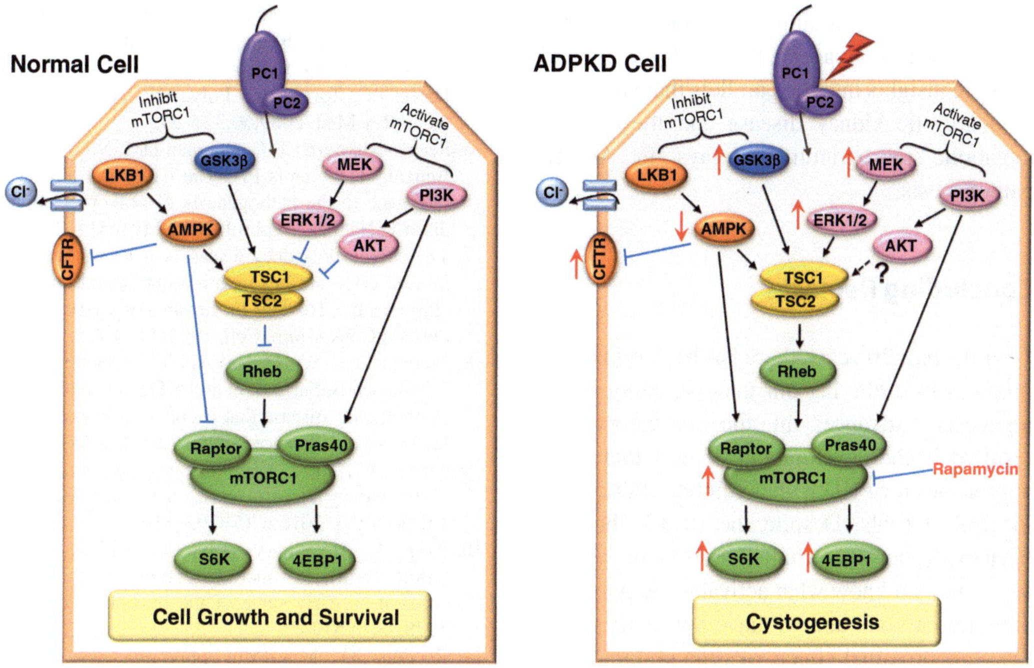

Fig. 4.3 Overview of metabolic reprogramming in ADPKD. Schematic diagram showing a subset of signaling pathways that converge on the mammalian target of rapamycin (mTOR) to control cell metabolism. mTOR is a conserved serine/threonine kinase that integrates information about cellular energetics to regulate pathways that control growth and survival. mTOR exists in two distinct complexes, mTORC1 and mTORC2; only the former is depicted here. The TSC1-TSC2 complex acting thru Rheb (see text) is the primary negative regulator of mTORC1. Under normal conditions (left panel), there are various positive (e.g., MAPK/ERK1/2 and Akt) and negative inputs at the level of TSC1/TSC2 (e.g., AMPK and GSK3β) that either increase or decrease mTOR signaling, respectively. Disruption of the polycystin complex (right panel) is associated with upregulation of the MAPK/ERK pathway and decreased levels of AMPK which result in upregulation of mTOR. AMPK negatively regulates CFTR, so reduction in AMPK may result in an increase in fluid-driven chloride secretion. Overexpression of PC1 results in increased levels of p-AKT^{473} but whether the converse is true in PC1-deficient cells is less clear and may hint at complicated cross talk between mTORC1 and mTORC2 [157, 158, 178]. Most of the data supporting this diagram has been generated in *Pkd1* mutant cells and tissues, and the role of *Pkd2* has not been explored in depth

with the ultimate goal of restoring cellular ATP levels to ensure survival. mTOR is among the pathways negatively regulated by AMPK, which phosphorylates TSC and raptor, core components of the mTORC1 complex [187, 188]. In *Pkd1*$^{-/-}$ cells, LKB1 is phosphorylated at ERK specific sites, which results in inhibition of AMPK [178]. Presumably in this scenario, AMPK would be further inhibited by elevated rates of aerobic glycolysis yielding high levels of ATP and a decrease in the AMP to ATP intracellular ratio. Indeed, in several studies *Pkd1*$^{-/-}$ cells and kidneys appear to have reduced levels of phosphorylated (active) AMPK [178, 184, 185]. Consistent with this, agents that increase AMPK (and inhibit ERK) such as metformin have been shown to slow renal cystogenesis presumably by inhibition of mTOR and also of CFTR-mediated chloride secretion, which is also negatively regulated by AMPK [178, 189–191].

In addition to the LKB1-AMPK and mTOR pathways, other metabolic sensors such as sirtuin 1 have also been implicated in cystogenesis. Sirtuin1 (SIRT1), a deacetylase which senses NAD+ levels and, in turn, modulates the expression of metabolic genes, was found to be upregulated in *Pkd1* mutant kidneys [192, 193]. Inactivation of SIRT1 delayed the cystic phenotype and treatment with inhibitors led to delayed renal cyst growth in *Pkd1* mutants [192].

As our understanding of metabolism in neoplastic diseases advances, there will undoubtedly be more insights into the parallels that are present in polycystic kidney disease and the role that metabolic reprogramming plays in ADPKD pathogenesis.

Concluding Remarks

Over the past 20 years, there has been remarkable progress in furthering our understanding of cystogenesis. Advances in the laboratory have resulted in the development of new therapeutic approaches for PKD with a number of drugs now in clinical trials. Despite the strides that have been made, however, challenges remain. Notably, we do not yet know what activates the polycystin complex in vivo, and we have not distinguished the most proximal effects of gene mutation from secondary cellular abnormalities that arise from distorted cystic architecture in late stages of disease. Many of the pathogenic pathways that have been implicated in cyst progression, such as mTOR, cAMP, and calcium signaling, are complex and have varying regulatory functions contingent upon cell type, environment, and developmental stage. How the dysregulation of PKD signaling pathways arises, what the implication of these changes are, and how they fit into a larger more complete picture of disease pathogenesis will require further investigation. The authors apologize if any relevant publications were overlooked in this review.

References

1. Hildebrandt F, Attanasio M, Otto E. Nephronophthisis: disease mechanisms of a ciliopathy. J Am Soc Nephrol. 2009;20(1):23–35.
2. Onuchic LF, Furu L, Nagasawa Y, Hou X, Eggermann T, Ren Z, et al. PKHD1, the polycystic kidney and hepatic disease 1 gene, encodes a novel large protein containing multiple immunoglobulin-like plexin-transcription-factor domains and parallel beta-helix 1 repeats. Am J Hum Genet. 2002;70(5):1305–17.
3. Ward CJ, Hogan MC, Rossetti S, Walker D, Sneddon T, Wang X, et al. The gene mutated in autosomal recessive polycystic kidney disease encodes a large, receptor-like protein. Nat Genet. 2002;30(3):259–69.
4. Zaghloul NA, Katsanis N. Mechanistic insights into Bardet-Biedl syndrome, a model ciliopathy. J Clin Invest. 2009;119(3):428–37.
5. Harris PC, Torres VE. Polycystic kidney disease. Annu Rev Med. 2009;60:321–37.
6. Seeger-Nukpezah T, Geynisman DM, Nikonova AS, Benzing T, Golemis EA. The hallmarks of cancer: relevance to the pathogenesis of polycystic kidney disease. Nat Rev Nephrol. 2015;11(9):515–34.
7. The polycystic kidney disease 1 gene encodes a 14 kb transcript and lies within a duplicated region on chromosome 16. The European Polycystic Kidney Disease Consortium. Cell. 1994;78(4):725.
8. Mochizuki T, Wu G, Hayashi T, Xenophontos SL, Veldhuisen B, Saris JJ, et al. PKD2, a gene for polycystic kidney disease that encodes an integral membrane protein. Science. 1996;272(5266):1339–42.
9. Chebib FT, Torres VE. Autosomal dominant polycystic kidney disease: core curriculum 2016. Am J Kidney Dis. 2016;67(5):792–810.
10. Baert L. Hereditary polycystic kidney disease (adult form): a microdissection study of two cases at an early stage of the disease. Kidney Int. 1978;13(6):519–25.
11. Reeders ST. Multilocus polycystic disease. Nat Genet. 1992;1(4):235–7.
12. Qian F, Watnick TJ. Somatic mutation as mechanism for cyst formation in autosomal dominant polycystic kidney disease. Mol Genet Metab. 1999;68(2):237–42.
13. Qian F, Watnick TJ, Onuchic LF, Germino GG. The molecular basis of focal cyst formation in human autosomal dominant polycystic kidney disease type I. Cell. 1996;87(6):979–87.
14. Pei Y, Watnick T, He N, Wang K, Liang Y, Parfrey P, et al. Somatic PKD2 mutations in individual kidney and liver cysts support a "two-hit" model of cystogenesis in type 2 autosomal dominant polycystic kidney disease. J Am Soc Nephrol. 1999;10(7):1524–9.
15. Watnick T, He N, Wang K, Liang Y, Parfrey P, Hefferton D, et al. Mutations of PKD1 in ADPKD2 cysts suggest a pathogenic effect of trans-heterozygous mutations. Nat Genet. 2000;25(2):143–4.
16. Brasier JL, Henske EP. Loss of the polycystic kidney disease (PKD1) region of chromosome 16p13 in renal cyst cells supports a loss-of-function model for cyst pathogenesis. J Clin Invest. 1997;99(2):194–9.
17. Torra R, Badenas C, San Millan JL, Perez-Oller L, Estivill X, Darnell A. A loss-of-function model for cystogenesis in human autosomal dominant polycystic kidney disease type 2. Am J Hum Genet. 1999;65(2):345–52.
18. Watnick TJ, Torres VE, Gandolph MA, Qian F, Onuchic LF, Klinger KW, et al. Somatic mutation in individual liver cysts supports a two-hit model of cystogenesis in autosomal dominant polycystic kidney disease. Mol Cell. 1998;2(2):247–51.
19. Wu G, D'Agati V, Cai Y, Markowitz G, Park JH, Reynolds DM, et al. Somatic inactivation of

Pkd2 results in polycystic kidney disease. Cell. 1998;93(2):177–88.
20. Piontek KB, Huso DL, Grinberg A, Liu L, Bedja D, Zhao H, et al. A functional floxed allele of Pkd1 that can be conditionally inactivated in vivo. J Am Soc Nephrol. 2004;15(12):3035–43.
21. Garcia-Gonzalez MA, Outeda P, Zhou Q, Zhou F, Menezes LF, Qian F, et al. Pkd1 and Pkd2 are required for normal placental development. PLoS One. 2010;5(9).
22. Ma M, Tian X, Igarashi P, Pazour GJ, Somlo S. Loss of cilia suppresses cyst growth in genetic models of autosomal dominant polycystic kidney disease. Nat Genet. 2013;45(9):1004–12.
23. Rossetti S, Kubly VJ, Consugar MB, Hopp K, Roy S, Horsley SW, et al. Incompletely penetrant PKD1 alleles suggest a role for gene dosage in cyst initiation in polycystic kidney disease. Kidney Int. 2009;75(8):848–55.
24. Jiang ST, Chiou YY, Wang E, Lin HK, Lin YT, Chi YC, et al. Defining a link with autosomal-dominant polycystic kidney disease in mice with congenitally low expression of Pkd1. Am J Pathol. 2006;168(1):205–20.
25. Lantinga-van Leeuwen IS, Dauwerse JG, Baelde HJ, Leonhard WN, van de Wal A, Ward CJ, et al. Lowering of Pkd1 expression is sufficient to cause polycystic kidney disease. Hum Mol Genet. 2004;13(24):3069–77.
26. Gallagher AR, Germino GG, Somlo S. Molecular advances in autosomal dominant polycystic kidney disease. Adv Chronic Kidney Dis. 2010;17(2): 118–30.
27. Piontek K, Menezes LF, Garcia-Gonzalez MA, Huso DL, Germino GG. A critical developmental switch defines the kinetics of kidney cyst formation after loss of Pkd1. Nat Med. 2007;13(12):1490–5.
28. Lantinga-van Leeuwen IS, Leonhard WN, van der Wal A, Breuning MH, de Heer E, Peters DJ. Kidney-specific inactivation of the Pkd1 gene induces rapid cyst formation in developing kidneys and a slow onset of disease in adult mice. Hum Mol Genet. 2007;16(24):3188–96.
29. Takakura A, Contrino L, Beck AW, Zhou J. Pkd1 inactivation induced in adulthood produces focal cystic disease. J Am Soc Nephrol. 2008;19(12):2351–63.
30. Takakura A, Contrino L, Zhou X, Bonventre JV, Sun Y, Humphreys BD, et al. Renal injury is a third hit promoting rapid development of adult polycystic kidney disease. Hum Mol Genet. 2009;18(14):2523–31.
31. Leonhard WN, Happe H, Peters DJ. Variable cyst development in autosomal dominant polycystic kidney disease: the biologic context. J Am Soc Nephrol. 2016;27(12):3530–8.
32. Patel V, Li L, Cobo-Stark P, Shao X, Somlo S, Lin F, et al. Acute kidney injury and aberrant planar cell polarity induce cyst formation in mice lacking renal cilia. Hum Mol Genet. 2008;17(11):1578–90.
33. Watnick T, Germino G. From cilia to cyst. Nat Genet. 2003;34(4):355–6.
34. Calvet JP. Ciliary signaling goes down the tubes. Nat Genet. 2003;33(2):113–4.
35. Yoder BK, Hou X, Guay-Woodford LM. The polycystic kidney disease proteins, polycystin-1, polycystin-2, polaris, and cystin, are co-localized in renal cilia. J Am Soc Nephrol. 2002;13(10):2508–16.
36. Pazour GJ, San Agustin JT, Follit JA, Rosenbaum JL, Witman GB. Polycystin-2 localizes to kidney cilia and the ciliary level is elevated in orpk mice with polycystic kidney disease. Curr Biol. 2002;12(11):R378–80.
37. Reiter JF, Leroux MR. Genes and molecular pathways underpinning ciliopathies. Nat Rev Mol Cell Biol. 2017;18(9):533–47.
38. Pedersen LB, Rosenbaum JL. Intraflagellar transport (IFT) role in ciliary assembly, resorption and signalling. Curr Top Dev Biol. 2008;85:23–61.
39. Jin H, White SR, Shida T, Schulz S, Aguiar M, Gygi SP, et al. The conserved Bardet-Biedl syndrome proteins assemble a coat that traffics membrane proteins to cilia. Cell. 2010;141(7):1208–19.
40. Satir P, Pedersen LB, Christensen ST. The primary cilium at a glance. J Cell Sci. 2010;123(Pt 4):499–503.
41. Singla V, Reiter JF. The primary cilium as the cell's antenna: signaling at a sensory organelle. Science. 2006;313(5787):629–33.
42. Hildebrandt F, Benzing T, Katsanis N. Ciliopathies. N Engl J Med. 2011;364(16):1533–43.
43. Harris PC, Torres VE. Genetic mechanisms and signaling pathways in autosomal dominant polycystic kidney disease. J Clin Invest. 2014;124(6):2315–24.
44. Ma M, Gallagher AR, Somlo S. Ciliary mechanisms of cyst formation in polycystic kidney disease. Cold Spring Harb Perspect Biol. 2017;9:a028209.
45. Koulen P, Cai Y, Geng L, Maeda Y, Nishimura S, Witzgall R, et al. Polycystin-2 is an intracellular calcium release channel. Nat Cell Biol. 2002;4(3): 191–7.
46. Hanaoka K, Qian F, Boletta A, Bhunia AK, Piontek K, Tsiokas L, et al. Co-assembly of polycystin-1 and -2 produces unique cation-permeable currents. Nature. 2000;408(6815):990–4.
47. Gonzalez-Perrett S, Kim K, Ibarra C, Damiano AE, Zotta E, Batelli M, et al. Polycystin-2, the protein mutated in autosomal dominant polycystic kidney disease (ADPKD), is a Ca2+-permeable nonselective cation channel. Proc Natl Acad Sci U S A. 2001;98(3):1182–7.
48. Vassilev PM, Guo L, Chen XZ, Segal Y, Peng JB, Basora N, et al. Polycystin-2 is a novel cation channel implicated in defective intracellular Ca(2+) homeostasis in polycystic kidney disease. Biochem Biophys Res Commun. 2001;282(1):341–50.
49. Kottgen M. TRPP2 and autosomal dominant polycystic kidney disease. Biochim Biophys Acta. 2007;1772(8):836–50.
50. Chen XZ, Segal Y, Basora N, Guo L, Peng JB, Babakhanlou H, et al. Transport function of the naturally occurring pathogenic polycystin-2

mutant, R742X. Biochem Biophys Res Commun. 2001;282(5):1251–6.
51. Cantiello HF. Regulation of calcium signaling by polycystin-2. Am J Physiol Ren Physiol. 2004;286(6):F1012–29.
52. Delmas P, Nauli SM, Li X, Coste B, Osorio N, Crest M, et al. Gating of the polycystin ion channel signaling complex in neurons and kidney cells. FASEB J. 2004;18(6):740–2.
53. Shen PS, Yang X, DeCaen PG, Liu X, Bulkley D, Clapham DE, et al. The structure of the polycystic kidney disease channel PKD2 in lipid nanodiscs. Cell. 2016;167(3):763–73. e11
54. Grieben M, Pike AC, Shintre CA, Venturi E, El-Ajouz S, Tessitore A, et al. Structure of the polycystic kidney disease TRP channel polycystin-2 (PC2). Nat Struct Mol Biol. 2017;24(2):114–22.
55. Wilkes M, Madej MG, Kreuter L, Rhinow D, Heinz V, De Sanctis S, et al. Molecular insights into lipid-assisted Ca2+ regulation of the TRP channel polycystin-2. Nat Struct Mol Biol. 2017;24(2):123–30.
56. Qian F, Germino FJ, Cai Y, Zhang X, Somlo S, Germino GG. PKD1 interacts with PKD2 through a probable coiled-coil domain. Nat Genet. 1997;16(2):179–83.
57. Berridge MJ, Bootman MD, Roderick HL. Calcium signalling: dynamics, homeostasis and remodelling. Nat Rev Mol Cell Biol. 2003;4(7):517–29.
58. Busch T, Kottgen M, Hofherr A. TRPP2 ion channels: critical regulators of organ morphogenesis in health and disease. Cell Calcium. 2017;66:25–32.
59. Geng L, Okuhara D, Yu Z, Tian X, Cai Y, Shibazaki S, et al. Polycystin-2 traffics to cilia independently of polycystin-1 by using an N-terminal RVxP motif. J Cell Sci. 2006;119(Pt 7):1383–95.
60. Kottgen M, Benzing T, Simmen T, Tauber R, Buchholz B, Feliciangeli S, et al. Trafficking of TRPP2 by PACS proteins represents a novel mechanism of ion channel regulation. EMBO J. 2005;24(4):705–16.
61. Kottgen M, Walz G. Subcellular localization and trafficking of polycystins. Pflugers Arch. 2005;451(1):286–93.
62. Streets AJ, Moon DJ, Kane ME, Obara T, Ong AC. Identification of an N-terminal glycogen synthase kinase 3 phosphorylation site which regulates the functional localization of polycystin-2 in vivo and in vitro. Hum Mol Genet. 2006;15(9):1465–73.
63. Praetorius HA, Spring KR. Bending the MDCK cell primary cilium increases intracellular calcium. J Membr Biol. 2001;184(1):71–9.
64. Praetorius HA, Spring KR. Removal of the MDCK cell primary cilium abolishes flow sensing. J Membr Biol. 2003;191(1):69–76.
65. Nauli SM, Alenghat FJ, Luo Y, Williams E, Vassilev P, Li X, et al. Polycystins 1 and 2 mediate mechanosensation in the primary cilium of kidney cells. Nat Genet. 2003;33(2):129–37.
66. Nauli SM, Rossetti S, Kolb RJ, Alenghat FJ, Consugar MB, Harris PC, et al. Loss of polycystin-1 in human cyst-lining epithelia leads to ciliary dysfunction. J Am Soc Nephrol. 2006;17(4):1015–25.
67. Spasic M, Jacobs CR. Primary cilia: cell and molecular mechanosensors directing whole tissue function. Semin Cell Dev Biol. 2017;71:42–52.
68. Patel A, Honore E. Polycystins and renovascular mechanosensory transduction. Nat Rev Nephrol. 2010;6(9):530–8.
69. Kottgen M, Buchholz B, Garcia-Gonzalez MA, Kotsis F, Fu X, Doerken M, et al. TRPP2 and TRPV4 form a polymodal sensory channel complex. J Cell Biol. 2008;182(3):437–47.
70. DeCaen PG, Delling M, Vien TN, Clapham DE. Direct recording and molecular identification of the calcium channel of primary cilia. Nature. 2013;504(7479):315–8.
71. Delling M, DeCaen PG, Doerner JF, Febvay S, Clapham DE. Primary cilia are specialized calcium signalling organelles. Nature. 2013;504(7479):311–4.
72. Delling M, Indzhykulian AA, Liu X, Li Y, Xie T, Corey DP, et al. Primary cilia are not calcium-responsive mechanosensors. Nature. 2016;531(7596):656–60.
73. Kleene SJ, Kleene NK. The native TRPP2-dependent channel of murine renal primary cilia. Am J Physiol Ren Physiol. 2017;312(1):F96–F108.
74. Cai Y, Maeda Y, Cedzich A, Torres VE, Wu G, Hayashi T, et al. Identification and characterization of polycystin-2, the PKD2 gene product. J Biol Chem. 1999;274(40):28557–65.
75. Li Y, Santoso NG, Yu S, Woodward OM, Qian F, Guggino WB. Polycystin-1 interacts with inositol 1,4,5-trisphosphate receptor to modulate intracellular Ca2+ signaling with implications for polycystic kidney disease. J Biol Chem. 2009;284(52):36431–41.
76. Santoso NG, Cebotaru L, Guggino WB. Polycystin-1, 2, and STIM1 interact with IP(3)R to modulate ER Ca release through the PI3K/Akt pathway. Cell Physiol Biochem. 2011;27(6):715–26.
77. Li Y, Wright JM, Qian F, Germino GG, Guggino WB. Polycystin 2 interacts with type I inositol 1,4,5-trisphosphate receptor to modulate intracellular Ca2+ signaling. J Biol Chem. 2005;280(50):41298–306.
78. Anyatonwu GI, Estrada M, Tian X, Somlo S, Ehrlich BE. Regulation of ryanodine receptor-dependent calcium signaling by polycystin-2. Proc Natl Acad Sci U S A. 2007;104(15):6454–9.
79. Woodward OM, Li Y, Yu S, Greenwell P, Wodarczyk C, Boletta A, et al. Identification of a polycystin-1 cleavage product, P100, that regulates store operated Ca entry through interactions with STIM1. PLoS One. 2010;5(8):e12305.
80. Bagur R, Hajnoczky G. Intracellular Ca2+ sensing: its role in calcium homeostasis and signaling. Mol Cell. 2017;66(6):780–8.
81. Putney JW. Capacitative calcium entry: from concept to molecules. Immunol Rev. 2009;231(1):10–22.
82. Weber KH, Lee EK, Basavanna U, Lindley S, Ziegelstein RC, Germino GG, et al. Heterologous

expression of polycystin-1 inhibits endoplasmic reticulum calcium leak in stably transfected MDCK cells. Am J Physiol Ren Physiol. 2008;294(6):F1279–86.
83. Mekahli D, Sammels E, Luyten T, Welkenhuyzen K, van den Heuvel LP, Levtchenko EN, et al. Polycystin-1 and polycystin-2 are both required to amplify inositol-trisphosphate-induced Ca2+ release. Cell Calcium. 2012;51(6):452–8.
84. Qian Q, Hunter LW, Li M, Marin-Padilla M, Prakash YS, Somlo S, et al. Pkd2 haploinsufficiency alters intracellular calcium regulation in vascular smooth muscle cells. Hum Mol Genet. 2003;12(15):1875–80.
85. Geng L, Boehmerle W, Maeda Y, Okuhara DY, Tian X, Yu Z, et al. Syntaxin 5 regulates the endoplasmic reticulum channel-release properties of polycystin-2. Proc Natl Acad Sci U S A. 2008;105(41):15920–5.
86. Wegierski T, Steffl D, Kopp C, Tauber R, Buchholz B, Nitschke R, et al. TRPP2 channels regulate apoptosis through the Ca2+ concentration in the endoplasmic reticulum. EMBO J. 2009;28(5):490–9.
87. Torres VE, Harris PC. Strategies targeting cAMP signaling in the treatment of polycystic kidney disease. J Am Soc Nephrol. 2014;25(1):18–32.
88. Hughes J, Ward CJ, Peral B, Aspinwall R, Clark K, San Millan JL, et al. The polycystic kidney disease 1 (PKD1) gene encodes a novel protein with multiple cell recognition domains. Nat Genet. 1995;10(2):151–60.
89. Nims N, Vassmer D, Maser RL. Transmembrane domain analysis of polycystin-1, the product of the polycystic kidney disease-1 (PKD1) gene: evidence for 11 membrane-spanning domains. Biochemistry. 2003;42(44):13035–48.
90. Kim H, Xu H, Yao Q, Li W, Huang Q, Outeda P, et al. Ciliary membrane proteins traffic through the Golgi via a Rabep1/GGA1/Arl3-dependent mechanism. Nat Commun. 2014;5:5482.
91. Gainullin VG, Hopp K, Ward CJ, Hommerding CJ, Harris PC. Polycystin-1 maturation requires polycystin-2 in a dose-dependent manner. J Clin Invest. 2015;125(2):607–20.
92. Cai Y, Fedeles SV, Dong K, Anyatonwu G, Onoe T, Mitobe M, et al. Altered trafficking and stability of polycystins underlie polycystic kidney disease. J Clin Invest. 2014;124(12):5129–44.
93. Kim S, Nie H, Nesin V, Tran U, Outeda P, Bai CX, et al. The polycystin complex mediates Wnt/Ca(2+) signalling. Nat Cell Biol. 2016;18(7):752–64.
94. Halls ML, Cooper DM. Adenylyl cyclase signalling complexes – pharmacological challenges and opportunities. Pharmacol Ther. 2017;172:171–80.
95. Wallace DP. Cyclic AMP-mediated cyst expansion. Biochim Biophys Acta. 2011;1812(10):1291–300.
96. Lugnier C. Cyclic nucleotide phosphodiesterase (PDE) superfamily: a new target for the development of specific therapeutic agents. Pharmacol Ther. 2006;109(3):366–98.
97. Chang XB, Tabcharani JA, Hou YX, Jensen TJ, Kartner N, Alon N, et al. Protein kinase A (PKA) still activates CFTR chloride channel after mutagenesis of all 10 PKA consensus phosphorylation sites. J Biol Chem. 1993;268(15):11304–11.
98. Xu ZC, Yang Y, Hebert SC. Phosphorylation of the ATP-sensitive, inwardly rectifying K+ channel, ROMK, by cyclic AMP-dependent protein kinase. J Biol Chem. 1996;271(16):9313–9.
99. Snyder PM, Olson DR, Kabra R, Zhou R, Steines JC. cAMP and serum and glucocorticoid-inducible kinase (SGK) regulate the epithelial Na(+) channel through convergent phosphorylation of Nedd4-2. J Biol Chem. 2004;279(44):45753–8.
100. Brown D, Breton S, Ausiello DA, Marshansky V. Sensing, signaling and sorting events in kidney epithelial cell physiology. Traffic. 2009;10(3):275–84.
101. Yamaguchi T, Nagao S, Kasahara M, Takahashi H, Grantham JJ. Renal accumulation and excretion of cyclic adenosine monophosphate in a murine model of slowly progressive polycystic kidney disease. Am J Kidney Dis. 1997;30(5):703–9.
102. Torres VE, Wang X, Qian Q, Somlo S, Harris PC, Gattone VH 2nd. Effective treatment of an orthologous model of autosomal dominant polycystic kidney disease. Nat Med. 2004;10(4):363–4.
103. Gattone VH 2nd, Wang X, Harris PC, Torres VE. Inhibition of renal cystic disease development and progression by a vasopressin V2 receptor antagonist. Nat Med. 2003;9(10):1323–6.
104. Smith LA, Bukanov NO, Husson H, Russo RJ, Barry TC, Taylor AL, et al. Development of polycystic kidney disease in juvenile cystic kidney mice: insights into pathogenesis, ciliary abnormalities, and common features with human disease. J Am Soc Nephrol. 2006;17(10):2821–31.
105. Starremans PG, Li X, Finnerty PE, Guo L, Takakura A, Neilson EG, et al. A mouse model for polycystic kidney disease through a somatic in-frame deletion in the 5′ end of Pkd1. Kidney Int. 2008;73(12):1394–405.
106. Hopp K, Ward CJ, Hommerding CJ, Nasr SH, Tuan HF, Gainullin VG, et al. Functional polycystin-1 dosage governs autosomal dominant polycystic kidney disease severity. J Clin Invest. 2012;122(11):4257–73.
107. Yamaguchi T, Pelling JC, Ramaswamy NT, Eppler JW, Wallace DP, Nagao S, et al. cAMP stimulates the in vitro proliferation of renal cyst epithelial cells by activating the extracellular signal-regulated kinase pathway. Kidney Int. 2000;57(4):1460–71.
108. Belibi FA, Reif G, Wallace DP, Yamaguchi T, Olsen L, Li H, et al. Cyclic AMP promotes growth and secretion in human polycystic kidney epithelial cells. Kidney Int. 2004;66(3):964–73.
109. Chebib FT, Sussman CR, Wang X, Harris PC, Torres VE. Vasopressin and disruption of calcium signalling in polycystic kidney disease. Nat Rev Nephrol. 2015;11(8):451–64.
110. Rees S, Kittikulsuth W, Roos K, Strait KA, Van Hoek A, Kohan DE. Adenylyl cyclase 6 deficiency ameliorates polycystic kidney disease. J Am Soc Nephrol. 2014;25(2):232–7.

111. Sussman CR, Ward CJ, Leightner AC, Smith JL, Agarwal R, Harris PC, et al. Phosphodiesterase 1A modulates cystogenesis in zebrafish. J Am Soc Nephrol. 2014;25(10):2222–30.
112. Wang X, Yamada S, LaRiviere WB, Ye H, Bakeberg JL, Irazabal MV, et al. Generation and phenotypic characterization of Pde1a mutant mice. PLoS One. 2017;12(7):e0181087.
113. Putnam WC, Swenson SM, Reif GA, Wallace DP, Helmkamp GM Jr, Grantham JJ. Identification of a forskolin-like molecule in human renal cysts. J Am Soc Nephrol. 2007;18(3):934–43.
114. Parnell SC, Magenheimer BS, Maser RL, Rankin CA, Smine A, Okamoto T, et al. The polycystic kidney disease-1 protein, polycystin-1, binds and activates heterotrimeric G-proteins in vitro. Biochem Biophys Res Commun. 1998;251(2):625–31.
115. Gabow PA, Kaehny WD, Johnson AM, Duley IT, Manco-Johnson M, Lezotte DC, et al. The clinical utility of renal concentrating capacity in polycystic kidney disease. Kidney Int. 1989;35(2):675–80.
116. Seeman T, Dusek J, Vondrak K, Blahova K, Simkova E, Kreisinger J, et al. Renal concentrating capacity is linked to blood pressure in children with autosomal dominant polycystic kidney disease. Physiol Res. 2004;53(6):629–34.
117. de Bree FM, Burbach JP. Structure-function relationships of the vasopressin prohormone domains. Cell Mol Neurobiol. 1998;18(2):173–91.
118. Boertien WE, Meijer E, Zittema D, van Dijk MA, Rabelink TJ, Breuning MH, et al. Copeptin, a surrogate marker for vasopressin, is associated with kidney function decline in subjects with autosomal dominant polycystic kidney disease. Nephrol Dial Transplant. 2012;27(11):4131–7.
119. Zittema D, Boertien WE, van Beek AP, Dullaart RP, Franssen CF, de Jong PE, et al. Vasopressin, copeptin, and renal concentrating capacity in patients with autosomal dominant polycystic kidney disease without renal impairment. Clin J Am Soc Nephrol. 2012;7(6):906–13.
120. Wang X, Wu Y, Ward CJ, Harris PC, Torres VE. Vasopressin directly regulates cyst growth in polycystic kidney disease. J Am Soc Nephrol. 2008;19(1):102–8.
121. Wang X, Gattone V 2nd, Harris PC, Torres VE. Effectiveness of vasopressin V2 receptor antagonists OPC-31260 and OPC-41061 on polycystic kidney disease development in the PCK rat. J Am Soc Nephrol. 2005;16(4):846–51.
122. Hopp K, Hommerding CJ, Wang X, Ye H, Harris PC, Torres VE. Tolvaptan plus pasireotide shows enhanced efficacy in a PKD1 model. J Am Soc Nephrol. 2015;26(1):39–47.
123. Torres VE, Chapman AB, Devuyst O, Gansevoort RT, Grantham JJ, Higashihara E, et al. Tolvaptan in patients with autosomal dominant polycystic kidney disease. N Engl J Med. 2012;367(25):2407–18.
124. Yamaguchi T, Nagao S, Wallace DP, Belibi FA, Cowley BD, Pelling JC, et al. Cyclic AMP activates B-Raf and ERK in cyst epithelial cells from autosomal-dominant polycystic kidneys. Kidney Int. 2003;63(6):1983–94.
125. Hanaoka K, Guggino WB. cAMP regulates cell proliferation and cyst formation in autosomal polycystic kidney disease cells. J Am Soc Nephrol. 2000;11(7):1179–87.
126. Parker E, Newby LJ, Sharpe CC, Rossetti S, Streets AJ, Harris PC, et al. Hyperproliferation of PKD1 cystic cells is induced by insulin-like growth factor-1 activation of the Ras/Raf signalling system. Kidney Int. 2007;72(2):157–65.
127. Sebolt-Leopold JS, Herrera R. Targeting the mitogen-activated protein kinase cascade to treat cancer. Nat Rev Cancer. 2004;4(12):937–47.
128. Yamaguchi T, Wallace DP, Magenheimer BS, Hempson SJ, Grantham JJ, Calvet JP. Calcium restriction allows cAMP activation of the B-Raf/ERK pathway, switching cells to a cAMP-dependent growth-stimulated phenotype. J Biol Chem. 2004;279(39):40419–30.
129. Yamaguchi T, Hempson SJ, Reif GA, Hedge AM, Wallace DP. Calcium restores a normal proliferation phenotype in human polycystic kidney disease epithelial cells. J Am Soc Nephrol. 2006;17(1):178–87.
130. Sullivan LP, Wallace DP, Grantham JJ. Epithelial transport in polycystic kidney disease. Physiol Rev. 1998;78(4):1165–91.
131. Grantham JJ, Ye M, Gattone VH 2nd, Sullivan LP. In vitro fluid secretion by epithelium from polycystic kidneys. J Clin Invest. 1995;95(1):195–202.
132. Sullivan LP, Wallace DP, Grantham JJ. Chloride and fluid secretion in polycystic kidney disease. J Am Soc Nephrol. 1998;9(5):903–16.
133. Rajagopal M, Wallace DP. Chloride secretion by renal collecting ducts. Curr Opin Nephrol Hypertens. 2015;24(5):444–9.
134. Ye M, Grantham JJ. The secretion of fluid by renal cysts from patients with autosomal dominant polycystic kidney disease. N Engl J Med. 1993;329(5):310–3.
135. Riordan JR, Rommens JM, Kerem B, Alon N, Rozmahel R, Grzelczak Z, et al. Identification of the cystic fibrosis gene: cloning and characterization of complementary DNA. Science. 1989;245(4922):1066–73.
136. Saint-Criq V, Gray MA. Role of CFTR in epithelial physiology. Cell Mol Life Sci. 2017;74(1):93–115.
137. Brill SR, Ross KE, Davidow CJ, Ye M, Grantham JJ, Caplan MJ. Immunolocalization of ion transport proteins in human autosomal dominant polycystic kidney epithelial cells. Proc Natl Acad Sci U S A. 1996;93(19):10206–11.
138. Hanaoka K, Devuyst O, Schwiebert EM, Wilson PD, Guggino WB. A role for CFTR in human autosomal dominant polycystic kidney disease. Am J Phys. 1996;270(1 Pt 1):C389–99.
139. Davidow CJ, Maser RL, Rome LA, Calvet JP, Grantham JJ. The cystic fibrosis transmembrane conductance regulator mediates transepithelial fluid

secretion by human autosomal dominant polycystic kidney disease epithelium in vitro. Kidney Int. 1996;50(1):208–18.
140. Magenheimer BS, St John PL, Isom KS, Abrahamson DR, De Lisle RC, Wallace DP, et al. Early embryonic renal tubules of wild-type and polycystic kidney disease kidneys respond to cAMP stimulation with cystic fibrosis transmembrane conductance regulator/Na(+),K(+),2Cl(−) Co-transporter-dependent cystic dilation. J Am Soc Nephrol. 2006;17(12):3424–37.
141. Tradtrantip L, Sonawane ND, Namkung W, Verkman AS. Nanomolar potency pyrimido-pyrrolo-quinoxalinedione CFTR inhibitor reduces cyst size in a polycystic kidney disease model. J Med Chem. 2009;52(20):6447–55.
142. Snyder DS, Tradtrantip L, Yao C, Kurth MJ, Verkman AS. Potent, metabolically stable benzopyrimido-pyrrolo-oxazine-dione (BPO) CFTR inhibitors for polycystic kidney disease. J Med Chem. 2011;54(15):5468–77.
143. Persu A, Devuyst O, Lannoy N, Materne R, Brosnahan G, Gabow PA, et al. CF gene and cystic fibrosis transmembrane conductance regulator expression in autosomal dominant polycystic kidney disease. J Am Soc Nephrol. 2000;11(12):2285–96.
144. O'Sullivan DA, Torres VE, Gabow PA, Thibodeau SN, King BF, Bergstralh EJ. Cystic fibrosis and the phenotypic expression of autosomal dominant polycystic kidney disease. Am J Kidney Dis. 1998;32(6):976–83.
145. Xu N, Glockner JF, Rossetti S, Babovich-Vuksanovic D, Harris PC, Torres VE. Autosomal dominant polycystic kidney disease coexisting with cystic fibrosis. J Nephrol. 2006;19(4):529–34.
146. Lebeau C, Hanaoka K, Moore-Hoon ML, Guggino WB, Beauwens R, Devuyst O. Basolateral chloride transporters in autosomal dominant polycystic kidney disease. Pflugers Arch. 2002;444(6):722–31.
147. Buchholz B, Schley G, Faria D, Kroening S, Willam C, Schreiber R, et al. Hypoxia-inducible factor-1alpha causes renal cyst expansion through calcium-activated chloride secretion. J Am Soc Nephrol. 2014;25(3):465–74.
148. Buchholz B, Teschemacher B, Schley G, Schillers H, Eckardt KU. Formation of cysts by principal-like MDCK cells depends on the synergy of cAMP- and ATP-mediated fluid secretion. J Mol Med (Berl). 2011;89(3):251–61.
149. Brook-Carter PT, Peral B, Ward CJ, Thompson P, Hughes J, Maheshwar MM, et al. Deletion of the TSC2 and PKD1 genes associated with severe infantile polycystic kidney disease – a contiguous gene syndrome. Nat Genet. 1994;8(4):328–32.
150. Crino PB, Nathanson KL, Henske EP. The tuberous sclerosis complex. N Engl J Med. 2006;355(13):1345–56.
151. Zoncu R, Efeyan A, Sabatini DM. mTOR: from growth signal integration to cancer, diabetes and ageing. Nat Rev Mol Cell Biol. 2011;12(1):21–35.
152. Tee AR, Blenis J. mTOR, translational control and human disease. Semin Cell Dev Biol. 2005;16(1):29–37.
153. Laplante M, Sabatini DM. mTOR signaling in growth control and disease. Cell. 2012;149(2):274–93.
154. Wullschleger S, Loewith R, Hall MN. TOR signaling in growth and metabolism. Cell. 2006;124(3):471–84.
155. Huang J, Manning BD. The TSC1-TSC2 complex: a molecular switchboard controlling cell growth. Biochem J. 2008;412(2):179–90.
156. Tee AR, Fingar DC, Manning BD, Kwiatkowski DJ, Cantley LC, Blenis J. Tuberous sclerosis complex-1 and -2 gene products function together to inhibit mammalian target of rapamycin (mTOR)-mediated downstream signaling. Proc Natl Acad Sci U S A. 2002;99(21):13571–6.
157. Boletta A. Emerging evidence of a link between the polycystins and the mTOR pathways. PathoGenetics. 2009;2(1):6.
158. Distefano G, Boca M, Rowe I, Wodarczyk C, Ma L, Piontek KB, et al. Polycystin-1 regulates extracellular signal-regulated kinase-dependent phosphorylation of tuberin to control cell size through mTOR and its downstream effectors S6K and 4EBP1. Mol Cell Biol. 2009;29(9):2359–71.
159. Hartman TR, Liu D, Zilfou JT, Robb V, Morrison T, Watnick T, et al. The tuberous sclerosis proteins regulate formation of the primary cilium via a rapamycin-insensitive and polycystin 1-independent pathway. Hum Mol Genet. 2009;18(1):151–63.
160. Shillingford JM, Murcia NS, Larson CH, Low SH, Hedgepeth R, Brown N, et al. The mTOR pathway is regulated by polycystin-1, and its inhibition reverses renal cystogenesis in polycystic kidney disease. Proc Natl Acad Sci U S A. 2006;103(14):5466–71.
161. Zafar I, Ravichandran K, Belibi FA, Doctor RB, Edelstein CL. Sirolimus attenuates disease progression in an orthologous mouse model of human autosomal dominant polycystic kidney disease. Kidney Int. 2010;78(8):754–61.
162. Belibi F, Ravichandran K, Zafar I, He Z, Edelstein CL. mTORC1/2 and rapamycin in female Han:SPRD rats with polycystic kidney disease. Am J Physiol Ren Physiol. 2011;300(1):F236–44.
163. Wahl PR, Serra AL, Le Hir M, Molle KD, Hall MN, Wuthrich RP. Inhibition of mTOR with sirolimus slows disease progression in Han:SPRD rats with autosomal dominant polycystic kidney disease (ADPKD). Nephrol Dial Transplant. 2006;21(3):598–604.
164. Shillingford JM, Piontek KB, Germino GG, Weimbs T. Rapamycin ameliorates PKD resulting from conditional inactivation of Pkd1. J Am Soc Nephrol. 2010;21(3):489–97.
165. Tao Y, Kim J, Schrier RW, Edelstein CL. Rapamycin markedly slows disease progression in a rat model of polycystic kidney disease. J Am Soc Nephrol. 2005;16(1):46–51.

166. Wu M, Wahl PR, Le Hir M, Wackerle-Men Y, Wuthrich RP, Serra AL. Everolimus retards cyst growth and preserves kidney function in a rodent model for polycystic kidney disease. Kidney Blood Press Res. 2007;30(4):253–9.
167. Zafar I, Belibi FA, He Z, Edelstein CL. Long-term rapamycin therapy in the Han:SPRD rat model of polycystic kidney disease (PKD). Nephrol Dial Transplant. 2009;24(8):2349–53.
168. Kim HJ, Edelstein CL. Mammalian target of rapamycin inhibition in polycystic kidney disease: from bench to bedside. Kidney Res Clin Pract. 2012;31(3):132–8.
169. Serra AL, Poster D, Kistler AD, Krauer F, Raina S, Young J, et al. Sirolimus and kidney growth in autosomal dominant polycystic kidney disease. N Engl J Med. 2010;363(9):820–9.
170. Walz G, Budde K, Mannaa M, Nurnberger J, Wanner C, Sommerer C, et al. Everolimus in patients with autosomal dominant polycystic kidney disease. N Engl J Med. 2010;363(9):830–40.
171. Canaud G, Knebelmann B, Harris PC, Vrtovsnik F, Correas JM, Pallet N, et al. Therapeutic mTOR inhibition in autosomal dominant polycystic kidney disease: what is the appropriate serum level? Am J Transplant. 2010;10(7):1701–6.
172. Watnick T, Germino GG. mTOR inhibitors in polycystic kidney disease. N Engl J Med. 2010;363(9):879–81.
173. Shillingford JM, Leamon CP, Vlahov IR, Weimbs T. Folate-conjugated rapamycin slows progression of polycystic kidney disease. J Am Soc Nephrol. 2012;23(10):1674–81.
174. Grantham JJ. Polycystic kidney disease: neoplasia in disguise. Am J Kidney Dis. 1990;15(2):110–6.
175. Menezes LF, Zhou F, Patterson AD, Piontek KB, Krausz KW, Gonzalez FJ, et al. Network analysis of a Pkd1-mouse model of autosomal dominant polycystic kidney disease identifies HNF4alpha as a disease modifier. PLoS Genet. 2012;8(11):e1003053.
176. Menezes LF, Germino GG. Systems biology of polycystic kidney disease: a critical review. Wiley Interdiscip Rev Syst Biol Med. 2015;7(1):39–52.
177. Rhee J, Inoue Y, Yoon JC, Puigserver P, Fan M, Gonzalez FJ, et al. Regulation of hepatic fasting response by PPARgamma coactivator-1alpha (PGC-1): requirement for hepatocyte nuclear factor 4alpha in gluconeogenesis. Proc Natl Acad Sci U S A. 2003;100(7):4012–7.
178. Rowe I, Chiaravalli M, Mannella V, Ulisse V, Quilici G, Pema M, et al. Defective glucose metabolism in polycystic kidney disease identifies a new therapeutic strategy. Nat Med. 2013;19(4):488–93.
179. Chiaravalli M, Rowe I, Mannella V, Quilici G, Canu T, Bianchi V, et al. 2-deoxy-d-glucose ameliorates PKD progression. J Am Soc Nephrol. 2016;27(7):1958–69.
180. Vander Heiden MG, Cantley LC, Thompson CB. Understanding the Warburg effect: the metabolic requirements of cell proliferation. Science. 2009;324(5930):1029–33.
181. Ward PS, Thompson CB. Metabolic reprogramming: a cancer hallmark even warburg did not anticipate. Cancer Cell. 2012;21(3):297–308.
182. Rowe I, Boletta A. Defective metabolism in polycystic kidney disease: potential for therapy and open questions. Nephrol Dial Transplant. 2014;29(8):1480–6.
183. Menezes LF, Lin CC, Zhou F, Germino GG. Fatty acid oxidation is impaired in an orthologous mouse model of autosomal dominant polycystic kidney disease. EBioMedicine. 2016;5:183–92.
184. Warner G, Hein KZ, Nin V, Edwards M, Chini CC, Hopp K, et al. Food restriction ameliorates the development of polycystic kidney disease. J Am Soc Nephrol. 2016;27(5):1437–47.
185. Kipp KR, Rezaei M, Lin L, Dewey EC, Weimbs T. A mild reduction of food intake slows disease progression in an orthologous mouse model of polycystic kidney disease. Am J Physiol Renal Physiol. 2016;310(8):F726–F31.
186. Shackelford DB, Shaw RJ. The LKB1-AMPK pathway: metabolism and growth control in tumour suppression. Nat Rev Cancer. 2009;9(8):563–75.
187. Gwinn DM, Shackelford DB, Egan DF, Mihaylova MM, Mery A, Vasquez DS, et al. AMPK phosphorylation of raptor mediates a metabolic checkpoint. Mol Cell. 2008;30(2):214–26.
188. Inoki K, Zhu T, Guan KL. TSC2 mediates cellular energy response to control cell growth and survival. Cell. 2003;115(5):577–90.
189. Takiar V, Nishio S, Seo-Mayer P, King JD Jr, Li H, Zhang L, et al. Activating AMP-activated protein kinase (AMPK) slows renal cystogenesis. Proc Natl Acad Sci U S A. 2011;108(6):2462–7.
190. King JD Jr, Fitch AC, Lee JK, McCane JE, Mak DO, Foskett JK, et al. AMP-activated protein kinase phosphorylation of the R domain inhibits PKA stimulation of CFTR. Am J Phys Cell Phys. 2009;297(1):C94–101.
191. Hallows KR, Raghuram V, Kemp BE, Witters LA, Foskett JK. Inhibition of cystic fibrosis transmembrane conductance regulator by novel interaction with the metabolic sensor AMP-activated protein kinase. J Clin Invest. 2000;105(12):1711–21.
192. Zhou X, Fan LX, Sweeney WE Jr, Denu JM, Avner ED, Li X. Sirtuin 1 inhibition delays cyst formation in autosomal-dominant polycystic kidney disease. J Clin Invest. 2013;123(7):3084–98.
193. Li X. SIRT1 and energy metabolism. Acta Biochim Biophys Sin Shanghai. 2013;45(1):51–60.

Cilia and Polycystic Kidney Disease

5

Dawn E. Landis, Scott J. Henke, and Bradley K. Yoder

Introduction

Many pathways involved in renal cyst development are regulated by the cilium, and most proteins linked to cystic kidney phenotypes either localize to cilia or disrupt ciliary assembly or function [1–3]. Diseases that are associated with the dysfunction of cilia are classified as *ciliopathies* [4, 5]. Although the phenotypes of different ciliopathies can vary dramatically, many of the ciliopathies present with a cystic kidney phenotype [4]. A prime example is found in polycystic kidney disease (PKD), one of the most common genetic causes of kidney failure in humans [6]. The three main proteins associated with PKD localize to the primary cilium, and mutation of these proteins results in defects in multiple signaling pathways [1, 3]. Thus, to develop effective therapeutic strategies, it is important that we understand the mechanisms involved in cilia formation and maintenance and the diverse roles they may have in the kidney. Many studies utilizing model systems that range from single-celled eukaryotes to humans have led to several hypotheses to explain how loss of cilia function might contribute to cystogenesis. This chapter will discuss these hypotheses in light of mechanisms of ciliogenesis and the proposed roles for the cilium in the kidney.

D. E. Landis, PhD · S. J. Henke, BA
B. K. Yoder, PhD (✉)
Department of Cell, Developmental and Integrative Biology, University of Alabama at Birmingham Medical School, Birmingham, AL, USA
e-mail: dawn.landis@nih.gov; byoder@uab.edu

Cilia

Cilia are microtubule-based organelles that extend from the surface of most cell types in the mammalian body [7]. Cilia can be classified into two broad groups: motile and primary (immotile) cilia (Fig. 5.1a). Motile cilia have roles in movement of cells and to generate fluid flow across various cell types, while primary cilia are critical in many sensory functions, such as smell and vision, and have been implicated as mechanosensors and in reception of several secreted ligands [8–11]. The involvement of cilia in human health was originally observed decades ago when defects in motile cilia were linked to a disease called primary ciliary dyskinesia (PCD, OMIM #, 244400) named for primary movement defects in motile cilia and not primary cilia [12, 13]. In contrast to this long history documenting the clinical significance of motile cilia, primary immotile forms of cilia were long thought to be vestigial. A dramatic shift in cilia research occurred in the late 1990s and early 2000s when mutations involved in cilia formation revealed that primary cilia are critical for proper development and tissue function [14–16].

B. D. Cowley, Jr., J. J. Bissler (eds.), *Polycystic Kidney Disease*,
https://doi.org/10.1007/978-1-4939-7784-0_5

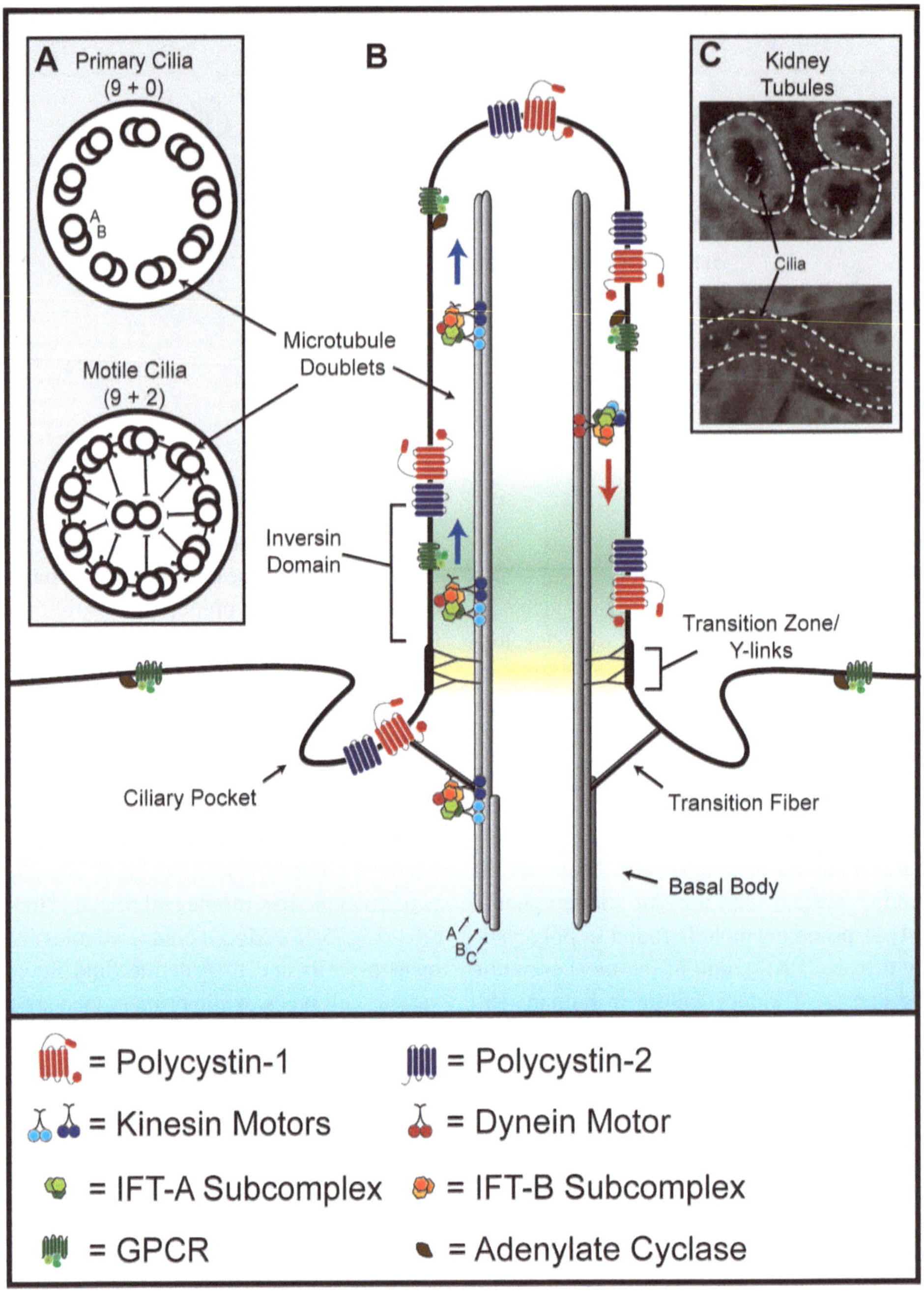

Fig. 5.1 Cilia structure, subdomains, and intraflagellar transport. (**a**) Cross sections of primary and motile cilia. Nine microtubule doublets are symmetrically distributed in the cilia axoneme. Motile cilia have an additional two microtubules which extend through the center of the axoneme, as well as a pair of inner dynein and outer dynein arms which connect with the neighboring microtubules to generate movement. (**b**) The cilium extends from the basal body which is composed of triplet (a, b, c) microtubules. Microtubule doublets (a and b) then form the core structure within the cilium and extend outward from the basal body at the cilium's base. The transition fibers, located just distal to the basal body, as well as the "Y-links" of the transition zone separate the cell's cytoplasm from that of the cilium. The intraflagellar transport (IFT) protein complex attaches to the transition fibers and is carried from the base of the cilium to its tip (anterograde movement, blue arrow) by kinesin motors and back again toward the base (retrograde movement, red arrow) by the dynein motor (Red arrow). Many receptors, signaling machinery, and channels, including polycystin-1 and polycystin-2 complex and GPCRs, are enriched in the ciliary compartment. (**c**) Cross and longitudinal sections, respectively, of kidney tubules showing cilia projecting from the tubule epithelial cells into the nephron lumen (tubules are outlined by white dotted lines)

Motile cilia are found on a few distinct cell types in mammals, and unlike solitary primary cilia, motile cilia are normally present on large numbers per cell. These types of motile cilia are found in the respiratory tracts, fallopian tubes, and the ependymal cells lining the ventricles in the brain. Motile cilia beat in a coordinated wave to move fluid across the epithelia. For example, cilia on the ependymal cells move cerebral spinal fluid through the ventricular system; cilia of the tracheal epithelium are used to move mucus and clear debris; and cilia of the fallopian tubes aid in the migration of the ova. As such, defects in the motility of these cilia as seen in PCD patients are associated with hydrocephalus, chronic respiratory infection, and infertility [17–19].

Interestingly, PCD patients also present with defects in left-right asymmetry, and some patients display a complete inversion of the internal organs called situs inversus [18, 20]. This situs defect is a clinical hallmark of a subset of PCD known as Kartagener's syndrome (OMIM# 242650) [18]. At the cellular level, situs inversus is due to the loss of nodal cilia function. Nodal cilia are another form of motile cilia located on an early developmental structure called the node [21]. The node acts as the organizer for gastrulation in mammals and is involved in specifying left-right body axis patterning [22]. Coordinated beating of nodal cilia creates extraembryonic fluid movement across the node's surface [23–25] that initiates increased Ca^{2+} signaling in the cells on the left side of the node [26]. This Ca^{2+} signal is dependent on polycystin-2 (PKD2), a ciliary localized calcium channel better known for its connection to renal cyst formation in PKD [27]. Mutations in Pkd2 in mice, zebrafish, and some human ADPKD patients with mutations with recessive hypomorphic mutations in PKD2 also result in situs inversus showing a link between situs defects observed in ciliopathies and cystic kidney patients [28–30].

Cilia Structure

The cilium membrane and its axonemal microtubules protrude from the cell surface and can be divided into multiple subdomains (Fig. 5.1b). At the base, anchoring the cilium to the cell cytoskeleton is the basal body from which the microtubule axoneme extends [31]. The basal body contains nine triplet microtubules (A, B, and C microtubule) arranged in a circle [31–34]. The basal body is docked to the cell membrane through transition fibers. Just distal to the transition fibers is the transition zone (TZ). The TZ along with the rest of the ciliary axoneme typically have nine pairs of microtubule doublets (A and B microtubules). The TZ is also defined by elaborate structures called "Y-links" that extend from the microtubule doublets at the junction between the A and B microtubule to the ciliary membrane. The Y-links are thought to connect to the membrane through the ciliary necklace, a protein aggregation of unknown composition located around the membrane at the level of the TZ [7, 35, 36]. The TZ subdomain can vary in length and structure depending on organism or even tissue. For example, the connecting cilium in the photoreceptor cells is an elongated TZ that is typically 500 nm compared to 200 nm for primary cilia of most mammalian cells [37]. Just distal to the TZ in the axoneme is another subdomain called the inversin compartment because of the localization of the protein inversin (Inv) to this region. When disrupted in mice, it causes renal cystic disease. Inv is required in renal development and left-right axis patterning. It is thought to inhibit the canonical Wnt pathway by targeting cytoplasmic disheveled (Dvl1) for degradation and may be required during renal development to oppose the repression of terminal differentiation of tubular epithelial cells caused by Wnt signaling. Inv is also involved in the organization of apical junctions in kidney cells. Electron microscopy studies indicate the inversin compartment is not structurally distinct from the rest of the cilium but is classified as a separate subdomain due to its unique protein composition [38, 39]. The functions of the transition zone, the ciliary necklace, transition fibers, and inversin compartments are still to be determined.

The cilia microtubule axoneme is the main extension of the cilia, and it is typically subdivided into the proximal and distal segment. The proximal segment is made up of nine doublet microtubules (A and B microtubules) arranged in a ring. A well-defined distal segment characterized by the presence of only single microtubules (A microtubule) is not typically present in most mammalian cells but is found in some organisms such as *C. elegans* (a nematode often used in cilia research) cilia as well as in mammalian olfactory cilia [31, 33, 40]. The functional significance of this singlet microtubule domain is not well known, but it is interesting in *C. elegans* that a specific microtubule motor protein (OSM3) is needed for transport along these microtubules [41]. The sub-compartmentalization of the cilia may provide specialization of the sensory and signaling activities of the cilium.

Regardless of whether it is a primary cilia or a motile cilia, both require a process called intraflagellar transport (IFT) for their assembly (Fig. 5.1b). IFT is the process by which structural subunits and other signaling and sensory machinery are actively transported bidirectionally (anterograde and retrograde) along the cilia axoneme by IFT proteins and their associated motor proteins [42]. IFT has been extensively analyzed in *Chlamydomonas* and *C. elegans* [42–47]. The motor proteins responsible for moving these particle trains include the heterotrimeric kinesin-2 motor that moves the IFT particle in the anterograde (base to tip) direction and the cytoplasmic dynein-2 motor involved in retrograde (tip to base) transport [43, 45]. In addition to their role in the cilium, several proteins involved in IFT have also been implicated in other functions such as trafficking proteins from the Golgi to the ciliary base, mitotic spindle function and genomic stability, and in immune synapse formation [48–53]. IFT proteins dock at the transition fibers at the base of the cilium and assemble into a large complex that travels along the cilium [54]. The IFT particle is comprised of two different molecular IFT sub-complexes, IFT-A and IFT-B [45, 46]. When proteins in complex B are mutated, anterograde movement of IFT is disrupted and cilia are not formed [55]. If complex A proteins are disrupted, retrograde movement is impaired and proteins accumulate in the distal portion of the axoneme, and cilia become stumpy and bulbous [56, 57]. Mutations affecting IFT proteins in mice are typically embryonic lethal, and those found in human patients are associated with severe *ciliopathies*. Interestingly, every IFT mutation identified in human patients thus far is hypomorphic, suggesting that the loss of IFT is not viable, similar to what was observed in IFT mutant mice [58, 59].

Ciliary Function

The protein composition of the primary cilia is unique from that of the rest of the cell even though the ciliary membrane and lumen is continuous with the cell's membrane. This distinct protein composition allows the primary cilium to function as a specialized signaling and sensory center. Examples of this specialization are the many G-protein-coupled receptors (GPCRs) such as somatostatin receptor 3 (SSTR3), serotonin receptor (5HT6), the olfactory receptors of olfactory sensory neurons, and rhodopsin in photoreceptors that localize to the cilium [60, 61]. In addition to GPCRs, there are many other types of signaling receptors and components enriched in the cilium, for instance, cyclic nucleotide gate channels (in the photoreceptors, olfactory neurons, and kidney collecting duct cells), adenylate cyclases 3 and 6, the polycystins, and hedgehog pathway components [62–74]. The importance of having these receptors and signaling machinery in the cilia for regulation of these pathways remains poorly defined.

There are several models that have been proposed for how the cilium may establish and maintain its unique complement of proteins. Some ciliary proteins have a ciliary targeting signal, although there appears to be no universal motif common to cilia proteins [61, 75]. Other studies have suggested a sequence similar to that found on proteins targeted to the nucleus [76]. Intriguingly, nuclear pore complex proteins have been localized to the base of the cilium and thus may function to regulate cilia entry [76–78]. While small proteins freely diffuse into the cilium, proteins larger than 9 nm are restricted from entering the cilium and require active transport for ciliary entry, similar to the mechanism of the nuclear pore complex [79]. Support for the active transport theory is established through experiments confirming the dependence of a kinesin motor involved in IFT (KIF17) ciliary localization on the gradient of the small GTPase (Ran) between the cilia and cytoplasm. Disrupting the Ran GTP/GDP gradient through expression of GTP-bound versions of Ran, which negatively affect association of importins (proteins involved in transported other proteins into the nucleus through binding to a specific recognition sequence) and their cargos, disrupts ciliary localization of KIF17 [76, 78, 80, 81]. Suggesting an alternate explanation to a nuclear pore complex at the base of the cilium are studies involving GFP monomers, dimers, and trimers expressed transgenically in frog rod cells. These data suggest that the differing ciliary permeability of these molecules is due to the steric hinderance from the outer segment disc membranes and due to active transport [82]. Another model proposes that cilia composition regulation may involve a selective protein retention mechanism that utilized PDZ protein domain-dependent interactions to retain certain proteins outside the cilium [83, 84]. Additionally, the structures found at the TZ may constitute a *ciliary* size diffusion barrier regulating what proteins are allowed access to the cilium or are retained within the cilium [36]. Using a chemically inducible diffusion trap at the base of the cilia, it was shown that proteins ranging in size from 3.2 to 7.9 nm were able to enter into the cilium, although their rate of entrance was inversely correlated with size, suggesting a molecular sieve at the base of the cilium [85]. Of further interest, multiple proteins involved in renal cystic disease syndromes, such as Nephronophthisis (NPHP) and Meckel-Gruber syndrome (MKS), localize to the TZ [36, 86–88]. Mutations in these NPHP and MKS proteins result in "leaky" cilia where nonciliary proteins are allowed access into the cilium and proteins that normally localized in the cilium fail to accumulate there. Most relevant to PKD is that polycystin-2 fails to be retained in the cilium of several of the transition zone mutants in mice [36, 89, 90].

The specialized nature of the cilium is thought to have an important role in allowing it to regulate numerous pathways. Several examples of pathways in which cilia have been implicated in regulating their activity are discussed further below and include mTOR, Wnt, PDGF, purinergic, Jak/STAT, and hedgehog (Hh).

Polycystic Kidney Disease

PKD is broadly classified as either autosomal recessive polycystic kidney disease (ARPKD) or autosomal dominant polycystic kidney disease (ADPKD). ADPKD is the more common form that typically begins showing symptoms in adulthood. In most cases the development of cystic kidneys in these patients results in eventual end-stage renal disease. Eighty-five percent of ADPKD are caused by mutations in PKD1, while the remaining 15% of cases are caused by mutations in PKD2 [6, 91]. Despite ADPKD being a dominantly inherited disease, it is recessive at the molecular level requiring a germline mutation and a subsequent somatic mutation or "second hit" in the second allele. Patients found with homozygous mutations in PKD1 develop a severe phenotype similar to ARPKD patients supporting the idea of a second hit mutation. This model is further supported by the clonal nature of the cells with the same second somatic mutation identified in epithelium within a single cyst [92, 93]. The "second hit" hypothesis helps explain the development of cysts later in life, variability of cyst formation with families, and the limited number of nephrons affected as these new mutations must be acquired over time. The factor that leads to cyst formation after loss of the second allele is not clear. In some studies it appears to be proliferation; however, in other studies, increased proliferation is a consequence of cyst formation and not a driving cause [94–96].

A second and less common form of the disease is autosomal recessive polycystic kidney disease (ARPKD). ARPKD is caused by mutations in PKHD1 [97]. This form of the disease is more severe as it develops earlier in life, frequently prenatally. Most neonates with ARPKD die shortly after birth of pulmonary hypoplasia. Of the patients that survive the neonatal period, 80% live past the age of 10 but develop end-stage renal disease by age 15 [98]. ARPKD patients also present with hepatic defects associated with ductal plate malformation and fibrosis. Although we've made substantial advances in care for ARPKD patients, the prognosis is poor and there is little treatment available aside from kidney transplantation [99].

Connections Between the Cilium and PKD

Although the connection between cilia and PKD is a recent discovery, Zimmerman first visualized primary cilia projecting from kidney epithelial cells and into the lumen of nephrons in 1898 [100] (Fig. 5.1c). An important advance connecting cilia dysfunction to PKD came from the development of the Oak Ridge Polycystic Kidney (ORPK) mouse. The ORPK mouse was generated in the lab of Dr. Richard Woychik during a large-scale transgene insertional mutagenesis project at the Oak Ridge National Laboratory [101]. In this particular case, a transgene inserted into an intron of the *Tg737* gene that was subsequently determined to encode the protein IFT88 [1, 16, 55]. This integration partially disrupted Ift88 expression and causes a hypomorphic mutation [102]. ORPK mice develop cysts in the kidney, liver, and pancreas, hydrocephalus, blindness, anosmia, polydactyly, cleft palate, and extra teeth, have scruffy fur with abnormal follicle formation, and are growth retarded. Scanning electron microscopy analysis of the kidney tubules of ORPK mice showed that the cilia were stunted and malformed [103]. The hypomorphic mutation in the ORPK mice was fortuitous in making the connection between cilia dysfunction, cyst development, and other ciliopathy phenotypes as a complete null allele of Ift88 was subsequently shown to cause body situs and neural tube defects that cause early embryonic lethality prior to kidney development [16, 102–104].

Another important breakthrough establishing the link between PKD and cilia was research done in *C. elegans* on the homologs of PKD1 (an interactor of PKD2 that is mutated in the majority of PKD patients) and PKD2 (the calcium channel mutated in the remaining cases of PKD). During a mutagenesis screen for male mating behavior defects, Barr et al. identified mutations in *lov-1* (the homolog of Pkd1) that resulted in the inability of males to sense and locate the hermaphrodite vulva (a cilia-dependent behavior) [105]. Lov-1 and Pkd-2 proteins were shown to localize to the cilia of the male-specific ciliated sensory neurons [3, 105, 106]. Subsequent studies then confirmed that mammalian PKD1 and PKD2 also localize to the primary cilium (as well as to several other sites in the cell) and that the loss of these proteins disrupts ciliary-related signaling while leaving the ciliary structure unaffected [2, 107].

Temporal Effects of Cilia Dysfunction and Cyst Progression

Studies using conditional cilia (IFT mutants), Pkd1, and Pkd2 mutant mouse lines have unexpectedly revealed that cilia dysfunction induced at different time points will cause dramatically different rates of cyst progression. In the case of Ift88 conditional mutants, cilia loss induced prior to p12 (juvenile-induced) causes cysts to form rapidly, within 3 weeks (Fig. 5.2). If cilia are lost after p12 (adult-induced mutants), cyst forms slowly and can take more than 6 months to form [108]. Similar results were obtained with the Pkd1 and Pkd2 mutant mouse lines [109–111]. These data raised the possibility that a proliferative environment, such as seen in the juvenile kidney, in combination with cilia dysfunction may be an important factor in determining the rate of cyst formation. Cell proliferation rates in the early postnatal kidney drop by around p14, coinciding with the time point where there is a switch from rapid to slow cyst progression [95]. An increase in proliferation rates in combination with changes in the orientation of cell division was raised as a possible mechanism that would lead to an increase in tubule diameter and eventual cyst formation (Fig. 5.3). This hypothesis is

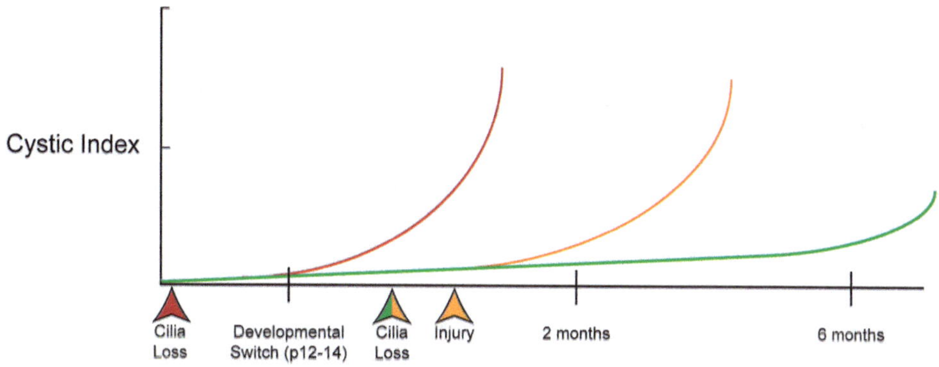

Fig. 5.2 Temporal effects of cilia loss on cyst progression. Disruption of cilia in the kidney prior to postnatal day 12 (p12) leads to rapid cyst development (red line) in mice. However, if cilia are disrupted after this period, the rate of cyst progression is protracted requiring months (green line) for cysts to develop. In adult-induced cilia mutants, rapid cyst formation similar to that observed in juvenile-induced cilia mice can be initiated by injury (orange line). (Red- and green-/orange-colored arrows indicate when cilia loss was induced for each paradigm. Orange arrow indicates timing of kidney injury)

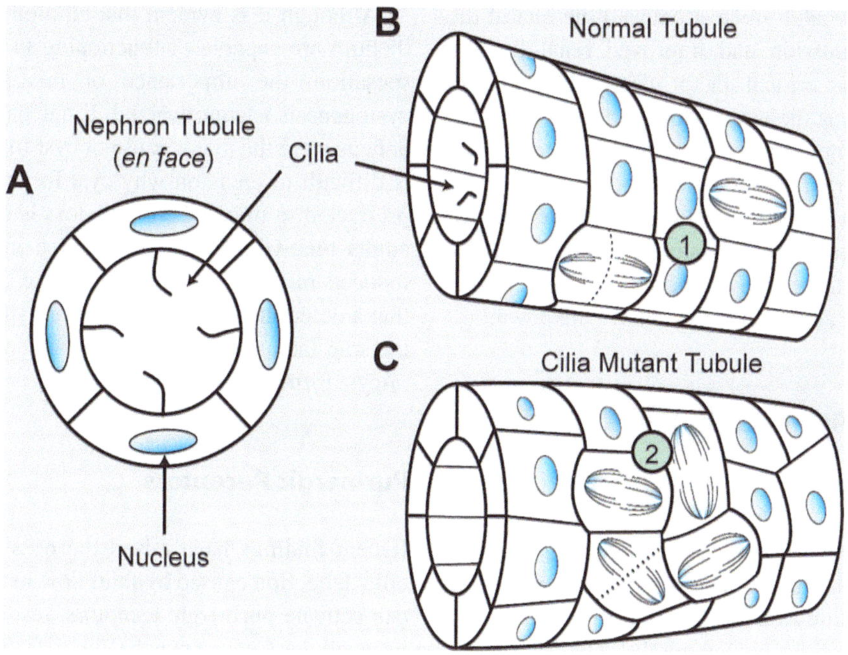

Fig. 5.3 Oriented cell division in the nephron. (**a**) Schematic of a nephron tubule depicting cilia on the apical side of the cells pointing toward the tubule's lumen. (**b**) A schematic of a tubule showing normal orientation of cell divisions with the mitotic spindles positioned parallel to the tubule's axis. This process contributes an increase in tubule length. (**c**) In PCP and cilia mutant tubules, the orientation of cell division is random (2) and does not contribute to elongation of the nephron. As such, disorganized cell divisions may cause spherical growth of the tubule that contributes an increase in tubule diameter and cyst development

supported by the rapid cyst development that occurs in adult-induced cilia mutant mice after ischemic reperfusion (IR). IR injury causes increased proliferation rates in the tubule epithelium similar to the proliferation rates in the juvenile-induced cilia mutants [112]. The rapid rate of cystogenesis that occurs in adults after IR injury could however be caused by other factors than proliferation, such as inflammation and cellular dedifferentiation, and reinitiation of developmental pathways. The direct connection between cilia loss, proliferation, and the rate of cyst initiation is uncertain as data showing that genetically maintaining high proliferation rates, at least in the proximal tubules of the kidney of adult-induced cilia mutants, was not sufficient to exacerbate the rate of cyst formation [96]. Thus, the cause for the divergent rates of cyst formation that occurs in the juvenile-induced versus adult-induced cilia and polycystin mutants is not yet known.

Another recent intriguing finding reported by Ma et al. was that in polycystin conditional mutants, the subsequent deletion of cilia in either juvenile or adult mice attenuated the rate of disease progression and improved renal function [113]. The critical factor determining disease severity was the amount of time the polycystins were absent prior to the involution of the cilium. These data led the authors to propose a polycystin-dependent inhibition and cilia-dependent activation of a rapid cyst-promoting signal [113]. The nature of these signals and interactions between the cilium and the polycystins are unknown.

Cilia Regulating Signaling and PKD

Cilia and Mechanosensation

Cilia extend off most epithelial cells of the nephron into the lumen leading to a model wherein cilia function as a mechanosensor to detect fluid flow through the kidney tubules. The first suggestion that cilia could be involved in mechanosensation was experiments showing that deflection of cilia on MDCK cells caused an increase in intercellular Ca^{2+} (Fig. 5.4) [114–116]. Importantly, the flow-induced Ca^{2+} response fails to occur in cells lacking the polycystin proteins or the cilium [115, 117, 118]. Similar mechanosensory roles for the cilium have been proposed on the early embryonic node, endothelium of blood vessels, and epithelium of the biliary and pancreatic ducts. During mammalian development, the embryonic node uses motile cilia to generate flow toward the left side of the embryo that also establishes a Ca^{2+} signal. This flow and the ability of cilia to sense it through Pkd2 are necessary for establishing the left-right axis [28, 119]. Cilia loss in murine biliary and pancreatic ductile epithelium leads to pancreatic cysts possibly through a similar mechanism as in the kidney [120].

In cultures of renal epithelium, flow-induced deflection of the cilium also prevents the proteolytic cleavage of the C-terminal tail of PC-1 (the protein product of the PKD1) by PC-2 (the protein product of PKD2) [121]. The C-terminal tail of PC-1 is critical for the complex interaction between Pkd1 and Pkd2 as well as multiple other proteins [122, 123].

Although it is evident that cilia on renal epithelium are capable of functioning in mechanosensation, the importance of this signal for cystogenesis is controversial. If mechanosensory defects were the major cause of cyst formation, it is difficult to envision why cyst formation is so protracted in mice where cilia loss is induced in adults relative to what is observed in juvenile-induced mice [95, 108, 110]. These data argue that a defect in the mechanosensory signal is not the sole factor determining the rate and severity of cyst formation and progression.

Purinergic Receptors

Recent findings have raised the possibility that cilia deflection caused by fluid flow in the kidney can activate purinergic receptors, resulting in an intracellular Ca^{+2} response (Fig. 5.4). Supporting this theory, the purinergic-dependent intracellular Ca^{+2} signal induced by flow was blocked using the P2YR pan inhibitor, suramin. Similarly, the response to flow is reduced in mouse mutants lacking the P2Y2 receptor, indicating this receptor as a likely candidate in the response even though these mice do not develop cysts [124, 125]. Recent data also suggests that fluid flow sensed through cilia and purinergic pathway activation stimulates clathrin- and dynamin-dependent

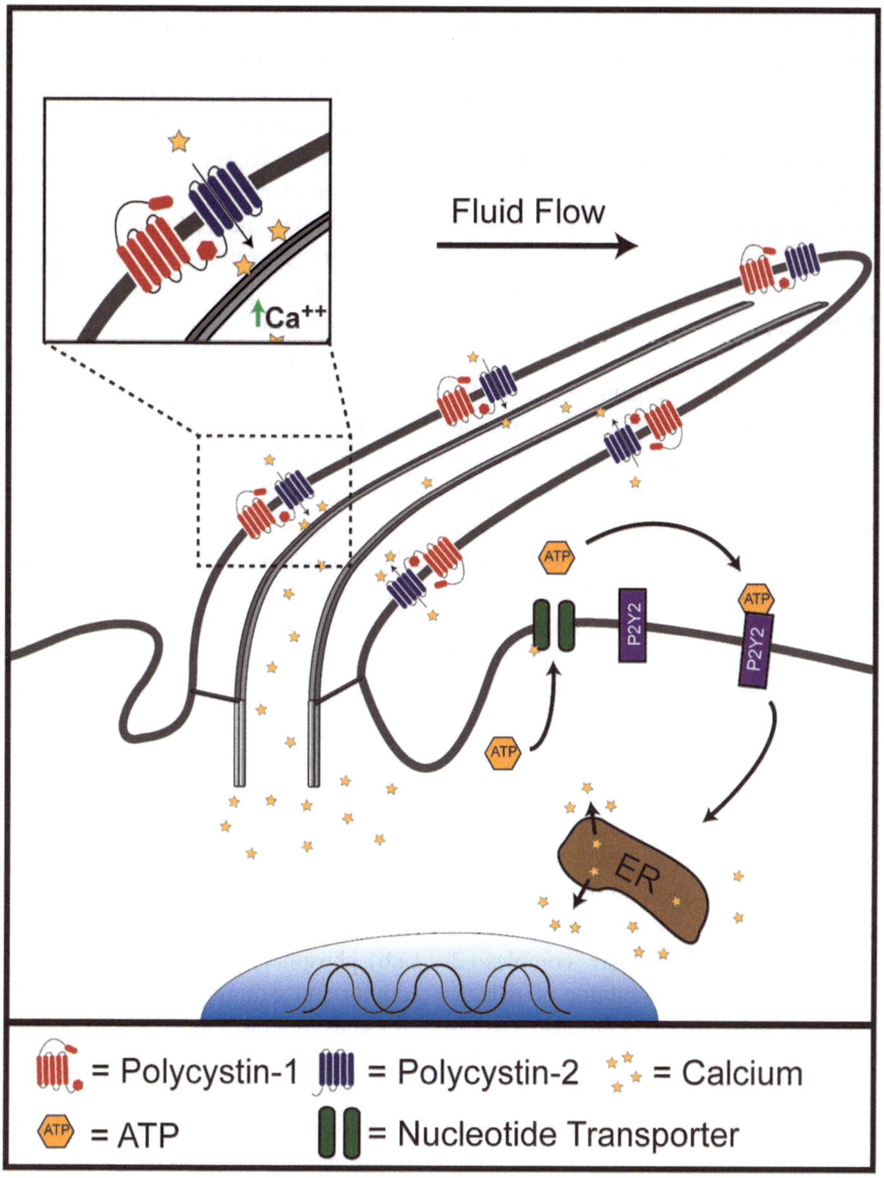

Fig. 5.4 Purinergic signaling and the cilium. Fluid flowing across the cell causes the cilium to bend and allows calcium to enter the cilium involving the polycystin-2 channel (inset). The ciliary calcium activates nucleotide transporters which release ATP into the extracellular environment. ATP then signals back onto the purinergic receptor (P2Y2) to signal the release of calcium from the endoplasmic reticulum

apical endocytosis in the proximal tubules [126]. Increasing apical endocytosis could aid in the retrieval of filtered proteins in the proximal tubule. This action is important in aiding the kidney in controlling resorption rates and fractional solute resorption across a wide range of glomerular filtration rates.

Control of ATP and Ca^{+2} levels through purinergic signaling is critical for regulating electrolyte and water transport in the nephron [127]. ATP inhibits ion transport from proximal to distal tubules causing a diuretic response. It has been shown that using antagonists to the purinergic receptor P2X7 in zebrafish morpholinos of PKD2 improves cystic phenotypes [128]. These antagonists reduce glomerular cysts and reduce pERK activity and cell proliferation. This suggests that purinergic receptor signaling through cilia may function to modulate the kidney's ability to absorb filtrate and could be a contributing factor in disease progression.

mTOR Pathway

The mammalian target of rapamycin (mTOR) signaling pathway allows a cell to incorporate environmental cues to regulate cell metabolism and growth, protein translation, autophagy, proliferation, and survival. mTOR acts as a serine/threonine phosphatidylinositol kinase-related kinase that is regulated by many different factors such as insulin, growth factors, amino acids, oxygen, and energy levels. The mTOR pathway has been implicated in many diseases such as cancer, obesity, neurodegeneration, and type 2 diabetes, and the pathway is markedly upregulated in cystic renal epithelium [129–131]. Mechanistic in vitro studies indicate that polycystin-1 regulates the mTOR pathway through its C-terminal tail that is proteolytically cleaved and released into the cytosol. This regulation also involves tuberous sclerosis complex 2 (TSC2) [132]. TSC2 is an inhibitor of mTOR activity, and mutations in TSC2 are also associated with cystic kidney pathology [133]. TSC2 is phosphorylated by AKT retaining it at the cell membrane where it regulates mTOR. The uncleaved membrane-bound C-terminal tail of PKD1 interacts with TSC2 and prevents its phosphorylation by AKT (Fig. 5.5). In the absence of phosphorylation, TSC2 is partitioned into the cytosol where it will no longer inhibit mTOR [132]. Thus, through TSC2, PKD1 can regulate mTOR activity. Importantly, nonfunctional humanized versions of PKD1 expressed in cell culture preventing its C-terminal tail from associating with TSC2 impair the inhibition of the mTOR pathway [132]. Disruption of this interaction through mutations in Pkd1 could be involved in cyst progression in some PKD patients.

Studies involving unilateral nephrectomy also support the hypothesis that cystic kidney formation could involve aberrant mTOR signaling through the cilium [134]. Mice with induced cilia loss that underwent unilateral nephrectomy showed an increase in cyst severity. When wild-type and adult-induced cilia mutants underwent unilateral nephrectomy, the cilia mutants showed significantly higher levels of mTOR in the remaining kidney compared to controls. This resulted in renal hypertrophy and rapid cyst formation in the cilia mutants [134].

mTor pathway activity may also be regulated through mechanosensation signals. In vitro assays demonstrated that cilia-mediated detection of the flow regulated cell size in part by inhibiting the mTOR pathway. In contrast to ciliated cells, when cilia mutant cells were cultured in the presence of flow, the cells did not adjust cell volume and were significantly larger than the ciliated control cells. The abnormal cell size phenotype was reversed by inhibitors of the mTOR pathway, confirming this was an mTOR-mediated phenotype. Unexpectedly this was not regulated by PKD1 or PKD2 but was mediated through Lkb1. Lkb1 is a kinase that also localizes to the cilium and is an inhibitor of the mTOR pathway through AMP-activated protein kinase (AMPK). Lkb1 phosphorylates AMPK that inhibits mTOR activity and is upregulated as a consequence of cilia sensing flow under normal conditions [135]. Since cilia on the cells of the kidney tubules in PKD patients may be unable to respond to flow, Lkb1 would also be deregulated leading to altered mTOR pathway activity.

Studies using mTOR inhibitors sirolimus (formerly rapamycin) and everolimus cause a reduction in cyst size and kidney volume in several mouse models [136, 137]. In human PKD trials, sirolimus was less efficacious in part due to the low dosage that was tolerable by humans without severe side effects [138]. In an attempt to circumvent this problem, trials with a folate-conjugated rapamycin, which is taken up through folate receptor-dependent endocytosis, directly targeting the drug to the kidney, and requires lower concentrations, strongly attenuated proliferation, growth of renal cysts, and preserved renal

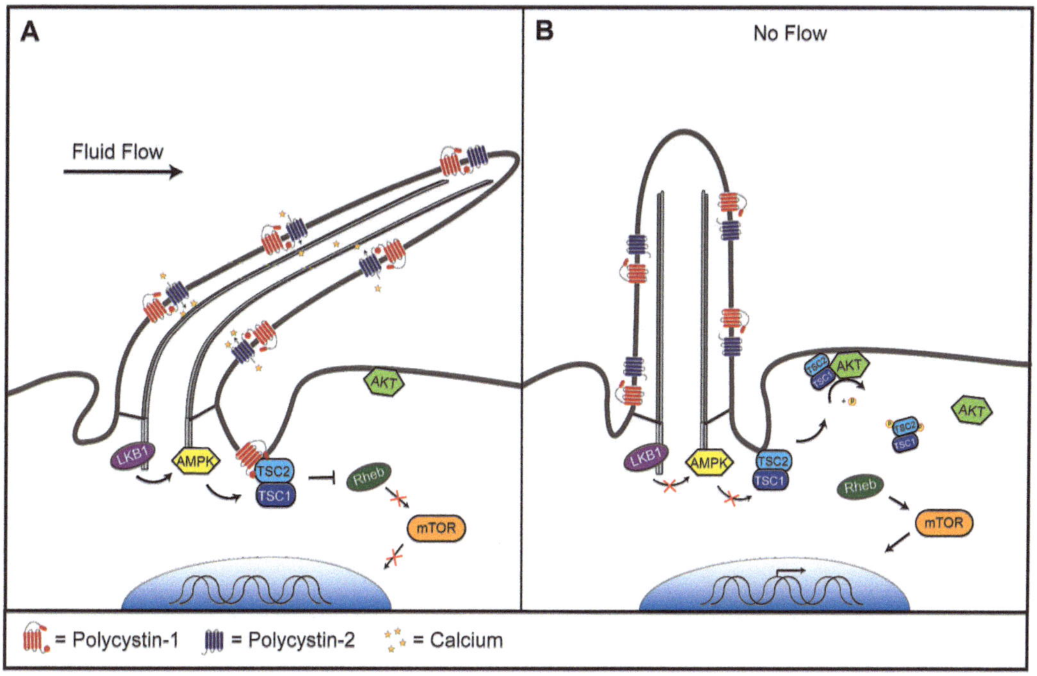

Fig. 5.5 Flow modulates polycystin-1 regulation of mTOR signaling. (**a**) LKB1 and AMPK localize to the base of the cilium. In the presence of flow, LKB1 phosphorylates and activates AMPK. AMPK subsequently activates TSC2 and downregulates the mTOR pathway. TSC2/polycystin-1 interaction prevents AKT from phosphorylating and deactivating TSC2 – further down regulating mTOR. (**b**) In the absence of flow, LKB1 does not activate AMPK, and the C-terminal tail of polycystin-1 is unavailable to prevent AKT from inactivating TSC2. Thus, Rheb is free to stimulate mTOR and activate the mTOR pathway

function in mouse models [139]. As renal cyst cells highly express folate receptors, this conjugated rapamycin inhibited mTOR activity in the kidney without affecting other organs. This study suggests using mTOR inhibitors that specifically target cystic cells may be useful means to treat PKD patients.

Jak/STAT Signaling and Immune Response

The Jak/STAT pathway is important for development and homeostasis in mammals. It is one of the main pathways that receive signals from cytokines and growth factors to alter transcription and affect many different cellular activities such as inflammation, cell proliferation, cell migration, differentiation, and apoptosis. Jak/STAT activation is critical for immune cell development and inflammation, hematopoiesis, mammary gland development, kidney development, stem cell maintenance, and organismal growth [140]. The Jak/STAT pathway is activated during kidney development for proper tubulogenesis, but down-regulated in adult kidneys (Fig. 5.6a). Deregulation of this pathway has been implicated in cancer, immune deficiency, and myeloproliferative disorders, and it is markedly upregulated in renal cystic epithelium [141].

PKD1 is able to regulate the Jak/STAT pathway through multiple mechanisms. One of the first links between the Jak/STAT pathway and PKD was that overexpression of PC-1 led to increased PC-2-dependent activation of STAT1 through phosphorylation of Ser727 and Tyr701 residues [142]. Additionally, the reverse was proven when PKD1 mutant mouse embryos were shown to have lower levels of activated STAT1. The C-terminal region of PC-1 can bind directly to JAK2 suggesting that STAT1 activation might be controlled by PC-1 through JAK2

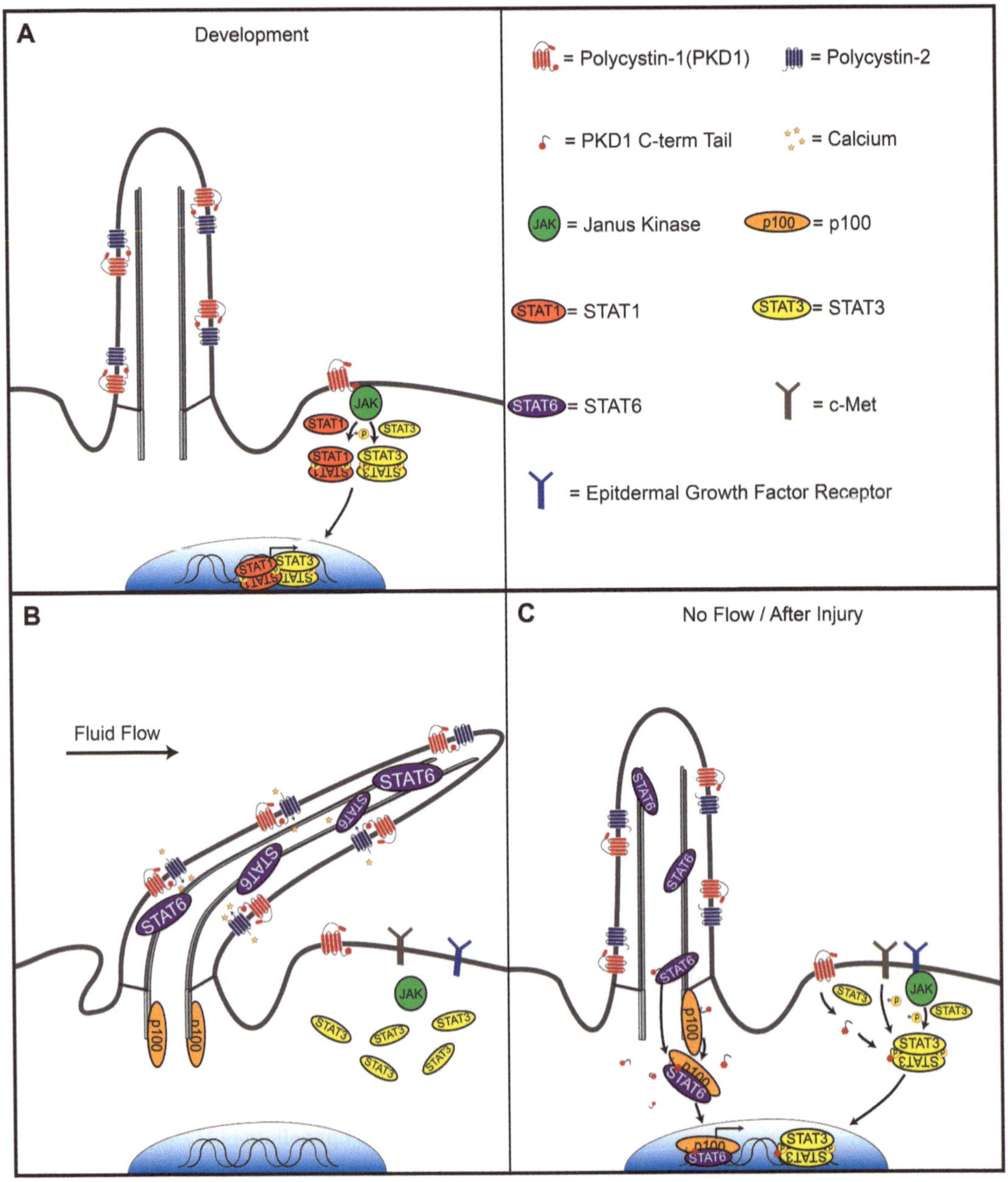

Fig. 5.6 Polycystin-1 is a regulator of Jak/STAT signaling. (**a**) During development JAK2 binds polycystin-1's C-terminal tail to phosphorylate STAT1 and STAT3. This activates STAT1 and STAT3 and causes them to travel to the nucleus. (**b**) Kidney epithelial cells in normal conditions have inactive STAT3 and STAT6 present. (**c**) Upon tubule injury, cytokines activate STAT3 and STAT6. After phosphorylation, STAT3 and STAT6 bind to the cleaved polycystin-1 tail and translocate to the nucleus

(Fig. 5.6a) [143]. Studies have also shown that STAT3 can also be regulated by PC-1 through two different mechanisms [144]. Membrane-bound PC-1 can activate STAT3 in a JAK2-dependent mechanism similar to STAT1. Further, the proteolytically cleaved C-terminal tail of PC-1 also functions as a coactivator of STAT1, STAT3, and STAT6 in response to cytokine signaling [144]. Finally, STAT6 and p100, another STAT coactivator, localize to cilia and the basal body, respectively, and in the absence of flow STAT6 and p100 translocate to the nucleus along with the C-terminal tail product of PC-1 to regulate downstream targets (Fig. 5.6c) [145]. Regulation of the Jak/STAT pathway has shown promise in controlling cystic kidney disease progression. Inhibition of STAT signaling genetically or through pharmacological approaches decreased cyst size and kidney volume and maintained better renal function [146].

Inflammatory Responses and Cystic Kidney Disease

Research has shown that an inflammatory response, which has strong ties to the Jak/STAT pathway and mTOR activity, can influence severity of cyst development and fibrosis in PKD and that this could be mediated through a cilia-dependent mechanism [91, 147, 148]. Cystic epithelial cells secrete macrophage chemoattractants such as MCP-1 (Ccl2) and Cxcl16 [149]. In fact, one of the best urinary biomarkers associated with cystic disease progression is MCP-1, as increased levels of this protein in urine have a negative correlation with cyst progression and future renal function decline [150]. These chemokines induce recruitment of myeloid cells including monocytes and neutrophils into the kidney similar to what occurs after renal injury. Once in the kidney, the monocytes normally become polarized into an M1 (proinflammatory) and M2 (anti-inflammatory/pro-fibrotic) fate. Interestingly, in the cystic kidney, there is a marked increase in the number of M2 macrophages [98]. This polarization change may occur in response to cytokine signals from the epithelium that are regulated by Stat3 and Stat6, expression of which could be controlled through cilia/polycystin function. In vitro experiments with cytokines expressed downstream of STAT3 and STAT6 show that renal epithelial cells from cysts will promote naïve monocyte differentiation toward an M2 fate and that these M2 macrophages subsequently increase proliferation in the epithelium of tubules [151]. Importantly, when macrophages are depleted from the cystic mouse models, the cystic phenotype is reduced and renal function is improved [98]. These experiments have increased interest in the area of the innate immune responses in the context of cyst development and progression. A current hypothesis is that cilia-mediated signals regulate resolution of an inflammatory or injury response. The slow and more focal nature of the cysts that form in the adult-induced cilia mutants may result in nephrons that have received an injury that occurs as part of normal renal function. In the absence of the cilium, this injury response is inappropriately regulated leading to excess proliferation and cyst formation.

Canonical WNT Signaling and Planar Cell Polarity

The planar cell polarity pathway (PCP) is a critical pathway regulating how cells orient in an appropriate direction and position within tissues. A classic example in mammalian development is the position of the stereocilia in the inner ear [152]. PCP is also important for proper orientation of cells undergoing division and for migration events such as convergent extension during gastrulation and has been implicated in tubulogenesis during renal development [153–155]. PCP involves the Wnt pathway, but in a β-catenin-independent manner, and as such is often referred to as one of the noncanonical Wnt pathways. Attenuation of noncanonical Wnt9b expression in mouse results in decreased tubule diameter size establishment and maintenance [156]. The PCP pathway regulates the cytoskeleton to orient the cell correctly. This is done through repositioning of the centrioles to the apical side of the cell and asymmetrically distributing polar proteins, such as Vangl, Van Gogh, Frizzled, and Flamingo through Rho-kinase family cascades [157, 158]. The activation of PCP in the kidney is regulated by the interaction of disheveled (Dvl) and inversin (Inv/NPHP2). The binding of a noncanonical ligand and flow will induce elevated levels of inversin which targets Dvl to the basal

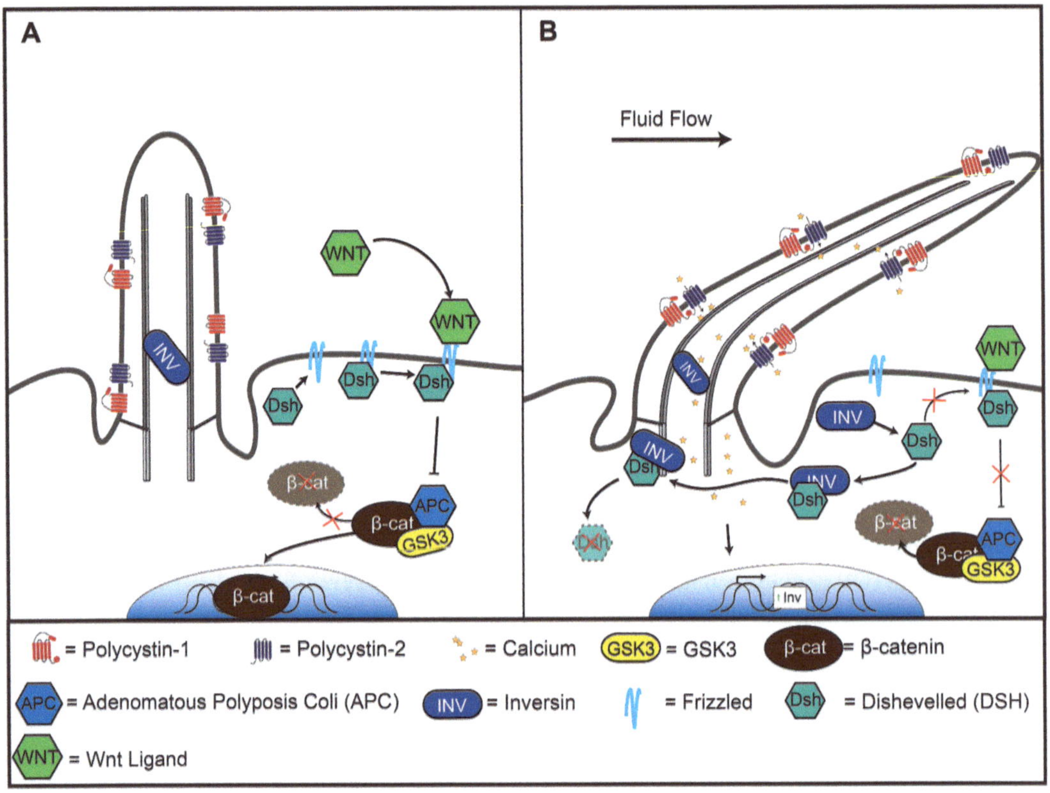

Fig. 5.7 Fluid flow shifts Wnt signaling from the canonical pathway to the noncanonical, PCP, pathway. (**a**) Low beta-catenin levels are maintained in the cell by the APC complex and GSK3 actively marking the β-catenin for degradation. However, when Wnt ligands bind the Frizzled receptor, disheveled is recruited to Frizzled and inhibits the APC complex and GSK3 from initiating the degradation of β-catenin. β-Catenin levels are therefore able to rise and enter the nucleus to regulate transcription. (**b**) Deflection of the cilia by flow induces an intracellular rise in calcium and leads to an increase in the transcription rate of inversin. When inversin levels are elevated, inversin is able to recruit free cytosolic disheveled to the basal body where it is marked for degradation. This lowers the amount of disheveled available to be recruited to Frizzled upon Wnt binding and diminishes the cell's response to Wnt ligands

body. This results in a modification of Dvl that causes degradation of cytosolic Dvl and the downregulation of the canonical Wnt pathway (Fig. 5.7). The downregulation of the canonical Wnt pathway allows an increased amount of activity in PCP.

Some of the PCP proteins, such as Vangl2, are critical for the proper apical localization of the primary cilium [159]. Mutations in several different ciliary proteins in zebrafish or mice result in phenotypes typical of those observed when the PCP pathway is disrupted [21, 160–162]. However, in some cases, such as those in the inner ear, the defects have been shown to be independent of the PCP proteins, as PCP proteins organize properly even though the cochlear stereociliary bundles are disorganized [163]. One hypothesis is that cilia are important for controlling the strength of the polarizing cues generated by noncanonical Wnt signaling as cilia mutants in some studies and kidneys of PKD patients were shown to have an increased level of sRFP4 (a protein that blocks Wnt from binding to Frizzled receptors) which results in blocking of some canonical Wnt components [164].

PCP is an essential pathway in the developing kidney, regulating cell migration and cell division [154]. Disruption of Wnt signaling in the developing kidney can cause severe malformation of the nephrons which is thought to contribute to cyst formation [156]. In mouse and rat nephrons, the mitotic spindle is typically oriented parallel to the nephron lumen allowing cell division to extend the tubule lengthwise instead of increasing its diameter (Fig. 5.3). In cystic animals this mitotic spindle orientation becomes random [165]. While divisions parallel to the kidney lumen would cause lengthening of the nephron, division perpendicular to this axis would result in expansion of the tubule. Thus cells dividing in a random orientation could result in the development of expanded tubules that ultimately develop into cysts. Some theories have merged the mechanosensation and PCP theories to suggest that the sensing of flow through the cilia is critical for the proper orientation of the mitotic spindles. Cilia mutants would be unable to properly sense the flow causing mitotic spindles to be misoriented and result in cyst formation. Some PCP mouse mutant models, such as FAT4 mutants, are known to develop kidney cysts [166, 167]. Despite many studies supporting a role for cilia and PCP in kidney cyst development, there are also several studies that raise concerns with this model. Mouse studies involving BBS7 mutant mice indicate that cilia may not be important for PCP [168]. Zebrafish morpholinos of BBS7 and Prickle2 suggest that loss of recruitment of some PCP proteins such as Prickle2 to the actin cytoskeleton is not dependent on BBS7, despite overlapping phenotypes in the knockdowns indicating PCP is independent of BBS [168]. IFT88 mutant zebrafish studies showed PCP was ciliary independent as cilia were not required to establish PCP in these mutants [163]. Also, mice with mutations in Pkhd1 have the misaligned mitotic spindles, but yet do not develop kidney cysts [169]. Thus, the importance of PCP and oriented cell divisions in the development of the cystic kidney phenotype and how cilia may regulate these processes are still being assessed.

Hedgehog Signaling and Cyst Formation

The hedgehog (Hh) pathway is arguably the most conclusively connected to the cilium. The receptor for Hh, Patched 1 (Ptch1), is localized to the cilia when the pathway is not active (Fig. 5.8a). When Hh binds Patched 1 (Ptch1), Ptch1 leaves the cilia, preventing it from repressing the entry or accumulation of Smoothened (Smo) into the cilium (Fig. 5.8b). Once Smo enters the cilium, it results in the conversion of transcription factors (Gli1/Gli2) into activators and prevents proteolytic processing of Gli3 into the repressor form. These transcription factors then translocate to the nucleus to activate Hh-responsive genes. The formation of the Gli activators and repressor does not occur properly in cilia mutants leading to dysregulation of the pathway [71]. Experiments to disrupt Hh signaling in mice cause severe defects in kidney development that include hydronephrosis, fewer nephrons, inhibited ureteric branching, and less glomeruli [155, 170–174]. It has also been shown that patients with Smith-Lemli-Opitz syndrome, which is thought to disrupt Hh signaling by affecting cholesterol biosynthesis, develop cystic kidneys [175]. Genetically deleting Gli2 in kidney explants from Thm1 (IFT139) mutants that have retrograde IFT defects and show elevated Hh pathway activity was able to decrease cyst severity [176]. This suggests that the overactivation of the Hh pathway in the Thm1 mutant mice is contributing to the cyst growth; however, it is intriguing that mutations in anterograde IFT proteins, such as IFT88, also develop cysts yet have a repressed Hh pathway. Thus, the level of Hh signaling may need to be tightly controlled with too much or too little pathway activity contributing to cyst formation. The Hh pathway is also important in regulating renal injury and repair processes [177, 178]. Thus, the increased cyst formation that occurs after injury may be related to defects in proper regulation of the Hh signal when cilia are not present. Although hedgehog has been linked to renal abnormalities and cilia are essential for normal Hh pathway regulation, defects in Hh

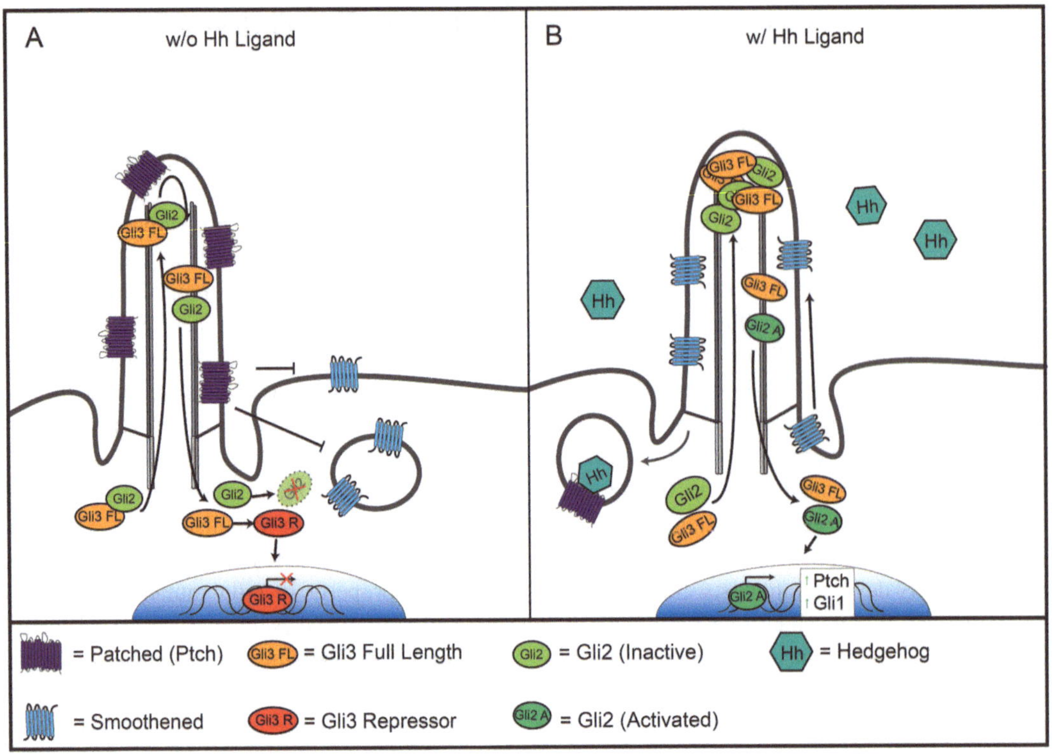

Fig. 5.8 Cilia and hedgehog signaling in developed kidneys. (**a**) In normal adult kidneys, the hedgehog (Hh) pathway is inactive. Without Hh binding to its receptor Patched, Smoothened, Gli2, and Gli3 do not accumulate in the cilium. Gli3 is processed into Gli3 repressor (Gli3R) and Gli2 is degraded. (**b**) During development and after injury, the hedgehog pathway is activated. Hedgehog ligand binds to Patched causing Patched to become internalized. Smoothened begins to accumulate in the cilium resulting in the activation of Gli2 and preventing the processing of Gli3 to its repressor form. The activated Gli transcription factors then enter the nucleus to induce expression of Patched and Gli1 and other Hh target genes

activity have not yet been directly linked to cyst formation in humans.

Cilia and Regulation of Water Reabsorption

Vasopressin signaling is one of the primary mechanisms for the human body to control water homeostasis. Vasopressin is a hormone produced in the hypothalamus and stored in the pituitary. It is released in response to dehydration or decreased blood volume. Vasopressin signaling causes vasoconstriction and triggers the retention of water in an attempt to correct these conditions. The increase of water retention by vasopressin signaling mostly occurs in the kidney tubules by increasing the water permeability of the collecting duct and distal tubule. The receptor for vasopressin (V2R) localizes to the basolateral membrane and in one report was detected in the cilium of renal tubule epithelium [179]. In the presence of vasopressin, V2R begins a signaling cascade that results in increased cAMP levels. This activates protein kinase A (PKA) that phosphorylates the water channel aquaporin 2 (AQP2) in the collecting duct of the kidney tubules [180]. This causes AQP2 to translocate to the apical cell surface increasing absorption of water from the renal filtrate (Fig. 5.9a). Cell culture from cilia mutant mice has shown that loss of cilia results in mislocalization of V2R from the basolateral membrane and an increase of AQP2 in the apical membrane [181] (Fig. 5.9b).

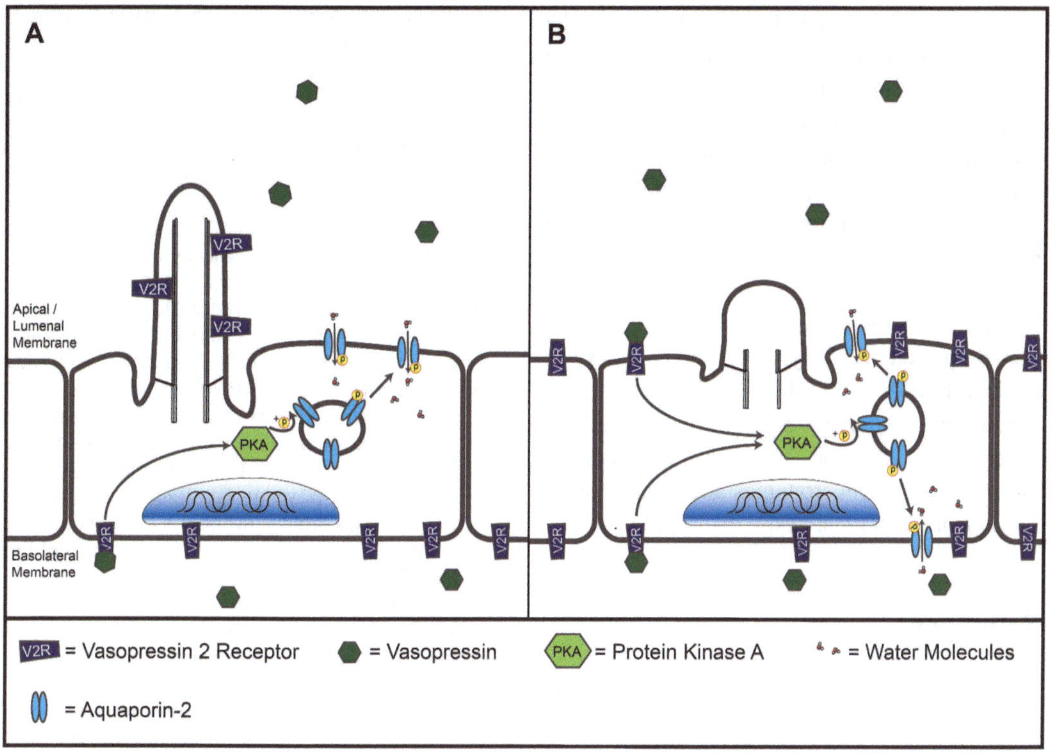

Fig. 5.9 The loss of cilia disrupts vasopressin localization and signaling. (**a**) Vasopressin 2 receptor (V2R) localizes to the basolateral membrane as well as to the cilium. Under normal conditions, only the V2Rs located on the basolateral membrane bind vasopressin and activate the pathway. V2R activation leads to increased cAMP which activates protein kinase A (PKA). PKA then phosphorylates aquaporin 2, which activates the channel and causes it to be transported to the apical membrane increasing water reabsorption. (**b**) When cilia are mutated or missing, V2Rs are no longer restricted to the cilium and can be found throughout the apical membrane and basolateral membranes. Interestingly, in these mutants apical and basolateral V2Rs can be activated by vasopressin and stimulate aquaporin 2 incorporation into either membrane

This mislocalization may interfere with the function of the pathway.

The connections of the vasopressin pathway in kidney functions and cystic diseases have been studied in depth. Patients with PKD as well as nearly all of the mouse cystic kidney disease models have increased levels of intracellular cAMP and difficulty concentrating urine [182–185]. Mouse studies using V2R antagonists to treat cystic kidneys have shown promise as they have reduced intracellular cAMP levels and attenuation of cyst progression [186]. A phase III clinical trial investigating the effect of the V2R antagonist tolvaptan in ADPKD patients has shown that this treatment blunts kidney growth, reduces associated symptoms, and slows kidney function decline when given over 3 years, but also caused aquaresis and adverse hepatic effects leading to a high discontinuation rate [187, 188]. Recent studies have shown that therapies that combine tolvaptan with other drugs such as rapamycin, AEZ-13, and pasireotide may be efficacious in treating cyst formation [189, 190].

Conclusion

The long understudied organelle, the primary cilium, is now the focus of intense research to dissect its diverse functions as a coordinator of multiple signaling pathways. There have been substantial advances made in the field especially the work showing a direct link between cilia dysfunction and cystic kidney disorders. However, the cilium's role in the kidney as a purely mechanosensor appears to have been an oversimplification. Current research has shown that the connection between cilia and PKD is complicated and probably involves multiple intertwined pathways. Future research will elucidate the precise roles for the cilium in these signaling pathways and their subsequent contributions to disease. Unfortunately, there are currently no curative treatments beyond kidney transplantation or prolonged dialysis for PKD. However, clinical trials based on the cilia-PKD connection are currently underway. Some of these treatments have provided hope that we will develop improved treatment strategies and quality of life for patients with renal cystic disorders.

References

1. Haycraft CJ, Swoboda P, Taulman PD, Thomas JH, Yoder BK. The C. elegans homolog of the murine cystic kidney disease gene Tg737 functions in a ciliogenic pathway and is disrupted in osm-5 mutant worms. Development. 2001;128(9):1493–505.
2. Yoder BK, Hou X, Guay-Woodford LM. The polycystic kidney disease proteins, polycystin-1, polycystin-2, polaris, and cystin, are co-localized in renal cilia. J Am Soc Nephrol: JASN. 2002;13(10):2508–16.
3. Qin H, Rosenbaum JL, Barr MM. An autosomal recessive polycystic kidney disease gene homolog is involved in intraflagellar transport in C. elegans ciliated sensory neurons. Curr Biol: CB. 2001;11. England:457–61.
4. Hildebrandt F, Benzing T, Katsanis N. Ciliopathies. N Engl J Med. 2011;364(16):1533–43.
5. Waters AM, Beales PL. Ciliopathies: an expanding disease spectrum. Pediatr Nephrol. 2011;26(7):1039–56.
6. Takiar V, Caplan MJ. Polycystic kidney disease: pathogenesis and potential therapies. Biochim Biophys Acta. 2011;1812. Netherlands: 2010 Elsevier B.V:1337–43.
7. Fisch C, Dupuis-Williams P. Ultrastructure of cilia and flagella – back to the future! Biol Cell. 2011;103. England:249–70.
8. Singla V, Reiter JF. The primary cilium as the cell's antenna: signaling at a sensory organelle. Science. 2006;313:629–33.
9. Mukhopadhyay S, Rohatgi R. G-protein-coupled receptors, hedgehog signaling and primary cilia. Semin Cell Dev Biol. 2014;33:63–72.
10. Berbari NF, O'Connor AK, Haycraft CJ, Yoder BK. The primary cilium as a complex signaling center. Curr Biol: CB. 2009;19. England:R526–35.
11. Pazour GJ, Witman GB. The vertebrate primary cilium is a sensory organelle. Curr Opin Cell Biol. 2003;15(1):105–10.
12. Rossman CM, Lee RM, Forrest JB, Newhouse MT. Nasal cilia in normal man, primary ciliary dyskinesia and other respiratory diseases: analysis of motility and ultrastructure. Eur J Respir Dis Suppl. 1983;127:64–70.
13. Escudier E, Duquesnoy P, Papon JF, Amselem S. Ciliary defects and genetics of primary ciliary dyskinesia. Paediatr Respir Rev. 2009;10(2):51–4.
14. Sharma N, Berbari NF, Yoder BK. Ciliary dysfunction in developmental abnormalities and diseases. Curr Top Dev Biol. 2008;85. United States:371–427.
15. Veland IR, Awan A, Pedersen LB, Yoder BK, Christensen ST. Primary cilia and signaling pathways in mammalian development, health and disease. Nephron Physiol. 2009;111. Switzerland:39–53.
16. Taulman PD, Haycraft CJ, Balkovetz DF, Yoder BK. Polaris, a protein involved in left-right axis patterning, localizes to basal bodies and cilia. Mol Biol Cell. 2001;12(3):589–99.
17. Veerman AJ, van Delden L, Feenstra L, Leene W. The immotile cilia syndrome: phase contrast light microscopy, scanning and transmission electron microscopy. Pediatrics. 1980;65(4):698–702.
18. Delp MH. Kartagener's triad; situs inversus, absent frontal sinuses with maxillary ethmoid and sphenoid infection, and bronchiectasis. J Kans Med Soc. 1946;47:93–6.
19. Lee L. Riding the wave of ependymal cilia: genetic susceptibility to hydrocephalus in primary ciliary dyskinesia. J Neurosci Res. 2013;91(9):1117–32.
20. Baccetti B, Afzelius BA. The biology of the sperm cell. Monogr Dev Biol. 1976;10:1–254.
21. Hirokawa N, Tanaka Y, Okada Y. Cilia, KIF3 molecular motor and nodal flow. Curr Opin Cell Biol. 2012;24(1):31–9.
22. Harvey RP. Links in the left/right axial pathway. Cell. 1998;94(3):273–6.
23. Nonaka S, Tanaka Y, Okada Y, Takeda S, Harada A, Kanai Y, et al. Randomization of left-right asymmetry due to loss of nodal cilia generating leftward flow of extraembryonic fluid in mice lacking KIF3B motor protein. Cell. 1998;95(6):829–37.
24. Okada Y, Nonaka S, Tanaka Y, Saijoh Y, Hamada H, Hirokawa N. Abnormal nodal flow precedes situs inversus in iv and inv mice. Mol Cell. 1999;4(4):459–68.
25. Takeda S, Yonekawa Y, Tanaka Y, Okada Y, Nonaka S, Hirokawa N. Left-right asymmetry and kinesin superfamily protein KIF3A: new insights in determination of laterality and mesoderm induction by kif3A−/− mice analysis. J Cell Biol. 1999;145(4):825–36.
26. Raya A, Kawakami Y, Rodriguez-Esteban C, Ibanes M, Rasskin-Gutman D, Rodriguez-Leon J, et al. Notch activity acts as a sensor for extracellular calcium during vertebrate left-right determination. Nature. 2004;427(6970):121–8.

27. Takao D, Nemoto T, Abe T, Kiyonari H, Kajiura-Kobayashi H, Shiratori H, et al. Asymmetric distribution of dynamic calcium signals in the node of mouse embryo during left-right axis formation. Dev Biol. 2013;376(1):23–30.
28. Bataille S, Demoulin N, Devuyst O, Audrezet MP, Dahan K, Godin M, et al. Association of PKD2 (polycystin 2) mutations with left-right laterality defects. Am J Kidney Dis: Off J Natl Kidney Found. 2011;58(3):456–60.
29. Schottenfeld J, Sullivan-Brown J, Burdine RD. Zebrafish curly up encodes a Pkd2 ortholog that restricts left-side-specific expression of southpaw. Development. 2007;134(8):1605–15.
30. Pennekamp P, Karcher C, Fischer A, Schweickert A, Skryabin B, Horst J, et al. The ion channel polycystin-2 is required for left-right axis determination in mice. Curr Biol. 2002;12(11):938–43.
31. Hoey DA, Downs ME, Jacobs CR. The mechanics of the primary cilium: an intricate structure with complex function. J Biomech. 2011. Elsevier Ltd. 45(1):17–26
32. Inglis PN, Ou G, Leroux MR, Scholey JM. The sensory cilia of Caenorhabditis elegans. WormBook: Online Rev C elegans Biol. 2007;8:1–22.
33. Ostrowski LE, Dutcher SK, Lo CW. Cilia and models for studying structure and function. Proc Am Thorac Soc. 2011;8(5):423–9.
34. Yamamoto M, Kataoka K. Electron microscopic observation of the primary cilium in the pancreatic islets. Arch Histologicum Japonicum = Nihon soshikigaku kiroku. 1986;49(4):449–57.
35. Williams CL, Masyukova SV, Yoder BK. Normal ciliogenesis requires synergy between the cystic kidney disease genes MKS-3 and NPHP-4. J Am Soc Nephrol: JASN. 2010;21. United States:782–93.
36. Williams CL, Li C, Kida K, Inglis PN, Mohan S, Semenec L, et al. MKS and NPHP modules cooperate to establish basal body/transition zone membrane associations and ciliary gate function during ciliogenesis. J Cell Biol. 2011;192. United States:1023–41.
37. Rohlich P. The sensory cilium of retinal rods is analogous to the transitional zone of motile cilia. Cell Tissue Res. 1975;161(3):421–30.
38. Shiba D, Yamaoka Y, Hagiwara H, Takamatsu T, Hamada H, Yokoyama T. Localization of Inv in a distinctive intraciliary compartment requires the C-terminal ninein-homolog-containing region. J Cell Sci. 2009;122(Pt 1):44–54.
39. Blacque OE, Sanders AA. Compartments within a compartment: what C. elegans can tell us about ciliary subdomain composition, biogenesis, function, and disease. Organogenesis. 2014;10(1):126–37.
40. Jauregui AR, Nguyen KC, Hall DH, Barr MM. The Caenorhabditis elegans nephrocystins act as global modifiers of cilium structure. J Cell Biol. 2008;180(5):973–88.
41. Mukhopadhyay S, Lu Y, Qin H, Lanjuin A, Shaham S, Sengupta P. Distinct IFT mechanisms contribute to the generation of ciliary structural diversity in C. elegans. EMBO J. 2007;26(12):2966–80.
42. Cole DG, Diener DR, Himelblau AL, Beech PL, Fuster JC, Rosenbaum JL. Chlamydomonas kinesin-II-dependent intraflagellar transport (IFT): IFT particles contain proteins required for ciliary assembly in Caenorhabditis elegans sensory neurons. J Cell Biol. 1998;141(4):993–1008.
43. Hao L, Acar S, Evans J, Ou G, Scholey JM. Analysis of intraflagellar transport in C. elegans sensory cilia. Methods Cell Biol. 2009;93:235–66.
44. Kozminski KG, Beech PL, Rosenbaum JL. The Chlamydomonas kinesin-like protein FLA10 is involved in motility associated with the flagellar membrane. J Cell Biol. 1995;131(6 Pt 1):1517–27.
45. Ou G, Blacque OE, Snow JJ, Leroux MR, Scholey JM. Functional coordination of intraflagellar transport motors. Nature. 2005;436(7050):583–7.
46. Scholey JM. Intraflagellar transport. Annu Rev Cell Dev Biol. 2003;19:423–43.
47. Ou G, Koga M, Blacque OE, Murayama T, Ohshima Y, Schafer JC, et al. Sensory ciliogenesis in Caenorhabditis elegans: assignment of IFT components into distinct modules based on transport and phenotypic profiles. Mol Biol Cell. 2007;18. United States:1554–69.
48. Delaval B, Bright A, Lawson ND, Doxsey S. The cilia protein IFT88 is required for spindle orientation in mitosis. Nat Cell Biol. 2011;13(4):461–8.
49. Jonassen JA, Sanagustin J, Baker SP, Pazour GJ. Disruption of IFT complex A causes cystic kidneys without mitotic spindle misorientation. J Am Soc Nephrol: JASN. 2012;23(4):641–51.
50. Keady BT, Le YZ, Pazour GJ. IFT20 is required for opsin trafficking and photoreceptor outer segment development. Mol Biol Cell. 2011;22(7):921–30.
51. Finetti F, Paccani SR, Riparbelli MG, Giacomello E, Perinetti G, Pazour GJ, et al. Intraflagellar transport is required for polarized recycling of the TCR/CD3 complex to the immune synapse. Nat Cell Biol. 2009;11(11):1332–9.
52. Follit JA, Tuft RA, Fogarty KE, Pazour GJ. The intraflagellar transport protein IFT20 is associated with the Golgi complex and is required for cilia assembly. Mol Biol Cell. 2006;17(9):3781–92.
53. Broekhuis JR, Rademakers S, Burghoorn J, Jansen G. SQL-1, homologue of the Golgi protein GMAP210, modulates intraflagellar transport in C. elegans. J Cell Sci. 2013;126(Pt 8):1785–95.
54. Deane JA, Cole DG, Seeley ES, Diener DR, Rosenbaum JL. Localization of intraflagellar transport protein IFT52 identifies basal body transitional fibers as the docking site for IFT particles. Curr Biol. 2001;11(20):1586–90.
55. Pazour GJ, Dickert BL, Vucica Y, Seeley ES, Rosenbaum JL, Witman GB, et al. Chlamydomonas IFT88 and its mouse homologue, polycystic kidney disease gene tg737, are required for assembly of cilia and flagella. J Cell Biol. 2000;151(3):709–18.

56. Blacque OE, Li C, Inglis PN, Esmail MA, Ou G, Mah AK, et al. The WD repeat-containing protein IFTA-1 is required for retrograde intraflagellar transport. Mol Biol Cell. 2006;17(12):5053–62.
57. Piperno G, Siuda E, Henderson S, Segil M, Vaananen H, Sassaroli M. Distinct mutants of retrograde intraflagellar transport (IFT) share similar morphological and molecular defects. J Cell Biol. 1998;143(6):1591–601.
58. Halbritter J, Bizet AA, Schmidts M, Porath JD, Braun DA, Gee HY, et al. Defects in the IFT-B component IFT172 cause Jeune and Mainzer-Saldino syndromes in humans. Am J Hum Genet. 2013;93(5):915–25.
59. Schmidts M, Vodopiutz J, Christou-Savina S, Cortes CR, McInerney-Leo AM, Emes RD, et al. Mutations in the gene encoding IFT dynein complex component WDR34 cause Jeune asphyxiating thoracic dystrophy. Am J Hum Genet. 2013;93(5):932–44.
60. Berbari NF, Lewis JS, Bishop GA, Askwith CC, Mykytyn K. Bardet-Biedl syndrome proteins are required for the localization of G protein-coupled receptors to primary cilia. Proc Natl Acad Sci U S A. 2008;105(11):4242–6.
61. Berbari NF, Johnson AD, Lewis JS, Askwith CC, Mykytyn K. Identification of ciliary localization sequences within the third intracellular loop of G protein-coupled receptors. Mol Biol Cell. 2008;19(4):1540–7.
62. Wojtyniak M, Brear AG, O'Halloran DM, Sengupta P. Cell- and subunit-specific mechanisms of CNG channel ciliary trafficking and localization in C. elegans. J Cell Sci. 2013;126(Pt 19):4381–95.
63. Jenkins PM, Zhang L, Thomas G, Martens JR. PACS-1 mediates phosphorylation-dependent ciliary trafficking of the cyclic-nucleotide-gated channel in olfactory sensory neurons. J Neurosci: Off J Soc Neurosci. 2009;29(34):10541–51.
64. Nakamura T, Gold GH. A cyclic nucleotide-gated conductance in olfactory receptor cilia. Nature. 1987;325(6103):442–4.
65. Guadiana SM, Semple-Rowland S, Daroszewski D, Madorsky I, Breunig JJ, Mykytyn K, et al. Arborization of dendrites by developing neocortical neurons is dependent on primary cilia and type 3 adenylyl cyclase. J Neurosci: Off J Soc Neurosci. 2013;33(6):2626–38.
66. Iwanaga T, Miki T, Takahashi-Iwanaga H. Restricted expression of somatostatin receptor 3 to primary cilia in the pancreatic islets and adenohypophysis of mice. Biomed Res. 2011;32(1):73–81.
67. Kwon RY, Temiyasathit S, Tummala P, Quah CC, Jacobs CR. Primary cilium-dependent mechanosensing is mediated by adenylyl cyclase 6 and cyclic AMP in bone cells. FASEB J: Off Publ Fed Am Soc Exp Biol. 2010;24(8):2859–68.
68. Lazard D, Barak Y, Lancet D. Bovine olfactory cilia preparation: thiol-modulated odorant-sensitive adenylyl cyclase. Biochim Biophys Acta. 1989;1013(1):68–72.
69. Sklar PB, Anholt RR, Snyder SH. The odorant-sensitive adenylate cyclase of olfactory receptor cells. Differential stimulation by distinct classes of odorants. J Biol Chem. 1986;261(33):15538–43.
70. Wang Z, Phan T, Storm DR. The type 3 adenylyl cyclase is required for novel object learning and extinction of contextual memory: role of cAMP signaling in primary cilia. J Neurosci: Off J Soc Neurosci. 2011;31(15):5557–61.
71. Corbit KC, Aanstad P, Singla V, Norman AR, Stainier DY, Reiter JF. Vertebrate Smoothened functions at the primary cilium. Nature. 2005;437(7061):1018–21.
72. Haycraft CJ, Banizs B, Aydin-Son Y, Zhang Q, Michaud EJ, Yoder BK. Gli2 and Gli3 localize to cilia and require the intraflagellar transport protein polaris for processing and function. PLoS Genet. 2005;1(4):e53.
73. Huangfu D, Anderson KV. Cilia and Hedgehog responsiveness in the mouse. Proc Natl Acad Sci U S A. 2005;102(32):11325–30.
74. May SR, Ashique AM, Karlen M, Wang B, Shen Y, Zarbalis K, et al. Loss of the retrograde motor for IFT disrupts localization of Smo to cilia and prevents the expression of both activator and repressor functions of Gli. Dev Biol. 2005;287(2):378–89.
75. Ward HH, Brown-Glaberman U, Wang J, Morita Y, Alper SL, Bedrick EJ, et al. A conserved signal and GTPase complex are required for the ciliary transport of polycystin-1. Mol Biol Cell. 2011;22. United States:3289–305.
76. Verhey KJ, Dishinger J, Kee HL. Kinesin motors and primary cilia. Biochem Soc Trans. 2011;39. England:1120–5.
77. Kee HL, Dishinger JF, Blasius TL, Liu CJ, Margolis B, Verhey KJ. A size-exclusion permeability barrier and nucleoporins characterize a ciliary pore complex that regulates transport into cilia. Nat Cell Biol. 2012;14(4):431–7.
78. Kee HL, Verhey KJ. Molecular connections between nuclear and ciliary import processes. Cilia. 2013;2(1):11.
79. Breslow DK, Koslover EF, Seydel F, Spakowitz AJ, Nachury MV. An in vitro assay for entry into cilia reveals unique properties of the soluble diffusion barrier. J Cell Biol. 2013;203(1):129–47.
80. Dishinger JF, Kee HL, Jenkins PM, Fan S, Hurd TW, Hammond JW, et al. Ciliary entry of the kinesin-2 motor KIF17 is regulated by importin-beta2 and RanGTP. Nat Cell Biol. 2010;12(7):703–10.
81. Fan S, Whiteman EL, Hurd TW, McIntyre JC, Dishinger JF, Liu CJ, et al. Induction of Ran GTP drives ciliogenesis. Mol Biol Cell. 2011;22(23):4539–48.
82. Najafi M, Maza NA, Calvert PD. Steric volume exclusion sets soluble protein concentrations in photoreceptor sensory cilia. Proc Natl Acad Sci U S A. 2012;109(1):203–8.
83. Francis SS, Sfakianos J, Lo B, Mellman I. A hierarchy of signals regulates entry of membrane proteins into the ciliary membrane domain in epithelial cells. J Cell Biol. 2011;193(1):219–33.

84. Duning K, Rosenbusch D, Schluter MA, Tian Y, Kunzelmann K, Meyer N, et al. Polycystin-2 activity is controlled by transcriptional coactivator with PDZ binding motif and PALS1-associated tight junction protein. J Biol Chem. 2010;285(44):33584–8.
85. Lin YC, Niewiadomski P, Lin B, Nakamura H, Phua SC, Jiao J, et al. Chemically inducible diffusion trap at cilia reveals molecular sieve-like barrier. Nat Chem Biol. 2013;9(7):437–43.
86. Benzing T, Schermer B. Transition zone proteins and cilia dynamics. Nat Genet. 2011;43. United States:723–4.
87. Omran H. NPHP proteins: gatekeepers of the ciliary compartment. J Cell Biol. 2010;190. United States:715–7.
88. Winkelbauer ME, Schafer JC, Haycraft CJ, Swoboda P, Yoder BK. The C. elegans homologs of nephrocystin-1 and nephrocystin-4 are cilia transition zone proteins involved in chemosensory perception. J Cell Sci. 2005;118. England:5575–87.
89. Garcia-Gonzalo FR, Corbit KC, Sirerol-Piquer MS, Ramaswami G, Otto EA, Noriega TR, et al. A transition zone complex regulates mammalian ciliogenesis and ciliary membrane composition. Nat Genet. 2011;43(8):776–84.
90. Reiter JF, Skarnes WC. Tectonic, a novel regulator of the hedgehog pathway required for both activation and inhibition. Genes Dev. 2006;20(1):22–7.
91. Grantham JJ, Mulamalla S, Swenson-Fields KI. Why kidneys fail in autosomal dominant polycystic kidney disease. Nat Rev Nephrol. 2011;7(10):556–66.
92. Nauli SM, Rossetti S, Kolb RJ, Alenghat FJ, Consugar MB, Harris PC, et al. Loss of polycystin-1 in human cyst-lining epithelia leads to ciliary dysfunction. J Am Soc Nephrol: JASN. 2006;17(4):1015–25.
93. Qian F, Watnick TJ, Onuchic LF, Germino GG. The molecular basis of focal cyst formation in human autosomal dominant polycystic kidney disease type I. Cell. 1996;87(6):979–87.
94. AbouAlaiwi WA, Takahashi M, Mell BR, Jones TJ, Ratnam S, Kolb RJ, et al. Ciliary polycystin-2 is a mechanosensitive calcium channel involved in nitric oxide signaling cascades. Circ Res. 2009;104(7):860–9.
95. Leeuwen ISL-V, Leonhard WN, Avd W, Breuning MH, Heer ED, Peters DJM. Kidney-specific inactivation of the Pkd1 gene induces rapid cyst formation in developing kidneys and a slow onset of disease in adult mice. Hum Mol Genet. 2007;16:3188–96.
96. Sharma N, Malarkey EB, Berbari NF, O'Connor AK, GBV H, Mrug M, et al. Proximal tubule proliferation is insufficient to induce rapid cyst formation after cilia disruption. J Am Soc Nephrol. 2013;24:456–64.
97. Ward CJ, Hogan MC, Rossetti S, Walker D, Sneddon T, Wang X, et al. The gene mutated in autosomal recessive polycystic kidney disease encodes a large, receptor-like protein. Nat Genet. 2002;30(3):259–69.
98. Karihaloo A, Koraishy F, Huen SC, Lee Y, Merrick D, Caplan MJ, et al. Macrophages promote cyst growth in polycystic kidney disease. J Am Soc Nephrol: JASN. 2011;22(10):1809–14.
99. Rossetti S, Harris PC. Genotype-phenotype correlations in autosomal dominant and autosomal recessive polycystic kidney disease. J Am Soc Nephrol: JASN. 2007;18(5):1374–80.
100. Wheatley DN. Landmarks in the first hundred years of primary (9+0) cilium research. Cell Biol Int. 2005;29(5):333–9.
101. Moyer JH, Lee-Tischler MJ, Kwon HY, Schrick JJ, Avner ED, Sweeney WE, et al. Candidate gene associated with a mutation causing recessive polycystic kidney disease in mice. Science. 1994;264(5163):1329–33.
102. Murcia NS, Richards WG, Yoder BK, Mucenski ML, Dunlap JR, Woychik RP. The Oak Ridge Polycystic Kidney (orpk) disease gene is required for left-right axis determination. Development. 2000;127(11):2347–55.
103. Yoder BK, Tousson A, Millican L, Wu JH, Bugg CE Jr, Schafer JA, et al. Polaris, a protein disrupted in orpk mutant mice, is required for assembly of renal cilium. Am J Physiol Renal Physiol. 2002;282(3):F541–52.
104. Lehman JM, Michaud EJ, Schoeb TR, Aydin-Son Y, Miller M, Yoder BK. The oak ridge polycystic kidney mouse: modeling ciliopathies of mice and men. Dev Dyn: Off Publ Am Assoc Anatomists. 2008;237(8):1960–71.
105. Barr MM, Sternberg PW. A polycystic kidney-disease gene homologue required for male mating behaviour in C. elegans. Nature. 1999;401(6751):386–9.
106. Barr MM, DeModena J, Braun D, Nguyen CQ, Hall DH, Sternberg PW. The Caenorhabditis elegans autosomal dominant polycystic kidney disease gene homologs lov-1 and pkd-2 act in the same pathway. Curr Biol: CB. 2001;11(17):1341–6.
107. Ward CJ, Yuan D, Masyuk TV, Wang X, Punyashthiti R, Whelan S, et al. Cellular and subcellular localization of the ARPKD protein; fibrocystin is expressed on primary cilia. Hum Mol Genet. 2003;12(20):2703–10.
108. Davenport JR, Watts AJ, Roper VC, Croyle MJ, van Groen T, Wyss JM, et al. Disruption of intraflagellar transport in adult mice leads to obesity and slow-onset cystic kidney disease. Curr Biol: CB. 2007;17(18):1586–94.
109. Piontek KB, Huso DL, Grinberg A, Liu L, Bedja D, Zhao H, et al. A functional floxed allele of Pkd1 that can be conditionally inactivated in vivo. J Am Soc Nephrol. 2004;15:3035–43.
110. Piontek K, Menezes LF, Garcia-Gonzalez MA, Huso DL, Germino GG. A critical developmental switch defines the kinetics of kidney cyst formation after loss of Pkd1. Nat Med. 2007;13(12):1490–5.
111. Kim I, Ding T, Fu Y, Li C, Cui L, Li A, et al. Conditional mutation of Pkd2 causes cystogenesis and upregulates beta-catenin. J Am Soc Nephrol: JASN. 2009;20(12):2556–69.
112. Patel V, Li L, Cobo-Stark P, Shao X, Somlo S, Lin F, et al. Acute kidney injury and aberrant planar cell

polarity induce cyst formation in mice lacking renal cilia. Hum Mol Genet. 2008;17:1578–90.
113. Ma M, Tian X, Igarashi P, Pazour GJ, Somlo S. Loss of cilia suppresses cyst growth in genetic models of autosomal dominant polycystic kidney disease. Nat Genet. 2013;45(9):1004–12.
114. Praetorius HA, Frokiaer J, Nielsen S, Spring KR. Bending the primary cilium opens Ca2+–sensitive intermediate-conductance K+ channels in MDCK cells. J Membr Biol. 2003;191(3):193–200.
115. Praetorius HA, Spring KR. Removal of the MDCK cell primary cilium abolishes flow sensing. J Membr Biol. 2003;191(1):69–76.
116. Praetorius HA, Spring KR. The renal cell primary cilium functions as a flow sensor. Curr Opin Nephrol Hypertens. 2003;12(5):517–20.
117. Nauli SM, Alenghat FJ, Luo Y, Williams E, Vassilev P, Li X, et al. Polycystins 1 and 2 mediate mechanosensation in the primary cilium of kidney cells. Nat Genet. 2003;33(2):129–37.
118. Xu C, Rossetti S, Jiang L, Harris PC, Brown-Glaberman U, Wandinger-Ness A, et al. Human ADPKD primary cyst epithelial cells with a novel, single codon deletion in the PKD1 gene exhibit defective ciliary polycystin localization and loss of flow-induced Ca2+ signaling. Am J Physiol Renal Physiol. 2007;292(3):F930–45.
119. Yoshiba S, Shiratori H, Kuo IY, Kawasumi A, Shinohara K, Nonaka S, et al. Cilia at the node of mouse embryos sense fluid flow for left-right determination via Pkd2. Science. 2012;338(6104):226–31.
120. Cano DA, Sekine S, Hebrok M. Primary cilia deletion in pancreatic epithelial cells results in cyst formation and pancreatitis. Gastroenterology. 2006;131(6):1856–69.
121. Chauvet V, Tian X, Husson H, Grimm DH, Wang T, Hiesberger T, et al. Mechanical stimuli induce cleavage and nuclear translocation of the polycystin-1 C terminus. J Clin Invest. 2004;114(10):1433–43.
122. Casuscelli J, Schmidt S, DeGray B, Petri ET, Celic A, Folta-Stogniew E, et al. Analysis of the cytoplasmic interaction between polycystin-1 and polycystin-2. Am J Physiol Renal Physiol. 2009;297(5):F1310–5.
123. Oatley P, Talukder MM, Stewart AP, Sandford R, Edwardson JM. Polycystin-2 induces a conformational change in polycystin-1. Biochemistry. 2013;52(31):5280–7.
124. Mamenko M, Zaika O, Jin M, O'Neil RG, Pochynyuk O. Purinergic activation of Ca2+-permeable TRPV4 channels is essential for mechano-sensitivity in the aldosterone-sensitive distal nephron. PLoS One. 2011;6(8):e22824.
125. Cressman VL, Lazarowski E, Homolya L, Boucher RC, Koller BH, Grubb BR. Effect of loss of P2Y(2) receptor gene expression on nucleotide regulation of murine epithelial Cl(−) transport. J Biol Chem. 1999;274(37):26461–8.
126. Raghavan V, Rbaibi Y, Pastor-Soler NM, Carattino MD, Weisz OA. Shear stress-dependent regulation of apical endocytosis in renal proximal tubule cells mediated by primary cilia. Proc Natl Acad Sci U S A. 2014;111(23):8506–11.
127. Burnstock G, Evans LC, Bailey MA. Purinergic signalling in the kidney in health and disease. Purinergic Signal. 2014;10(1):71–101.
128. Chang MY, Lu JK, Tian YC, Chen YC, Hung CC, Huang YH, et al. Inhibition of the P2X7 receptor reduces cystogenesis in PKD. J Am Soc Nephrol: JASN. 2011;22(9):1696–706.
129. Shillingford JM, Murcia NS, Larson CH, Low SH, Hedgepeth R, Brown N, et al. The mTOR pathway is regulated by polycystin-1, and its inhibition reverses renal cystogenesis in polycystic kidney disease. Proc Natl Acad Sci U S A. 2006;103(14):5466–71.
130. Fischer DC, Jacoby U, Pape L, Ward CJ, Kuwertz-Broeking E, Renken C, et al. Activation of the AKT/mTOR pathway in autosomal recessive polycystic kidney disease (ARPKD). Nephrol Dial Transplant: Off Publ Eur Dial Transplant Assoc – Eur Renal Assoc. 2009;24(6):1819–27.
131. Becker JU, Opazo Saez A, Zerres K, Witzke O, Hoyer PF, Schmid KW, et al. The mTOR pathway is activated in human autosomal-recessive polycystic kidney disease. Kidney Blood Press Res. 2010;33(2):129–38.
132. Dere R, Wilson PD, Sandford RN, Walker CL. Carboxy terminal tail of polycystin-1 regulates localization of TSC2 to repress mTOR. PLoS One. 2010;5(2):e9239.
133. Ong AC, Harris PC, Davies DR, Pritchard L, Rossetti S, Biddolph S, et al. Polycystin-1 expression in PKD1, early-onset PKD1, and TSC2/PKD1 cystic tissue. Kidney Int. 1999;56(4):1324–33.
134. Bell PD, Fitzgibbon W, Sas K, Stenbit AE, Amria M, Houston A, et al. Loss of primary cilia upregulates renal hypertrophic signaling and promotes cystogenesis. J Am Soc Nephrol: JASN. 2011;22(5):839–48.
135. Boehlke C, Kotsis F, Patel V, Braeg S, Voelker H, Bredt S, et al. Primary cilia regulate mTORC1 activity and cell size through Lkb1. Nat Cell Biol. 2010;12(11):1115–22.
136. Serra AL, Poster D, Kistler AD, Krauer F, Raina S, Young J, et al. Sirolimus and kidney growth in autosomal dominant polycystic kidney disease. N Engl J Med. 2010;363(9):820–9.
137. Walz G, Budde K, Mannaa M, Nurnberger J, Wanner C, Sommerer C, et al. Everolimus in patients with autosomal dominant polycystic kidney disease. N Engl J Med. 2010;363(9):830–40.
138. Canaud G, Knebelmann B, Harris PC, Vrtovsnik F, Correas JM, Pallet N, et al. Therapeutic mTOR inhibition in autosomal dominant polycystic kidney disease: what is the appropriate serum level? Am J Transplant Off J Am Soc Transplant Am Soc Transplant Surg. 2010;10(7):1701–6.
139. Shillingford JM, Leamon CP, Vlahov IR, Weimbs T. Folate-conjugated rapamycin slows progression of polycystic kidney disease. J Am Soc Nephrol: JASN. 2012;23(10):1674–81.

140. Chuang PY, He JC. JAK/STAT signaling in renal diseases. Kidney Int. 2010;78. United States:231–4.
141. Wang H, Yang Y, Sharma N, Tarasova NI, Timofeeva OA, Winkler-Pickett RT, et al. STAT1 activation regulates proliferation and differentiation of renal progenitors. Cell Signal. 2010;22(11):1717–26.
142. Bhunia AK, Piontek K, Boletta A, Liu L, Qian F, Xu PN, et al. PKD1 induces p21(waf1) and regulation of the cell cycle via direct activation of the JAK-STAT signaling pathway in a process requiring PKD2. Cell. 2002;109(2):157–68.
143. Kim H, Kang AY, Ko AR, Park HC, So I, Park JH, et al. Calpain-mediated proteolysis of polycystin-1 C-terminus induces JAK2 and ERK signal alterations. Exp Cell Res. 2014;320(1):62–8.
144. Talbot JJ, Shillingford JM, Vasanth S, Doerr N, Mukherjee S, Kinter MT, et al. Polycystin-1 regulates STAT activity by a dual mechanism. Proc Natl Acad Sci U S A. 2011;108(19):7985–90.
145. Low SH, Vasanth S, Larson CH, Mukherjee S, Sharma N, Kinter MT, et al. Polycystin-1, STAT6, and P100 function in a pathway that transduces ciliary mechanosensation and is activated in polycystic kidney disease. Dev Cell. 2006;10(1):57–69.
146. Olsan EE, Mukherjee S, Wulkersdorfer B, Shillingford JM, Giovannone AJ, Todorov G, et al. Signal transducer and activator of transcription-6 (STAT6) inhibition suppresses renal cyst growth in polycystic kidney disease. Proc Natl Acad Sci U S A. 2011;108(44):18067–72.
147. Zeier M, Fehrenbach P, Geberth S, Mohring K, Waldherr R, Ritz E. Renal histology in polycystic kidney disease with incipient and advanced renal failure. Kidney Int. 1992;42(5):1259–65.
148. Ibrahim S. Increased apoptosis and proliferative capacity are early events in cyst formation in autosomal-dominant, polycystic kidney disease. Sci World J. 2007;7:1757–67.
149. Zheng D, Wolfe M, Cowley BD Jr, Wallace DP, Yamaguchi T, Grantham JJ. Urinary excretion of monocyte chemoattractant protein-1 in autosomal dominant polycystic kidney disease. J Am Soc Nephrol: JASN. 2003;14(10):2588–95.
150. Meijer E, Boertien WE, Nauta FL, Bakker SJ, van Oeveren W, Rook M, et al. Association of urinary biomarkers with disease severity in patients with autosomal dominant polycystic kidney disease: a cross-sectional analysis. Am J Kidney Dis: Off J Natl Kidney Found. 2010;56(5):883–95.
151. Lee S, Huen S, Nishio H, Nishio S, Lee HK, Choi BS, et al. Distinct macrophage phenotypes contribute to kidney injury and repair. J Am Soc Nephrol: JASN. 2011;22(2):317–26.
152. May-Simera H, Kelley MW. Examining planar cell polarity in the mammalian cochlea. Methods Mol Biol. 2012;839:157–71.
153. McNeill H. Planar cell polarity and the kidney. J Am Soc Nephrol: JASN. 2009;20(10):2104–11.
154. Carroll TJ, Yu J. The kidney and planar cell polarity. Curr Top Dev Biol. 2012;101:185–212.
155. Goggolidou P. Wnt and planar cell polarity signaling in cystic renal disease. Organogenesis. 2014;10(1):86–95.
156. Karner CM, Chirumamilla R, Aoki S, Igarashi P, Wallingford JB, Carroll TJ. Wnt9b signaling regulates planar cell polarity and kidney tubule morphogenesis. Nat Genet. 2009;41(7):793–9.
157. Adler PN, Krasnow RE, Liu J. Tissue polarity points from cells that have higher frizzled levels towards cells that have lower frizzled levels. Curr Biol. 1997;7(12):940–9.
158. Vinson CR, Adler PN. Directional non-cell autonomy and the transmission of polarity information by the frizzled gene of Drosophila. Nature. 1987;329(6139):549–51.
159. Borovina A, Superina S, Voskas D, Ciruna B. Vangl2 directs the posterior tilting and asymmetric localization of motile primary cilia. Nat Cell Biol. 2010;12(4):407–12.
160. Cui C, Chatterjee B, Lozito TP, Zhang Z, Francis RJ, Yagi H, et al. Wdpcp, a PCP protein required for ciliogenesis, regulates directional cell migration and cell polarity by direct modulation of the actin cytoskeleton. PLoS Biol. 2013;11(11):e1001720.
161. Jones C, Roper VC, Foucher I, Qian D, Banizs B, Petit C, et al. Ciliary proteins link basal body polarization to planar cell polarity regulation. Nat Genet. 2008;40(1):69–77.
162. Ross AJ, May-Simera H, Eichers ER, Kai M, Hill J, Jagger DJ, et al. Disruption of Bardet-Biedl syndrome ciliary proteins perturbs planar cell polarity in vertebrates. Nat Genet. 2005;37(10):1135–40.
163. Borovina A, Ciruna B. IFT88 plays a cilia- and PCP-independent role in controlling oriented cell divisions during vertebrate embryonic development. Cell Rep. 2013;5(1):37–43.
164. Romaker D, Puetz M, Teschner S, Donauer J, Geyer M, Gerke P, et al. Increased expression of secreted frizzled-related protein 4 in polycystic kidneys. J Am Soc Nephrol: JASN. 2009;20(1):48–56.
165. Fischer E, Legue E, Doyen A, Nato F, Nicolas JF, Torres V, et al. Defective planar cell polarity in polycystic kidney disease. Nat Genet. 2006;38(1):21–3.
166. Mao Y, Mulvaney J, Zakaria S, Yu T, Morgan KM, Allen S, et al. Characterization of a Dchs1 mutant mouse reveals requirements for Dchs1-Fat4 signaling during mammalian development. Development. 2011;138(5):947–57.
167. Saburi S, Hester I, Fischer E, Pontoglio M, Eremina V, Gessler M, et al. Loss of Fat4 disrupts PCP signaling and oriented cell division and leads to cystic kidney disease. Nat Genet. 2008;40(8):1010–5.
168. Mei X, Westfall TA, Zhang Q, Sheffield VC, Bassuk AG, Slusarski DC. Functional characterization of Prickle2 and BBS7 identify overlapping phenotypes yet distinct mechanisms. Dev Biol. 2014;392(2):245–55.
169. Nishio S, Tian X, Gallagher AR, Yu Z, Patel V, Igarashi P, et al. Loss of oriented cell division does

not initiate cyst formation. J Am Soc Nephrol: JASN. 2010;21(2):295–302.
170. Tripathi P, Guo Q, Wang Y, Coussens M, Liapis H, Jain S, et al. Midline signaling regulates kidney positioning but not nephrogenesis through Shh. Dev Biol. 2010;340(2):518–27.
171. Cain JE, Islam E, Haxho F, Blake J, Rosenblum ND. GLI3 repressor controls functional development of the mouse ureter. J Clin Invest. 2011;121(3):1199–206.
172. Cain JE, Islam E, Haxho F, Chen L, Bridgewater D, Nieuwenhuis E, et al. GLI3 repressor controls nephron number via regulation of Wnt11 and Ret in ureteric tip cells. PLoS One. 2009;4(10):e7313.
173. Hu MC, Mo R, Bhella S, Wilson CW, Chuang PT, Hui CC, et al. GLI3-dependent transcriptional repression of Gli1, Gli2 and kidney patterning genes disrupts renal morphogenesis. Development. 2006;133(3):569–78.
174. Yu J, Carroll TJ, McMahon AP. Sonic hedgehog regulates proliferation and differentiation of mesenchymal cells in the mouse metanephric kidney. Development. 2002;129(22):5301–12.
175. Cohen MM Jr. Hedgehog signaling update. Am J Med Genet A. 2010;152A(8):1875–914.
176. Tran PV, Talbott GC, Turbe-Doan A, Jacobs DT, Schonfeld MP, Silva LM, et al. Downregulating hedgehog signaling reduces renal cystogenic potential of mouse models. J Am Soc Nephrol: JASN. 2014;25:2201–12.
177. Ozturk H, Tuncer MC, Buyukbayram H. Nitric oxide regulates expression of sonic hedgehog and hypoxia-inducible factor-1alpha in an experimental model of kidney ischemia-reperfusion. Ren Fail. 2007;29(3):249–56.
178. Zhou D, Li Y, Zhou L, Tan RJ, Xiao L, Liang M, et al. Sonic hedgehog is a novel tubule-derived growth factor for interstitial fibroblasts after kidney injury. J Am Soc Nephrol. 2014;25:2187–200.
179. Raychowdhury MK, Ramos AJ, Zhang P, McLaughin M, Dai XQ, Chen XZ, et al. Vasopressin receptor-mediated functional signaling pathway in primary cilia of renal epithelial cells. Am J Physiol Renal Physiol. 2009;296(1):F87–97.
180. Nedvetsky PI, Tamma G, Beulshausen S, Valenti G, Rosenthal W, Klussmann E. Regulation of aquaporin-2 trafficking. Handb Exp Pharmacol. 2009;190:133–57.
181. Saigusa T, Reichert R, Guare J, Siroky BJ, Gooz M, Steele S, et al. Collecting duct cells that lack normal cilia have mislocalized vasopressin-2 receptors. Am J Physiol Renal Physiol. 2012;302(7):F801–8.
182. Marion V, Schlicht D, Mockel A, Caillard S, Imhoff O, Stoetzel C, et al. Bardet-Biedl syndrome highlights the major role of the primary cilium in efficient water reabsorption. Kidney Int. 2011;79(9):1013–25.
183. Calvet JP. Strategies to inhibit cyst formation in ADPKD. Clin J Am Soc Nephrol. 2008;3(4):1205–11.
184. D'Angelo A, Mioni G, Ossi E, Lupo A, Valvo E, Maschio G. Alterations in renal tubular sodium and water transport in polycystic kidney disease. Clin Nephrol. 1975;3(3):99–105.
185. Yamaguchi T, Nagao S, Kasahara M, Takahashi H, Grantham JJ. Renal accumulation and excretion of cyclic adenosine monophosphate in a murine model of slowly progressive polycystic kidney disease. Am J Kidney Dis. 1997;30(5):703–9.
186. Chen NX, Moe SM, Eggleston-Gulyas T, Chen X, Hoffmeyer WD, Bacallao RL, et al. Calcimimetics inhibit renal pathology in rodent nephronophthisis. Kidney Int. 2011;80(6):612–9.
187. Aihara M, Fujiki H, Mizuguchi H, Hattori K, Ohmoto K, Ishikawa M, et al. Tolvaptan delays the onset of end-stage renal disease in a polycystic kidney disease model by suppressing increases in kidney volume and renal injury. J Pharmacol Exp Ther. 2014;349(2):258–67.
188. Torres VE, Chapman AB, Devuyst O, Gansevoort RT, Grantham JJ, Higashihara E, et al. Tolvaptan in patients with autosomal dominant polycystic kidney disease. N Engl J Med. 2012;367(25):2407–18.
189. Hopp K, Hommerding CJ, Wang X, Ye H, Harris PC, Torres VE. Tolvaptan plus pasireotide shows enhanced efficacy in a PKD1 model. J Am Soc Nephrol: JASN. 2014;26:39–47.
190. Sabbatini M, Russo L, Cappellaio F, Troncone G, Bellevicine C, De Falco V, et al. Effects of combined administration of rapamycin, tolvaptan, and AEZ-131 on the progression of polycystic disease in PCK rats. Am J Physiol Renal Physiol. 2014;306(10):F1243–50.

The Role of Inflammation and Fibrosis in Cystic Kidney Disease

6

James C. Harms, Cheng Jack Song, and Michal Mrug

In addition to renal cysts, interstitial inflammation and fibrosis are among the most notable hallmarks of cystic kidney diseases. While cyst formation and expansion are believed to play a principal role in renal pathobiology of polycystic kidney diseases (PKDs), interstitial inflammation and fibrosis used to be mostly attributed to advanced end-stage organ-like changes with limited impact on overall pathobiology of PKD progression. However, seminal studies by Cowley and Grantham have indicated that pro-inflammatory mediators may play a key role in the development of interstitial inflammation and renal function loss seen in PKD [1, 2]. Subsequent analyses, primarily in rodent models, provided compelling support for a complex interplay among immune responses and cyst formation and demonstrated relevance of such interactions in the progression of cystic kidney diseases. Therefore, abnormal PKD-associated immune responses and fibrosis are now recognized as key components of a complex multidirectional relationship that, together with abnormal injury and tissue repair, as well as renal tubular and vascular epithelial function, defines the pathobiology of renal cystic disease progression (Fig. 6.1).

J. C. Harms, MD
Division of Nephrology, Department of Medicine, University of Alabama at Birmingham, Birmingham, AL, USA
e-mail: jcharms@uabmc.edu

C. J. Song, BS
Department of Cell, Developmental and Integrative Biology, University of Alabama at Birmingham, Birmingham, AL, USA
e-mail: song1c@uab.edu

M. Mrug, MD (✉)
Division of Nephrology, Department of Medicine, University of Alabama at Birmingham, Birmingham, AL, USA

Department of Veterans Affairs Medical Center, Birmingham, AL, USA
e-mail: mmrug@uab.edu

Inflammatory Pathways Associated with PKD

Activation of Inflammation in PKD

The PKD-associated immune response was observed across a spectrum of stages of PKD progression. Since the pathobiology of these individual stages differs substantially (e.g., in degree of renal cystic burden, vascular dysfunction, interstitial and extracellular matrix changes, and proportion of normally functioning nephrons), it is conceivable that immune responses and their triggers also differ across individual stages of the renal cystic disease.

Perhaps the earliest PKD-induced immune changes are triggered by the loss of PKD protein function in renal epithelial cells, which may occur even before the immune pathway activation by PKD-associated renal injury (Fig. 6.2).

B. D. Cowley, Jr., J. J. Bissler (eds.), *Polycystic Kidney Disease*,
https://doi.org/10.1007/978-1-4939-7784-0_6

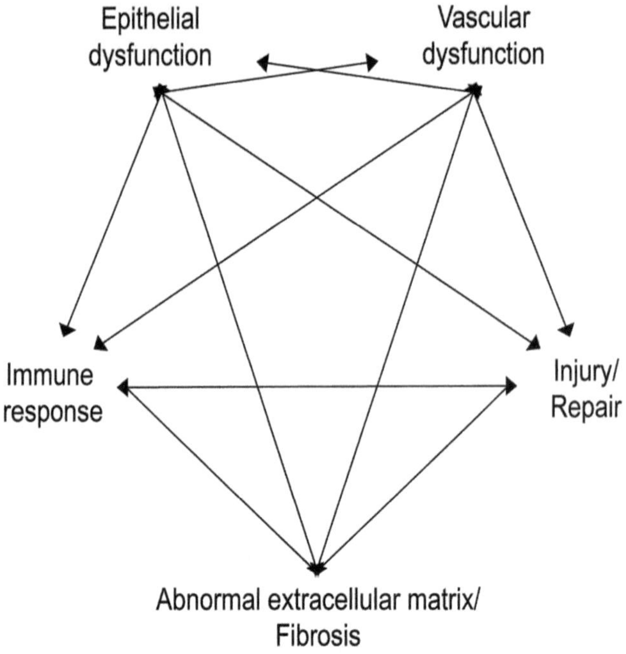

Fig. 6.1 Complex relationship of immune responses and fibrosis in the pathogenesis of renal cystic disorders. Polycystic kidney disease-associated epithelial and vascular dysfunction, abnormal immune responses, injury and repair, as well as extracellular matrix abnormalities and fibrosis are likely key components of a complex multidirectional relationship that defines the pathobiology of renal cystic disease progression

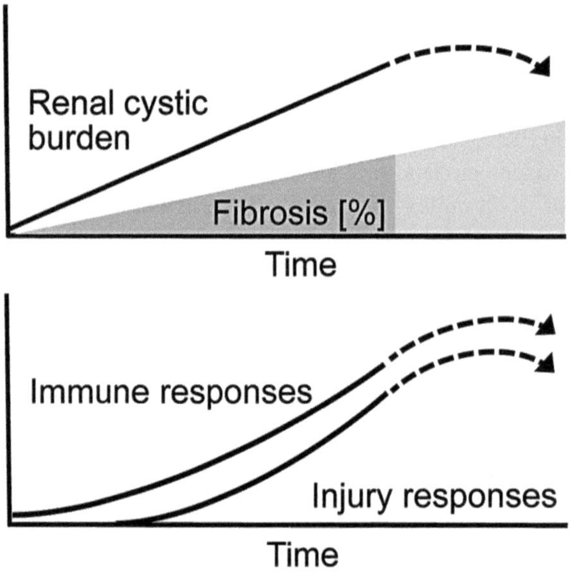

Fig. 6.2 Changes in renal cystic burden, fibrosis, and immune and injury responses over time. Renal cystic disease burden (e.g., as reflected by total kidney volume) increases over time in human studies (upper panel; solid line). In some animal studies (dashed line), the kidney size does not increase or may decrease in advanced stages of the disease progression, while the tissue becomes progressively more fibrotic. Abnormal immune responses represent one of the early hallmark features of renal cystic disease and may precede frank injury-like responses. Abnormalities in both immune and injury responses increase over time (solid line); however, in advanced stages of the disease, the progression magnitude of some of these responses may be reduced due to a loss of functional renal parenchyma (dashed line)

Several studies support this hypothesis. For example, polycystin-1-deficient tubular cell lines overexpress macrophage chemoattractants *Mcp1* and *Cxcl16* [3], while polycystin-2 or *Kif3a* deficiency in inner medullary collecting duct cell lines dysregulates expression of *Mcp1* and complement factor C3 [4, 5]. Similar to the polycystin-1-deficient cell lines, renal cystic epithelia isolated from ADPKD patients overexpress multiple immunomodulators including cytokines and complement system factors [6]. In addition, increased expression of *Mcp1* or monocyte/macrophage marker *Cd14* was observed before significant changes occurred in the expression of renal injury markers such as *Lcn2* (a neutrophil gelatinase-associated lipocalin; NGAL) [7].

Additional factors contribute to the induction of immune responses later, especially after the formation of renal cysts. Among these factors, renal tubular obstruction is most notable. However, renal tubules can be obstructed even in precystic kidneys by casts of sloughed off tubular epithelial cells. The importance of renal cyst-related obstruction increases along time with progressively worsening renal cystic burden. In addition, consequences of tubular obstruction may be related to the location of individual cysts. Since a single collecting duct drains ~2800 upstream nephrons, an inner medullary cyst that compresses six adjacent collecting ducts may potentially obstruct drainage from 16,800 upstream tubules (reviewed in [8]). The response of the renal parenchyma to such an alteration of tubular flow in cystic kidney diseases likely closely resembles studies of experimental urinary obstruction [9]. Parallels between cystic kidney disease and urinary obstruction include increased production of chemokines, pro- and anti-inflammatory cytokines, and paracrine and autocrine immunomodulating products [10, 11]. In addition to the obstruction of tubular flow, renal cysts can lead to compression of and diminished flow in the surrounding microvasculature. Functional relevance of such effects is suggested by impaired renal vascular architecture observed in PKD animal models and PKD patients [12]. The PKD-induced impairment in renal vascular flow leads to regional hypoxia and cellular injury, which have been denoted by increased expression of hemoxygenase [13] and shown to be exacerbated by reductions in superoxide dismutase [14]. Cellular responses to such injury trigger complex immune responses. While these immune responses play an important role in tissue repair and recovery from acute kidney injury (e.g., [15]), their chronic activation may lead to fibrotic changes and irreversible renal parenchyma loss. Recurrent activation of the injury-induced inflammatory pathways by chronic and progressive cystic kidney disease may thus explain prominent renal fibrosis seen in advanced stages of PKD. In addition, the chronic obstruction and vascular changes triggered by expanding renal cysts may induce ineffective repair (reviewed in [8]) that is in part regulated by inflammatory cells and their mediators [3].

Another potential cause of enhanced PKD-associated inflammatory responses is increased susceptibility to renal injury, e.g., in unilateral ischemia/reperfusion injury (IRI) that leads to excessive renal infiltration by macrophages and neutrophils in *Pkd2*$^{+/-}$ heterozygous mice [16]. Follow-up cytokine assays indicated that the observed enhancement of *Pkd2*-associated post-IRI interstitial inflammation is mediated by elevated levels of Cxcl1 and IL-1β [16]; IL-1β was found in 70% cyst fluids from patients with ADPKD [17].

Finally, systemic inflammatory changes induced by advanced renal dysfunction may modulate immune responses in PKD kidneys especially among individuals approaching end-stage renal disease. Such associations were observed in animal studies where expression of immune factors (e.g., *Mcp1* or *Cd14*) increased exponentially in advanced stages of cystic disease progression despite progressive loss of functional renal parenchyma that expresses these inflammatory factors [18]. Comparable studies in humans are complicated due to a lack of kidney tissues available for such analyses.

Inflammatory Signaling Pathways in PKD

Recent genome-wide expression analyses provided comprehensive assessment of biological processes associated with PKD. Among these studies, a global gene expression analysis of renal cystic epithelia from patients with *PKD1* mutations revealed that among the 100 most upregulated gene sets, 11 were associated with the Jak-STAT pathway and 3 with NF-κB signaling [19]. Therefore, these two pathways likely play a central role in the modulation of the immune responses of cystic epithelial cells. Since these pathways also play a central role in modulating of immune activity of other renal cell types (e.g., endothelial cells, fibroblasts, myeloid lineage cells), it is likely that the Jak-STAT and NF-κB signaling pathways are altered in multiple cell types found in PKD kidneys.

The Jak-STAT system represents one of the most important pathways in immune signaling. It is activated by several cytokines and growth factors including the key immunomodulators IL-6 and interferon gamma (IFNγ). Binding of these ligands to their receptors activates Janus kinase (Jak) that in turn transduces these cytokine-mediated signals through phosphorylation of STAT (signal transducer and activator of transcription). Dimers of phosphorylated STAT translocate to the nucleus to selectively activate transcription of specific genes [20]. Importantly, both Jak1 and Jak2 are activated by mutated polycystin-1 and polycystin-2 proteins [21]; polycystin-1 also regulates STAT3 [21]. Therefore, the abnormal activity of Jak-STAT signaling and its ensuing immunomodulatory effects may represent the initial PKD mutation-induced alteration of immune responses.

The NF-κB protein complexes regulate transcription of genes involved in many biological processes including inflammation, as well as growth and apoptosis [22, 23]. The NF-κB proteins are located in the cytoplasm of the cell, and once activated, they undergo phosphorylation and enter the nucleus, where they activate transcription of many important regulators of immune responses including MCP-1, TNFα, IL-1α and β, and IL-6 [22, 23]. Several studies demonstrated upregulated NF-κB activation in human PKD and its animal and cell line models. For example, increased NF-κB activity in *Pkd1*-deficient cells was shown by multiple approaches including luciferase assay, increased expression of NF-κB protein p65, and presence of p65 in $Pkd1^{-/-}$ cyst-derived epithelial cells [24]. In addition, phosphorylated NK-κB was identified in cyst-derived epithelial cell nuclei and in tubules surrounding cysts in mutant *Pkd2* mice and human ADPKD kidneys [25]. Importantly, experimental inhibition of NF-κB activity in animal PKD models had important functional consequences – reduction of renal cystic indices [24]. While the exact mechanisms underlying these effects of NF-κB inhibition remain unknown, they may include alterations of renal development or repair. This speculation is supported by NF-κB inhibition-induced downregulation of nephron development regulators (e.g., Pax2) and planar cell polarity regulators (e.g., *Wnt7a* and *Wnt7b*) in the context of *Pkd2* deficiency [24, 26–28]; macrophage-derived Wnt7b is critical for kidney repair [29]. NF-κB is also involved in interactions with primary apical cilia as suggested by IL-1-induced primary cilia elongation [30, 31]. Together, these data point to a central role of the NF-κB pathway in modulation of PKD-associated immune responses.

Immune Cell Infiltrates in PKD

Macrophages

Renal interstitial inflammatory infiltrates are among most notable hallmarks of PKD. Among these infiltrating inflammatory cells, macrophages represent the most extensively studied cell type. However, rather than belonging to a uniform cell population, macrophages consist of highly heterogeneous cell types that may have specific roles in the pathobiology of PKD progression. For example, yolk sac-derived resident macrophages (characterized in humans by $CD16^{+}$ expression and in mice by $F4/80^{high}$ and $Cd11b^{low}$ expression) may be involved in disease progression from the earliest stages of renal cystic disease. These cells may provide critical supportive roles in renal tissue that resemble the effects of microglia on proper function of the brain (reviewed in [32]); microglia is another type of yolk sac-derived resident macrophage that operates in brain tissue (reviewed in [33]). For example, the resident renal macrophages play a central role in ureteric bud branching during kidney development [34]. Also, after injury, these cells cross endothelial vessels and are thought to monitor surrounding cells for injury [35]. The other distinct population of renal macrophages expresses $CD16^{-}$ in humans and $F4/80^{low}$ and $Cd11b^{high}$ (Myb-dependent population) in mice. These macrophages (or their earlier differentiation stage – monocytes) are derived from bone marrow. They infiltrate renal tissue after an injury (e.g., after renal ischemia-reperfusion injury; IRI) and at least initially differentiate into inflammatory macrophages [35, 36]. As the magnitude of injury-like responses increases in the cystic kidney increases over time (Fig. 6.2), these macrophages may elicit prominent effects on renal cystic disease progression in more advanced stages of the disease (Fig. 6.3).

In addition to the division of macrophages by their origin (the yolk sac-derived resident vs bone marrow-derived infiltrating macrophages), macrophage populations can also be defined by their "activation" pathway [37]. For example, the $Ly6C^{high}$ macrophages express IL-1β and Cxcl2 and are associated with the "classical" macrophage activation that is often designated as M1 activation. In contrast, the $Ly6C^{low}$ macrophages share gene expression characteristics with the alternative (or M2) macrophage activation pathway. The "classical" or "innate" M1 pathway is typically also associated with IFNγ activation and pathogen recognition by pattern recognition receptors (e.g., LPS by CD14-TLR4 complex). The $Ly6C^{high}$ monocytes are the major infiltrating cell subtype inducing injury after both IRI and unilateral ureteric obstruction (UUO) [35, 38]. The impact of these extrarenal cells is further enhanced by phenotypic and physiologic changes that these infiltrating cells trigger in macrophages and other mononuclear phagocytes that are already present in renal tissue [39–41]. In contrast to the M1 macrophages, the classification of the "alternative" M2 pathway is emerging to be more complex and likely involves several M2 macrophage subtypes (reviewed in [42]). However, at least a subset of M2 macrophages is believed to slow the production of pro-inflammatory cytokines and participate in tissue repair and fibrosis [35]. There is also another model suggesting that M1 macrophages are engaged in cleanup of necrotic or apoptotic cells

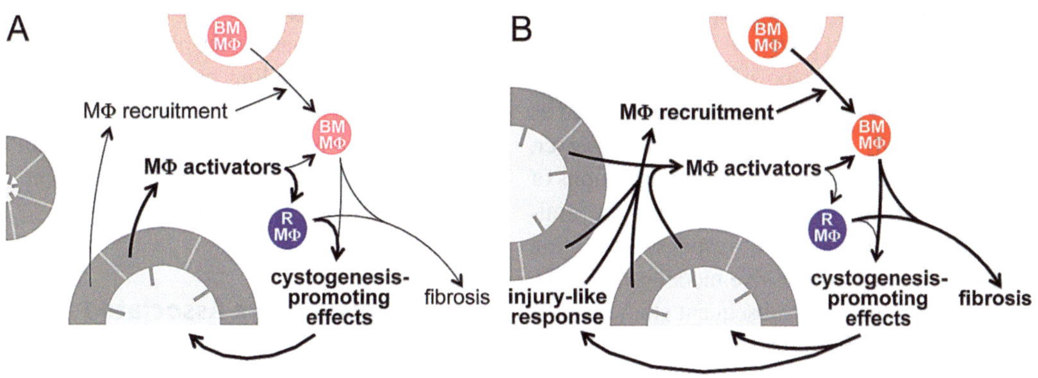

Fig. 6.3 Hypothetical differences in immunomodulatory responses in early and late stages of renal cystic disease progression. (**a**) In early stages, some immunomodulators released by affected renal tubular epithelial cells may promote cystogenesis through activation of immune cells that are already present in renal tissue; such cells likely include yolk sac-derived resident macrophages (R MΦ). (**b**) In more advanced stages of the disease progression, an injury-like response enhances recruitment of bone marrow-derived peripheral macrophages (BM MΦ) from blood; such cells likely become a dominant force in macrophage-enhanced cystogenesis and fibrosis seen in more advanced stages of cystic kidney disease

through phagocytosis. Once the M1 macrophages engulf these cells, they become M2-like macrophages. Then those M2 macrophages will secrete the anti-inflammatory cytokines to enhance the resolution of inflammation and to promote healing (reviewed in [43]).

While it remains to be determined whether the recruitment of macrophages to renal tissues is enhanced from the earliest stages of renal cystic disease progression, CD68-positive macrophages were observed in the renal interstitium in both early and late stages of ADPKD [44, 45] as well as in ARPKD [7, 46]. While in some cases recruitment of macrophages may be explained by cystic kidney infection [45], the presence of macrophages in adult ADPKD and newborn ADPKD patients without renal infections [47] further supports the idea that renal macrophage accumulation is an intrinsic feature of PKD rather than an antimicrobial response [37]. Similarly, multiple animal models including orthologous ADPKD and ARPKD models demonstrated accumulation of inflammatory cells in the renal interstitium suggesting it is a common factor in cystic renal diseases [37]. However, in some non-orthologous models, the cyst formation preceded the appearance of interstitial macrophages (e.g., in Lewis polycystic kidney (LPK) rat or in a *pcy* mouse) [48]. In contrast, CD68-positive macrophages have been detected in postnatal week 3 in heterozygous Han:SPRD-*Cy* rats when cystic dilatations were minimal [1, 49].

The predominant type of interstitial macrophages found in PKD kidneys is characterized as the alternatively activated M2 type (however, these studies did not consider the contributions of yolk sac-derived macrophages). The predominant M2 macrophage-like response was first noted in a rapidly progressive model of ARPKD, the *Cys1*^{cpk} mouse [7]. Subsequent studies in the orthologous *Pkd1*$^{fl/fl}$ *Pkhd1*-Cre mouse model validated the presence of alternatively activated macrophages in cystic kidney by demonstrating the predominance of Ly6C^{low} cells in cystic kidney infiltrates [35, 50]. Functional relevance of these macrophages in cystic disease progression was demonstrated by their depletion with liposomal clodronate in *Pkd1*$^{fl/fl}$ *Pkhd1*-Cre mice and *Cys1*^{cpk} mice [3, 51] This intervention decreased the circulating monocyte numbers and improved cystic indices as well as renal function in treated animals [50]. Reduction of proliferation in cystic kidneys with depletion of macrophages suggests that the tissue repair-promoting M2 macrophages enhance cystic disease progression at least in part as stimulators of cystic epithelial cell proliferation [8, 15].

Other Interstitial Inflammatory Cells in Cystic Kidneys

While macrophages are among the most extensively studied components of renal interstitial infiltrates, renal interstitium of ADPKD patients includes also CD45$^+$ and CD4$^+$ lymphocytes [44, 45]. Lymphocytes have also been identified in multiple mouse and rat PKD models [48, 52, 53]. Lymphocytes have been shown in other inflammatory renal states, such as IRI, to produce chemokines including TNFα and IFNγ, which may stimulate cystic disease progression-promoting inflammatory effects in PKD [37].

In addition to macrophages and lymphocytes, PKD was also associated with multiple other inflammatory cell types including mast cells, dendritic cells, and neutrophils (reviewed in [37]). These cells may promote cystic disease progression by enhancing immune and injury responses. For example, mast cells, which form a part of the renal interstitial infiltrates in ADPKD [54], produce chymases that play multiple roles in host defense including promotion of inflammation, chemotaxis, tissue remodeling, regulation of transcription of genes encoding specific immunomodulating factors, and conversion of angiotensin I to angiotensin II [55].

Immunomodulators Associated with PKD

As stated above, interstitial inflammation was found in PKD patients without a history of infection, indicating that it is likely an intrinsic component of PKD pathophysiology. Without an infectious nidus or presence of injury, PKD mutation-induced activation of immune signaling pathways (e.g., Jak-STAT or NF-κB) is likely central to initiation of PKD-associated immune responses. These intrinsic changes include the expression of chemokines, cytokines, and other immunomodulators that enhance recruitment of and activation of macrophages and inflammatory cells participating in multiple aspects of renal cystic disease progression and pathogenesis (e.g., initiation of cystogenesis and subsequent progressive growth of renal cysts, extracellular matrix changes, and fibrosis). While many immune response factors have been associated with PKD (reviewed in [37]), the most extensively studied ones include monocyte chemoattractant protein 1 (MCP-1), tumor necrosis alpha (TNFα), and complement component C3.

MCP-1 in PKD

MCP-1, a chemokine, mediates recruitment of monocytes and other inflammatory responses [56, 57]. This chemokine is secreted by multiple cell types including tubular epithelial cells and interstitial cells including different types of macrophages [58]. It has been implicated in the pathogenesis of many renal diseases (reviewed in [59, 60]) and recognized as a potential biomarker of acute kidney injury [61]. In ADPKD, increased levels of MCP-1 were found in renal cyst fluid (vs urine) [2]. Additionally, MCP-1 was associated with worse renal function [2, 62], higher height-adjusted total kidney volume (TKV), and PKD1 (vs PKD2) genotype [62]. In multivariable models, elevated MCP-1 was strongly associated with declining glomerular filtration rate (GFR) and served as a predictor of stage 3 chronic kidney disease [62–64]. On the basis of these findings, urinary MCP1 may be considered a marker of disease progression in patients with ADPKD.

TNFα in PKD

TNFα is a canonical immune cytokine that activates inflammatory signaling and plays important roles in multiple biological processes and clinical conditions (reviewed in [65]). It has been also implicated in the pathogenesis of PKD, where it interferes with processing and membrane presentation of polycystin-2 [66]. In ADPKD, TNFα is present in renal cysts, in half of them at concentrations similar to that of synovial fluid in psoriatic arthritis, and its intracystic levels correlated with the size of renal cysts [17, 66, 67]. TNFα enhanced cystogenesis in co-culture of *Pkd2*$^{-/-}$ and wild-type embryonic kidney explants, and intraperitoneal TNFα administration increased renal cystic disease severity in *Pkd2*$^{-/-}$ mice [66]. Importantly, TNFα inhibition with etanercept attenuated cytogenesis in *Pkd2*$^{-/-}$ mice [66]; however, this treatment was ineffective in animal models with established cystic kidney disease (*Pkhd1*^{PCK} rat and PKD2 $^{(ws25/w183)}$ mouse) [68].

Complement System in PKD

The complement system is activated by three independent pathways that converge on C3 [69]. C3 convertase cleaves C5, activating the common complement pathway (C6–C9). In addition, complement component split products have multiple biologic effects [70]. For example, activated C3 fragment C3b binds via its reactive thioester to cell surface carbohydrates or immune aggregates and has opsonic and immunoregulatory functions. Further cleavage of C3b generates iC3b, a major ligand for complement receptor 3 [CR3, also called macrophage receptor 1; Mac-1 [71]], an essential regulator of key cellular functions in monocytic/macrophage cells including their survival and alternative (M2; repair and fibrosis-promoting) activation [72] that appears to play a central role in cystic disease progression in PKD models [3].

The first association of abnormal complement system activation with the pace of cystic disease progression was based on genome-wide expression studies in the *Cys1*^{cpk} model of ARPKD [7]. Similarly, transcriptomic analyses of epithelial cells from *PKD1* renal cysts showed increased expression of multiple complement system genes [19]. Both of these studies identified *C3* among the most highly overexpressed complement genes, and subsequent mass spectrometry analyses have identified C3 as the most abundant protein in the cyst fluid from *Pkd1*-deficient mice and as one of the most abundant proteins in cyst fluid from ADPKD patients [73, 74]. While C3 is expressed in inactive form, cyst fluid and urine from ADPKD patients contained C3 fragments that were activated [75]. Functional relevance of C3 in PKD pathogenesis was demonstrated in crosses of PKD models with C3-deficient ($C3^{-/-}$) mice [5, 76], by administration of nonselective C3 inhibitors in several PKD models [77–79], and by association of hypoactive C3 variants with slower progression to ESRD among PKD patients [80].

Complex Pathobiology of Immune Effects in PKD

Initially, immune changes associated with PKD were attributed to various consequences of advanced renal cystic disease and were therefore expected to alter only this stage of the disease progression (e.g., inflammatory infiltrates in advanced disease stages in the Han:SPRD-*Cy* rat are concurrent with severe interstitial fibrosis and cyst formation [81]). However, overexpression of a large number of innate immune factors was also observed in juvenile mice with a rapid (vs slow) pace of renal cystic disease progression, e.g., in the $Cys1^{cpk}$ mouse model of ARPKD where a variability of cystic disease progression pace was induced by different admixtures of two genetic backgrounds [7]. These data suggested that immune responses have functionally relevant roles in the pathogenesis of renal cystic disease progression. This hypothesis was further supported by cystogenesis-promoting effects of TNFα in co-cultures of both $Pkd2^{+/-}$ heterozygous and wild-type kidneys [66]. In addition to potentially leading to worsening cystogenesis, abnormal immune responses in PKD may also further renal injury after it is already initiated. It may also contribute to adverse changes in extracellular matrix and facilitate the development of interstitial fibrosis. For example, in UUO, the $Ly6C^{low}$ macrophages, that are also present in transgenic *Pkd1* and *Pkd2* kidneys [50], express markers of pro-fibrotic activity (such as Ccl17, Ccl22, Igf-1, and PDGF-B) [38].

Immune responses may also mediate disease progression by affecting the primary cilia and/or function of primary cilia-associated proteins [37]. For example, exposure to IL-1 leads to cilia elongation, which could amplify the production of PGE2, a prostanoid with potent immunomodulatory properties [30]. Also, collecting duct cells treated with TNFα had diminished expression of polycystin-2 in the primary cilium but increased polycystin-2 expression in the nuclei [66]. TNFα also disrupted the interaction between polycystin-1 and polycystin-2, which normally forms a complex that mediates mechanosensory responses, and disruption of this interaction could potentially enhance cystogenesis [37, 82].

While multiple sources point to adverse effects of immune responses in the pathogenesis of cystic disease progression, immune responses may also have restorative potential. Cowley et al. suggested chemoattractants induced by cyst formation may be a signal to repair the renal parenchyma [1]. For example, the PKD-associated alternatively activated $Ly6C^{low}$ cells [50] were linked with protective pro-angiogenic factors in skeletal injury and anti-inflammatory markers in cardiac injury [83, 84]. However, the activation of reparative pathways in PKD may have dual protective and disease-promoting outcomes. While macrophage activity is not always predictable based on phenotype [85], the repair-promoting M2 macrophages may directly stimulate PKD progression by enhancing the proliferation of renal cystic epithelia [3]. Chronic activation of such responses in cystic kidneys may lead to “futile” repair that further exacerbates the rate of disease progression by enhancing cyst formation and interstitial fibrosis (reviewed in [86]). Further studies are needed to clarify these complex relationships.

Potential Immune Function-Modulating Therapies for PKD

While there is no FDA-approved therapy available for treatment of PKD, several drugs are or have been evaluated as potential PKD therapeutics in clinical studies (at this point the vasopressin receptor 2 antagonist tolvaptan [85] is in the most advanced phase 3b of clinical testing). Unfortunately, so far most clinical studies that may have altered immune responses did not demonstrate substantial efficacy in slowing the disease progression (e.g., in the case of everolimus, lisinopril, and telmisartan [87–89]). A potential exception is treatment with somatostatin agonists (somatostatin receptor is also expressed on lymphocytes and macrophages), because in initial studies it appeared to reduce the pace of ADPKD progression [90, 91]. However, it should be noted that the primary effect of somatostatin agonists may be due to inhibition of cyclic adenosine 3′,5′ phosphate production through activation of a G-inhibitory receptor.

A number of anti-inflammatory compounds ameliorated disease progression in animal models of PKD. Glucocorticoids administered to DBA/FG-pcy mice reduced cystic indices, improved renal function, and diminished interstitial infiltration of monocytes [92]. Rosmarinic acid that covalently binds C3 complement has reduced cystic indices and slowed renal function loss in *Pkd1* mouse and in Han:SPRD-*Cy* rat models [78]. Similarly, mycophenolate mofetil administered to Han:SPRD-*Cy* rats reduced cyst area, improved renal function, and decreased inflammation and fibrosis [93]. Additional promising cystic disease progression-inhibiting effects were noted with other drugs that have immunomodulating properties, such as COX-2 inhibitors [94], PPARγ agonists [95], or vasopressin V2 receptor antagonists [96]. However, Cowley et al. have reported that some immunosuppressants such as azathioprine or cyclosporine failed to improve renal disease in Han:SPRD-*Cy* rats, indicating that potential therapeutic benefits in PKD may be tied to targeting only a subset of specific immune pathways [37].

While many studies that targeted immune pathways in animal models appear promising, it remains to be determined if similar effects can be achieved in PKD patients. Differences in pharmacokinetics, use of excessive drug doses in animal models, and differences in immune responses between rodents and humans are examples of factors that may be at least in part responsible for a failure of promising candidate therapeutics in clinical studies. For example, angiotensin receptor blockade (ARB) administered to DBA/2FG-pcy mice reduced cyst areas [97]; however, it failed to slow disease progression in clinical testing [87]. Similarly, mTOR inhibition with sirolimus administered to Han:SPRD-*Cy* rats diminished cyst areas, improved renal function, and reduced inflammation and fibrosis in animal models [93], but did not induce significant changes in disease progression in two ADPKD clinical trials [88, 89]. Therefore, although some immune function-modulating drugs appear attractive as therapeutics in preclinical studies in animal PKD models, their effects will require a critical review before a subsequent evaluation in clinical trials.

Renal Fibrosis in PKD

Progressive tubulointerstitial fibrosis is recognized as a common mechanism by which renal injuries of diverse etiologies lead to end-stage renal disease. Therefore, similar to many other disorders, interstitial fibrosis is a hallmark of advanced cystic kidney diseases. Functional relevance of fibrotic changes in PKD is suggested by a strong association between the degree of fibrosis and rate of disease progression to ESRD [44, 98, 99]. However, the mechanisms underlying the pathogenesis of fibrosis in renal disorders are likely complex and incompletely understood even in genetically well-defined disorders like PKD.

PKD-Associated Changes in Extracellular Matrix (ECM)

The hallmark of tubulointerstitial fibrosis is accumulation of ECM proteins such as collagen I. Similar to many renal disorders, ECM abnormalities were also found in kidneys from PKD patients and from orthologous and non-orthologous animal PKD models [100–104]. These changes included abnormal ECM deposition in basement membranes and in the interstitium. While ECM changes were often described in end-stage kidneys, abnormal renal ECM composition and increased thickness of basement membranes were also observed in pre-dialysis ADPKD patients [105]. The ADPKD-associated changes include abnormalities in ECM production, composition, and turnover and include differences in the content of collagen types I and III, basement membrane collagen type IV, fibronectin, and heparin sulfate proteoglycan (HSPG) [101]. Similarly, abnormal expression of interstitial collagen type I, III, and IV genes was identified. These abnormalities were most commonly noted in the basement membrane structures surrounding cysts and interstitial fibroblasts [105].

Regulation of ECM Production in PKD

While many factors regulate the activity of pro-fibrotic pathways, recent studies in animal models indicate that polycystins regulate the production of ECM directly and that inadequate regulation of this process is responsible for PKD-associated vascular abnormalities [106]. Importantly, upregulation of the central regulator of ECM production transforming growth factor β (TGFβ) [105] was caused simply by *Pkd1* haploinsufficiency, and the loss of *PKD1* alone was also sufficient to induce a heightened responsiveness to TGFβ [107]. These observations may explain the enhanced TGFβ pathway signaling seen in PKD patients and *Pkd1* animal models. Similarly, polycystins regulated collagen production in zebra fish [108]. Together, these data suggest that the hallmark PKD-associated ECM changes represent an evolutionary conserved direct consequence of polycystin dysfunction.

In addition to the direct effects of cystoproteins on expression and responsiveness to TGFβ, PKD-related changes in ECM production were associated with other interstitial fibrosis modulators. They include epithelial growth factor (EGF), fibroblast growth factor-1 (FGF-1), and hepatocyte growth factor [100, 109–111]. While levels of these pro-fibrotic factors increased in PKD over time and their highest levels were often found in end-stage or near-end-stage PKD kidneys (e.g., in the case of TGFβ and FGF-1 [107, 110]), pro-fibrotic factors may alter the pathobiology of even very early stages of PKD progression. For example, overexpression of the bone morphogenic protein receptor activin receptor-like kinase (ALK)-3, as well as *Bmp-7* knockout, triggers the formation of renal cysts in mice [112, 113]. Importantly, in complementary studies BMP-7 treatment attenuated renal cystic disease progression in the *Nek8*^{jck} mouse model, and soluble activin type IIB receptor treatment effectively blocked cyst formation in a mouse *Pkd1* model [114, 115]. Similarly, EGF is another important regulator of cystic epithelial cell proliferation [100, 109], and targeting its pathway is currently being explored for therapeutic development in PKD.

Regulation of ECM Turnover in PKD

Interstitial fibrosis is a consequence of increased ECM production; however, inadequate matrix degradation represents another key regulator of the fibrogenic process [116]. Among many factors that influence ECM turnover, matrix metalloproteinases (MMPs) and tissue inhibitors of metalloproteinases (TIMPs) were perhaps most extensively studied in multiple renal disorders, including PKD. Consistent with extensive ECM changes observed in cystic kidneys, abnormal renal expression of MMPs and TIMPs was also described in PKD patients and several PKD models. Among many reported abnormalities in expression of multiple MMPs and TIMPs, several were consistently reported across different models of renal cystic disease. They include overexpression of MMP-2 in kidneys or tubules from ADPKD and ARPKD mouse models (e.g., mutant *Pkd1* mice, *Cys1*^{cpk} mice [107, 117]) and MMP-14 overexpression in kidneys from the *Pkd1* mouse model, the *Cys1*^{cpk} mice, and minimally cystic 3-week-old Han:SPRD-*Cy* rats [7, 107, 118]. In human studies, ADPKD-associated increases in serum levels of MMP-1, MMP-9, and TIMP-1 were noted [119]. In addition, expression of several MMPs was consistent in both pre-dialysis and end-stage ADPKD kidneys (e.g., MMP-2, MMP-3, MMP-9, TIMP-1 and TIMP-2, and plasminogen activator inhibitor-1 (PAI-1) [105]).

The functional consequences of changes in ECM turnover regulators in PKD are not fully understood. However, they likely include changes in multiple cellular functions, including proliferation and differentiation [105]. Their additional activities may resemble effects of a collagen I breakdown fragment proline-glycine-proline (PGP) in lungs. PGP is a key regulator of inflammatory neutrophil accumulation, a process that is central to the pathogenesis of chronic obstructive pulmonary disease [120]. Since one of the two MMPs that participate in the generation of PGP is also upregulated in ADPKD (MMP-9; [105]), PGP or other ECM collagen fragments may exert important immunoregulatory and disease progression-modulating effects also in PKD kidneys.

The interactions of cells with ECM or its breakdown products are mediated by specialized matrix receptors. They include chemokine receptors, as well as integrins and syndecans [121] that often interact with ECM components at focal adhesion complexes [122]. These complexes activate intracellular signaling pathways involved in regulation of major cellular regulatory processes, including gene expression [122, 123]. The complex interplay between ECM, its degradation fragments' receptors, signaling pathways, and ensuing selective transcriptional activation of specific genes provides a unique microenvironment that modulates local cellular responses [105]. Changes observed in ADPKD that point to specific abnormalities in interactions between cystic epithelial cells and ECM include increased expression of integrins α2β1, α8, αv, β4, syndecan-4, as well as integrin-associated focal adhesion kinase [103, 104, 124–126]. Some of these changes were identified in pre-dialysis ADKPD cystic epithelia. Induction of renal cyst formation in response to disruption of these pathways (e.g., by genetic targeting of β1 integrin in mice; [127]) and the fact that ECM receptors may localize on primary cilia (integrins α and β; [128]) point to functional relevance of cell-ECM interactions in the pathogenesis of PKD.

Roles of Specialized Cell Types in Regulation of ECM in PKD

Myofibroblasts are specialized cells that can exert large contractile forces, mediate wound healing, and substantially contribute to the expansion of ECM and development of tissue fibrosis [129]. A hallmark of the myofibroblast phenotype is the expression of cytoskeletal alpha smooth muscle actin (αSMA). While αSMA expressing interstitial cells were found in focal areas in early ADPKD kidneys, they become widespread in end-stage ADPKD kidneys [105]. αSMA-positive cells were also found in kidneys from several PKD models including *Pkd1*-deficient mice [107]. Similarly, expression of genes encoding smooth muscle proteins, a signature of myofibroblasts, was found in end-stage ADPKD kidneys and kidneys from Han:SPRD-*Cy* rats [19, 118]. Although the origin of renal PKD myofibroblasts remains unknown, it appears that these cells differentiate from several different precursors. For example, they may be derived from resident interstitial fibroblasts [110]. Such transformation may be regulated by TGFβ [130] or perhaps by PKD-related alteration of calcium flux [131]. Myofibroblasts may also differentiate from infiltrating bone marrow-derived inflammatory cells and fibrocytes (reviewed in [132]).

Fibroblasts may differentiate into myofibroblasts after appropriate stimulation. This stimulation may be enhanced in PKD as suggested by ADPKD and disease stage-specific differences in proliferative response to ECM-promoting factors such as TGFβ, platelet-derived growth factor (PDGF), FGF-1, and insulin-like growth factors (IGF) I and II [110]. These changes also included increased secretion of FGF-1 and overexpression of TGFβ, MMP-2, and heat shock protein 47 (HSP47). Similar changes in proliferative response and TGFβ pathway activation were observed in mouse embryonic fibroblasts with *Pkd1* defects [107, 133]. In addition, fibroblast differentiation to myofibroblasts may be modulated by macrophages that secrete growth factors including PDGF, FGF-2, insulin-like growth factor-binding protein 5, and galectin 3 [43].

Fibrocytes represent another ECM-producing cell type. They differentiate from peripheral blood leukocytes and express both hematopoietic (e.g., CD45) and stromal cell (e.g., collagen type I) markers, as well as multiple chemokine receptors [132]. Their differentiation is enhanced by cytokines associated with repair and fibrosis-promoting Th2-type immune response, and it is inhibited by pro-inflammatory Th1-type cytokines [134]. Since the pace of renal cystic disease progression was associated with the Th2-type immune response, fibrocyte differentiation may be enhanced in cystic kidneys and contribute to the PKD-associated ECM abnormalities.

Several inflammatory cell types are relevant to the regulation of ECM characteristics in PKD. They include macrophages, a heterogeneous group of cell types that differ by origin and activation. Among them, a subset of macrophages that are associated with Th2 cytokine-driven responses (an M2 type) promotes renal tissue repair and fibrosis (reviewed in [135, 136]). This subset of macrophages was associated with PKD [46, 51] but also with a rapid (vs slow) pace of renal cystic disease progression in the *Cys1*^{cpk} model of ARPKD [7]. The pro-fibrotic bone marrow-derived macrophages express CD11b, and this feature is often used for their identification [38]. However, some macrophage types may have opposite, fibrosis-attenuating effects [137]. In addition to macrophages, renal ECM abnormalities and fibrosis may be enhanced by CD11c-expressing dendritic cells [138, 139], lymphocytes [138], and mast cells [140].

Renal tubular and vascular epithelial cells or macrophages can also transition to a myofibroblast phenotype through a process called epithelial-mesenchymal transition (EMT) (reviewed in [141]). TGFβ1 is recognized as a potent EMT inducer. However, EMT likely makes negligible contributions to the pathogenesis of renal cystic disorder as suggested by studies in *Pkd1* mouse model of ADPKD [107].

Prognostic Value of ECM Abnormality Assessment in PKD

Since abnormal contents of collagen I- and III-derived fragments were recently identified in the urine of young, dialysis-independent ADPKD patients [142], ECM remodeling may play an important role in PKD pathogenesis and represents an attractive target for therapeutic development and for identification of predictive biomarkers. A follow-up study based on analyses of small urinary peptides (mostly urinary collagen fragments) by capillary electrophoresis-coupled mass spectrometry (CE-MS) provided further support for this hypothesis (urinary proteomic CE-MS score predicted ADPKD severity reflected by height-adjusted total kidney volume with $r = 0.415$ and $p < 0.0001$) [143].

References

1. Cowley BD Jr, Ricardo SD, Nagao S, Diamond JR. Increased renal expression of monocyte chemoattractant protein-1 and osteopontin in ADPKD in rats. Kidney Int. 2001;60(6):2087–96. PubMed PMID: 11737583.
2. Zheng D, Wolfe M, Cowley BD Jr, Wallace DP, Yamaguchi T, Grantham JJ. Urinary excretion of monocyte chemoattractant protein-1 in autosomal dominant polycystic kidney disease. J Am Soc Nephrol. 2003;14(10):2588–95. PubMed PMID: 14514736
3. Karihaloo A, Koraishy F, Huen SC, Lee Y, Merrick D, Caplan MJ, et al. Macrophages promote cyst growth in polycystic kidney disease. J Am Soc Nephrol. 2011.; Epub 2011/09/17. doi: ASN.2011010084 [pii] 10.1681/ASN.2011010084. PubMed PMID: 21921140.

4. Flores D, Battini L, Gusella GL, Rohatgi R. Fluid shear stress induces renal epithelial gene expression through polycystin-2-dependent trafficking of extracellular regulated kinase. Nephron Physiol. 2011;117(4):p27–36. Epub 2010/11/27. https://doi.org/10.1159/000321640. PubMed PMID: 21109758; PubMed Central PMCID: PMC2997441.
5. Zhou J, Ouyang X, Schoeb TR, Bolisetty S, Cui X, Mrug S, et al. Kidney injury accelerates cystogenesis via pathways modulated by heme oxygenase and complement. J Am Soc Nephrol. 2012;23(7):1161–71. Epub 2012/04/21. https://doi.org/10.1681/ASN.2011050442. PubMed PMID: 22518005; PubMed Central PMCID: PMC3380643.
6. Song XW, Di Giovanni V, He N, Wang KR, Ingram A, Rosenblum ND, et al. Systems biology of autosomal dominant polycystic kidney disease (ADPKD): computational identification of gene expression pathways and integrated regulatory networks. Hum Mol Genet. 2009;18(13):2328–43. https://doi.org/10.1093/Hmg/Ddp165. PubMed PMID: ISI:000266961400002.
7. Mrug M, Zhou J, Woo Y, Cui X, Szalai AJ, Novak J, et al. Overexpression of innate immune response genes in a model of recessive polycystic kidney disease. Kidney Int. 2008;73(1):63–76. Epub 2007/10/26. doi: 5002627 [pii] 10.1038/sj.ki.5002627. PubMed PMID: 17960140.
8. Grantham JJ, Mulamalla S, Swenson-Fields KI. Why kidneys fail in autosomal dominant polycystic kidney disease. Nat Rev Nephrol. 2011;7(10):556–66. Epub 2011/08/25. https://doi.org/10.1038/nrneph.2011.109. PubMed PMID: 21862990.
9. Chevalier RL. Obstructive nephropathy: lessons from cystic kidney disease. Nephron. 2000;84(1):6–12. Epub 2000/01/25. doi: 45532. PubMed PMID: 10644902.
10. Klahr S, Morrissey J. Obstructive nephropathy and renal fibrosis: the role of bone morphogenic protein-7 and hepatocyte growth factor. Kidney Int Suppl. 2003;87:S105–12. Epub 2003/10/09. PubMed PMID: 14531782.
11. Chevalier RL, Thornhill BA, Forbes MS, Kiley SC. Mechanisms of renal injury and progression of renal disease in congenital obstructive nephropathy. Pediatr Nephrol. 2010;25(4):687–97. Epub 2009/10/22. https://doi.org/10.1007/s00467-009-1316-5. PubMed PMID: 19844747.
12. Xu R, Franchi F, Miller B, Crane JA, Peterson KM, Psaltis PJ, et al. Polycystic kidneys have decreased vascular density: a micro-CT study. Microcirculation. 2013;20(2):183–9. Epub 2012/11/22. https://doi.org/10.1111/micc.12022. PubMed PMID: 23167921; PubMed Central PMCID: PMC3698948.
13. Maser RL, Vassmer D, Magenheimer BS, Calvet JP. Oxidant stress and reduced antioxidant enzyme protection in polycystic kidney disease. J Am Soc Nephrol: JASN. 2002;13(4):991–9. Epub 2002/03/26. PubMed PMID: 11912258
14. Menon V, Rudym D, Chandra P, Miskulin D, Perrone R, Sarnak M. Inflammation, oxidative stress, and insulin resistance in polycystic kidney disease. Clin J Am Soc Nephrol. 2011;6(1):7–13. Epub 2010/09/11. doi: CJN.04140510 [pii] 10.2215/CJN.04140510. PubMed PMID: 20829421; PubMed Central PMCID: PMC3022250.
15. Lee S, Huen S, Nishio H, Nishio S, Lee HK, Choi BS, et al. Distinct macrophage phenotypes contribute to kidney injury and repair. J Am Soc Nephrol. 2011;22(2):317–26. Epub 2011/02/04. doi: 22/2/317 [pii] 10.1681/ASN.2009060615. PubMed PMID: 21289217; PubMed Central PMCID: PMC3029904.
16. Prasad S, McDaid JP, Tam FW, Haylor JL, Ong AC. Pkd2 dosage influences cellular repair responses following ischemia-reperfusion injury. Am J Pathol. 2009;175(4):1493–503. Epub 2009/09/05. https://doi.org/10.2353/ajpath.2009.090227. PubMed PMID: 19729489; PubMed Central PMCID: PMC2751546.
17. Gardner KD Jr, Burnside JS, Elzinga LW, Locksley RM. Cytokines in fluids from polycystic kidneys. Kidney Int. 1991;39(4):718–24. Epub 1991/04/01. PubMed PMID: 2051729.
18. Zhou J, Ouyang X, Cui X, Schoeb TR, Smythies LE, Johnson MR, et al. Renal CD14 expression correlates with the progression of cystic kidney disease. Kidney Int. 2010;78(6):550–60. Epub 2010/06/18. doi: ki2010175 [pii] 10.1038/ki.2010.175. PubMed PMID: 20555320.
19. Song X, Di Giovanni V, He N, Wang K, Ingram A, Rosenblum ND, et al. Systems biology of autosomal dominant polycystic kidney disease (ADPKD): computational identification of gene expression pathways and integrated regulatory networks. Hum Mol Genet. 2009;18(13):2328–43. Epub 2009/04/07. https://doi.org/10.1093/hmg/ddp165. PubMed PMID: 19346236.
20. Schindler C, Levy DE, Decker T. JAK-STAT signaling: from interferons to cytokines. J Biol Chem 2007;282(28):20059–63. Epub 2007/05/16. https://doi.org/10.1074/jbc.R700016200. PubMed PMID: 17502367.
21. Bhunia AK, Piontek K, Boletta A, Liu L, Qian F, Xu PN, et al. PKD1 induces p21(waf1) and regulation of the cell cycle via direct activation of the JAK-STAT signaling pathway in a process requiring PKD2. Cell. 2002;109(2):157–68. Epub 2002/05/15. PubMed PMID: 12007403
22. Hayden MS, Ghosh S. NF-kappaB, the first quarter-century: remarkable progress and outstanding questions. Genes Dev. 2012;26(3):203–34. Epub 2012/02/04. https://doi.org/10.1101/gad.183434.111. PubMed PMID: 22302935; PubMed Central PMCID: PMC3278889.
23. Pahl HL. Activators and target genes of Rel/NF-kappaB transcription factors. Oncogene. 1999;18(49):6853–66. Epub 1999/12/22. https://doi.org/10.1038/sj.onc.1203239. PubMed PMID: 10602461.

24. Qin S, Taglienti M, Cai L, Zhou J, Kreidberg JA. c-Met and NF-kappaB-dependent overexpression of Wnt7a and -7b and Pax2 promotes cystogenesis in polycystic kidney disease. J Am Soc Nephrol: JASN. 2012;23(8):1309–18. Epub 2012/06/09. https://doi.org/10.1681/ASN.2011030277. PubMed PMID: 22677559; PubMed Central PMCID: PMC3402281.
25. Park EY, Seo MJ, Park JH. Effects of specific genes activating RAGE on polycystic kidney disease. Am J Nephrol. 2010;32(2):169–78. Epub 2010/07/08. https://doi.org/10.1159/000315859. PubMed PMID: 20606421.
26. Bacallao RL, McNeill H. Cystic kidney diseases and planar cell polarity signaling. Clin Genet. 2009;75(2):107–17. Epub 2009/02/14. https://doi.org/10.1111/j.1399-0004.2008.01148.x. PubMed PMID: 19215242.
27. Torres M, Gomez-Pardo E, Dressler GR, Gruss P. Pax-2 controls multiple steps of urogenital development. Development. 1995;121(12):4057–65. Epub 1995/12/01. PubMed PMID: 8575306.
28. Horster MF, Braun GS, Huber SM. Embryonic renal epithelia: induction, nephrogenesis, and cell differentiation. Physiol Rev. 1999;79(4):1157–91. Epub 1999/10/03. PubMed PMID: 10508232.
29. Lin SL, Li B, Rao S, Yeo EJ, Hudson TE, Nowlin BT, et al. Macrophage Wnt7b is critical for kidney repair and regeneration. Proc Natl Acad Sci U S A. 2010;107(9):4194–9. Epub 2010/02/18. https://doi.org/10.1073/pnas.0912228107. PubMed PMID: 20160075; PubMed Central PMCID: PMC2840080.
30. Wann AK, Knight MM. Primary cilia elongation in response to interleukin-1 mediates the inflammatory response. Cell Mol Life Sci CMLS. 2012;69(17):2967–77. Epub 2012/04/07. https://doi.org/10.1007/s00018-012-0980-y. PubMed PMID: 22481441; PubMed Central PMCID: PMC3417094.
31. Wann AK, Chapple JP, Knight MM. The primary cilium influences interleukin-1beta-induced NFkappaB signalling by regulating IKK activity. Cell Signal. 2014;26(8):1735–42. Epub 2014/04/15. https://doi.org/10.1016/j.cellsig.2014.04.004. PubMed PMID: 24726893; PubMed Central PMCID: PMC4064300.
32. Nayak D, Roth TL, McGavern DB. Microglia development and function. Annu Rev Immunol. 2014;32:367–402. Epub 2014/01/30. https://doi.org/10.1146/annurev-immunol-032713-120240. PubMed PMID: 24471431.
33. Gomez Perdiguero E, Klapproth K, Schulz C, Busch K, Azzoni E, Crozet L, et al. Tissue-resident macrophages originate from yolk-sac-derived erythro-myeloid progenitors. Nature. 2015;518(7540):547–51. Epub 2014/12/04. https://doi.org/10.1038/nature13989. PubMed PMID: 25470051.
34. Rae F, Woods K, Sasmono T, Campanale N, Taylor D, Ovchinnikov DA, et al. Characterisation and trophic functions of murine embryonic macrophages based upon the use of a Csf1r-EGFP transgene reporter. Dev Biol. 2007;308(1):232–46. Epub 2007/06/29. https://doi.org/10.1016/j.ydbio.2007.05.027. PubMed PMID: 17597598.
35. Rees AJ. Monocyte and macrophage biology: an overview. Semin Nephrol. 2010;30(3):216–33. Epub 2010/07/14. https://doi.org/10.1016/j.semnephrol.2010.03.002. PubMed PMID: 20620668.
36. Li L, Huang L, Sung SS, Vergis AL, Rosin DL, Rose CE, Jr., et al. The chemokine receptors CCR2 and CX3CR1 mediate monocyte/macrophage trafficking in kidney ischemia-reperfusion injury. Kidney Int. 2008;74(12):1526–37. Epub 2008/10/10. https://doi.org/10.1038/ki.2008.500. PubMed PMID: 18843253; PubMed Central PMCID: PMC2652647.
37. Ta MH, Harris DC, Rangan GK. Role of interstitial inflammation in the pathogenesis of polycystic kidney disease. Nephrology (Carlton). 2013;18(5):317–30. Epub 2013/03/02. https://doi.org/10.1111/nep.12045. PubMed PMID: 23448509.
38. Lin SL, Castano AP, Nowlin BT, Lupher ML, Jr., Duffield JS. Bone marrow Ly6Chigh monocytes are selectively recruited to injured kidney and differentiate into functionally distinct populations. J Immunol. 2009;183(10):6733–43. Epub 2009/10/30. https://doi.org/10.4049/jimmunol.0901473. PubMed PMID: 19864592.
39. Nelson PJ, Rees AJ, Griffin MD, Hughes J, Kurts C, Duffield J. The renal mononuclear phagocytic system. J Am Soc Nephrol: JASN. 2012;23(2):194–203. Epub 2011/12/03. https://doi.org/10.1681/ASN.2011070680. PubMed PMID: 22135312; PubMed Central PMCID: PMC3269181.
40. Lim AK, Tesch GH. Inflammation in diabetic nephropathy. Mediat Inflamm. 2012;2012:146154. Epub 2012/09/13. https://doi.org/10.1155/2012/146154. PubMed PMID: 22969168; PubMed Central PMCID: PMC3432398.
41. Praga M, Gonzalez E. Acute interstitial nephritis. Kidney Int. 2010;77(11):956–61. Epub 2010/03/26. https://doi.org/10.1038/ki.2010.89. PubMed PMID: 20336051.
42. Martinez FO, Gordon S. The M1 and M2 paradigm of macrophage activation: time for reassessment. F1000prime Reports. 2014;6:13. Epub 2014/03/29. https://doi.org/10.12703/P6-13. PubMed PMID: 24669294; PubMed Central PMCID: PMC3944738.
43. Huen SC, Cantley LG. Macrophage-mediated injury and repair after ischemic kidney injury. Pediatr Nephrol. 2015;30(2):199–209. Epub 2014/01/21. https://doi.org/10.1007/s00467-013-2726-y. PubMed PMID: 24442822.
44. Zeier M, Fehrenbach P, Geberth S, Mohring K, Waldherr R, Ritz E. Renal histology in polycystic kidney disease with incipient and advanced renal failure. Kidney Int. 1992;42(5):1259–65. PubMed PMID: 1453612.
45. Ibrahim S. Increased apoptosis and proliferative capacity are early events in cyst formation in autosomal-dominant, polycystic kidney disease. Sci World J. 2007;7:1757–67. Epub 2007/11/28. https://

doi.org/10.1100/tsw.2007.274. PubMed PMID: 18040538.
46. Mrug M, Zhou J, Guay-Woodford LM, Smythies LE. Renal macrophages in autosomal recessive polycystic kidney disease. Nephrology (Carlton). 2013;18(11):746. Epub 2014/02/28. https://doi.org/10.1111/nep.12153. PubMed PMID: 24571748.
47. Grantham JJ. Pathogenesis of autosomal dominant polycystic kidney disease: recent developments. Contrib Nephrol. 1997;122:1–9. Epub 1997/01/01. PubMed PMID: 9399029.
48. Takahashi H, Calvet JP, Dittemore-Hoover D, Yoshida K, Grantham JJ, Gattone VH 2nd. A hereditary model of slowly progressive polycystic kidney disease in the mouse. J Am Soc Nephrol: JASN. 1991;1(7):980–9. Epub 1991/01/01. PubMed PMID: 1883968.
49. Cowley BD Jr, Gudapaty S, Kraybill AL, Barash BD, Harding MA, Calvet JP, et al. Autosomal-dominant polycystic kidney disease in the rat. Kidney Int. 1993;43(3):522–34. Epub 1993/03/01. PubMed PMID: 8455352.
50. Karihaloo A, Koraishy F, Huen SC, Lee Y, Merrick D, Caplan MJ, et al. Macrophages promote cyst growth in polycystic kidney disease. J Am Soc Nephrol: JASN. 2011;22(10):1809–14. Epub 2011/09/17. https://doi.org/10.1681/ASN.2011010084. PubMed PMID: 21921140; PubMed Central PMCID: PMC3187181.
51. Swenson-Fields KI, Vivian CJ, Salah SM, Peda JD, Davis BM, van Rooijen N, et al. Macrophages promote polycystic kidney disease progression. Kidney Int. 2013;83(5):855–64. Epub 2013/02/21. https://doi.org/10.1038/ki.2012.446. PubMed PMID: 23423256.
52. Vogler C, Homan S, Pung A, Thorpe C, Barker J, Birkenmeier EH, et al. Clinical and pathologic findings in two new allelic murine models of polycystic kidney disease. J Am Soc Nephrol. 1999;10(12):2534–9. PubMed PMID: 10589692.
53. Kaspareit-Rittinghausen J, Rapp K, Deerberg F, Wcislo A, Messow C. Hereditary polycystic kidney disease associated with osteorenal syndrome in rats. Vet Pathol. 1989;26(3):195–201. Epub 1989/05/01. PubMed PMID: 2763410.
54. McPherson EA, Luo Z, Brown RA, LeBard LS, Corless CC, Speth RC, et al. Chymase-like angiotensin II-generating activity in end-stage human autosomal dominant polycystic kidney disease. J Am Soc Nephrol: JASN. 2004;15(2):493–500. Epub 2004/01/30. PubMed PMID: 14747398.
55. Ruiz-Ortega M, Ruperez M, Esteban V, Rodriguez-Vita J, Sanchez-Lopez E, Carvajal G, et al. Angiotensin II: a key factor in the inflammatory and fibrotic response in kidney diseases. Nephrol Dial Transplant: Off Publ Eur Dial Transplant Assoc – Eur Ren Assoc. 2006;21(1):16–20. Epub 2005/11/11. https://doi.org/10.1093/ndt/gfi265. PubMed PMID: 16280370.
56. Deshmane SL, Kremlev S, Amini S, Sawaya BE. Monocyte chemoattractant protein-1 (MCP-1): an overview. J Interferon Cytokine Res: Off J Int Soc Interferon Cytokine Res. 2009;29(6):313–26. Epub 2009/05/16. https://doi.org/10.1089/jir.2008.0027. PubMed PMID: 19441883; PubMed Central PMCID: PMC2755091.
57. Yadav A, Saini V, Arora S. MCP-1: chemoattractant with a role beyond immunity: a review. Clin Chim Acta; Int J Clin Chem. 2010;411(21–22):1570–9. Epub 2010/07/17. https://doi.org/10.1016/j.cca.2010.07.006. PubMed PMID: 20633546.
58. Cao Q, Wang Y, Wang XM, Lu J, Lee VW, Ye Q, et al. Renal F4/80+ CD11c+ mononuclear phagocytes display phenotypic and functional characteristics of macrophages in health and in adriamycin nephropathy. J Am Soc Nephrol. 2015;26(2):349–63. Epub 2014/07/12. https://doi.org/10.1681/ASN.2013121336. PubMed PMID: 25012165; PubMed Central PMCID: PMC4310657.
59. Segerer S, Nelson PJ, Schlondorff D. Chemokines, chemokine receptors, and renal disease: from basic science to pathophysiologic and therapeutic studies. J Am Soc Nephrol. 2000;11(1):152–76. Epub 2000/01/05. PubMed PMID: 10616852.
60. Viedt C, Orth SR. Monocyte chemoattractant protein-1 (MCP-1) in the kidney: does it more than simply attract monocytes? Nephrol Dial Transplant. 2002;17(12):2043–7. Epub 2002/11/28. PubMed PMID: 12454208.
61. Munshi R, Johnson A, Siew ED, Ikizler TA, Ware LB, Wurfel MM, et al. MCP-1 gene activation marks acute kidney injury. J Am Soc Nephrol. 2011;22(1):165–75. Epub 2010/11/13. https://doi.org/10.1681/ASN.2010060641. PubMed PMID: 21071523; PubMed Central PMCID: PMC3014045.
62. Grantham J, Torres V, Chapman A, Bae K, Tao C, Guay-Woodford L, et al. Urinary monocyte chemotactic protein-1 (MCP1) predicts progression in autosomal dominant polycystic kidney disease (ADPKD). J Am Soc Nehrol. 2010;21(Suppl):526A.
63. Chapman AB, Bost JE, Torres VE, Guay-Woodford L, Bae KT, Landsittel D, et al. Kidney volume and functional outcomes in autosomal dominant polycystic kidney disease. Clin J Am Soc Nephrol. 2012;7(3):479–86. Epub 2012/02/22. https://doi.org/10.2215/CJN.09500911. PubMed PMID: 22344503; PubMed Central PMCID: PMC3302672.
64. Mrug M, Mrug S, Landsittel D, Torres V, Bae K, Harris P, et al. Prediction of GFR endpoints in early autosomal dominant polycystic kidney disease. Am J Nephrol. 2013;24:59A.
65. Aggarwal BB, Gupta SC, Kim JH. Historical perspectives on tumor necrosis factor and its superfamily: 25 years later, a golden journey. Blood. 2012;119(3):651–65. Epub 2011/11/05. https://doi.org/10.1182/blood-2011-04-325225. PubMed PMID: 22053109; PubMed Central PMCID: PMC3265196.

66. Li X, Magenheimer BS, Xia S, Johnson T, Wallace DP, Calvet JP, et al. A tumor necrosis factor-alpha-mediated pathway promoting autosomal dominant polycystic kidney disease. Nat Med. 2008;14(8):863–8. PubMed PMID: 18552856.
67. Partsch G, Steiner G, Leeb BF, Dunky A, Broll H, Smolen JS. Highly increased levels of tumor necrosis factor-alpha and other proinflammatory cytokines in psoriatic arthritis synovial fluid. J Rheumatol. 1997;24(3):518–23. Epub 1997/03/01. PubMed PMID: 9058659.
68. Roix J, Saha S. TNF-alpha blockade is ineffective in animal models of established polycystic kidney disease. BMC Nephrol. 2013;14:233. Epub 2013/10/29. https://doi.org/10.1186/1471-2369-14-233. PubMed PMID: 24160989; PubMed Central PMCID: PMC4231369.
69. Zhou W, Farrar CA, Abe K, Pratt JR, Marsh JE, Wang Y, et al. Predominant role for C5b-9 in renal ischemia/reperfusion injury. J Clin Invest. 2000;105(10):1363–71. Epub 2000/05/17. https://doi.org/10.1172/JCI8621. PubMed PMID: 10811844; PubMed Central PMCID: PMC315463.
70. Bohana-Kashtan O, Ziporen L, Donin N, Kraus S, Fishelson Z. Cell signals transduced by complement. Mol Immunol. 2004;41(6–7):583–97. PubMed PMID: 15219997.
71. Ueda T, Rieu P, Brayer J, Arnaout MA. Identification of the complement iC3b binding site in the beta 2 integrin CR3 (CD11b/CD18). Proc Natl Acad Sci U S A. 1994;91(22):10680–4. PubMed PMID: 7524101.
72. Gordon S. Alternative activation of macrophages. Nat Rev Immunol. 2003;3(1):23–35. PubMed PMID: 12511873.
73. Bakun M, Niemczyk M, Domanski D, Jazwiec R, Perzanowska A, Niemczyk S, et al. Urine proteome of autosomal dominant polycystic kidney disease patients. Clin Proteomics 2012;9(1):13. Epub 2012/12/12. https://doi.org/10.1186/1559-0275-9-13. PubMed PMID: 23228063; PubMed Central PMCID: PMC3607978.
74. Wu Y, Xu J, Li S, Hsieh T, Lu T, Kong T. The role of complement C3 in focal inflammation and development of kidney cysts induced by Pkd1 inactivation. FASEB J. 2014;28(1 Suppl):690–3.
75. Mrug M, Zhou J, Mrug S, Guay-Woodford LM, Yoder BK, Szalai AJ. Complement C3 activation in cyst fluid and urine from autosomal dominant polycystic kidney disease patients. J Intern Med. 2014;276(5):539–40. Epub 2014/09/11. https://doi.org/10.1111/joim.12307. PubMed PMID: 25205519.
76. Fischer MB, Ma M, Goerg S, Zhou X, Xia J, Finco O, et al. Regulation of the B cell response to T-dependent antigens by classical pathway complement. J Immunol. 1996;157(2):549–56. PubMed PMID: 8752901.
77. Hong Y, Zhou W, Li K, Sacks SH. Triptolide is a potent suppressant of C3, CD40 and B7h expression in activated human proximal tubular epithelial cells. Kidney Int. 2002;62(4):1291–300. PubMed PMID: 12234299.
78. Su Z, Wang X, Gao X, Liu Y, Pan C, Hu H, et al. Excessive activation of the alternative complement pathway in autosomal dominant polycystic kidney disease. J Intern Med. 2014. Epub 2014/02/06. https://doi.org/10.1111/joim.12214. PubMed PMID: 24494798.
79. Mei C, Su Z, Wang X, Zhou J, Serra AL, Wuthrich RP. Excessive activation of the complement system in the progression of ADPKD. 2012;American Society of Nephrology meeting 2012:TH-PO639.
80. Mrug M, Zhou J, Mannon RB. C3 polymorphisms and outcomes of renal allografts. N Engl J Med. 2009;360(23):2477–8. Epub 2009/06/06. doi: 360/23/2477 [pii] 10.1056/NEJMc090635. PubMed PMID: 19494228.
81. Schafer K, Gretz N, Bader M, Oberbaumer I, Eckardt KU, Kriz W, et al. Characterization of the Han:SPRD rat model for hereditary polycystic kidney disease. Kidney Int. 1994;46(1):134–52. Epub 1994/07/01. PubMed PMID: 7933831.
82. Nauli SM, Alenghat FJ, Luo Y, Williams E, Vassilev P, Li X, et al. Polycystins 1 and 2 mediate mechanosensation in the primary cilium of kidney cells. Nat Genet. 2003;33(2):129–37. Epub 2003/01/07. https://doi.org/10.1038/ng1076. PubMed PMID: 12514735.
83. Arnold L, Henry A, Poron F, Baba-Amer Y, van Rooijen N, Plonquet A, et al. Inflammatory monocytes recruited after skeletal muscle injury switch into antiinflammatory macrophages to support myogenesis. J Exp Med. 2007;204(5):1057–69. Epub 2007/05/09. https://doi.org/10.1084/jem.20070075. PubMed PMID: 17485518; PubMed Central PMCID: PMC2118577.
84. Bogdan C, Vodovotz Y, Nathan C. Macrophage deactivation by interleukin 10. J Exp Med. 1991;174(6):1549–55. Epub 1991/12/01. PubMed PMID: 1744584; PubMed Central PMCID: PMC2119047.
85. Ricardo SD, van Goor H, Eddy AA. Macrophage diversity in renal injury and repair. J Clin Invest. 2008;118(11):3522–30. PubMed PMID: 18982158.
86. Weimbs T. Regulation of mTOR by polycystin-1: is polycystic kidney disease a case of futile repair? Cell Cycle. 2006;5(21):2425–9. Epub 2006/11/15. PubMed PMID: 17102641.
87. Torres VE, Abebe KZ, Chapman AB, Schrier RW, Braun WE, Steinman TI, et al. Angiotensin blockade in late autosomal dominant polycystic kidney disease. N Engl J Med. 2014;371(24):2267–76. Epub 2014/11/18. https://doi.org/10.1056/NEJMoa1402686. PubMed PMID: 25399731; PubMed Central PMCID: PMC4284824.
88. Walz G, Budde K, Mannaa M, Nurnberger J, Wanner C, Sommerer C, et al. Everolimus in patients with autosomal dominant polycystic kidney disease. N Engl J Med. 2010;363(9):830–40. Epub 2010/06/29. https://doi.org/10.1056/NEJMoa1003491. PubMed PMID: 20581392.

89. Serra AL, Poster D, Kistler AD, Krauer F, Raina S, Young J, et al. Sirolimus and kidney growth in autosomal dominant polycystic kidney disease. N Engl J Med. 2010;363(9):820–9. Epub 2010/06/29. https://doi.org/10.1056/NEJMoa0907419. PubMed PMID: 20581391.
90. Treille S, Bailly JM, Van Cauter J, Dehout F, Guillaume B. The use of lanreotide in polycystic kidney disease: a single-centre experience. Case Rep Nephrol Urol. 2014;4(1):18–24. Epub 2014/04/08. https://doi.org/10.1159/000358268. PubMed PMID: 24707279; PubMed Central PMCID: PMC3975724.
91. Caroli A, Perico N, Perna A, Antiga L, Brambilla P, Pisani A, et al. Effect of longacting somatostatin analogue on kidney and cyst growth in autosomal dominant polycystic kidney disease (ALADIN): a randomised, placebo-controlled, multicentre trial. Lancet 2013;382(9903):1485–95. Epub 2013/08/27. https://doi.org/10.1016/S0140-6736(13)61407-5. PubMed PMID: 23972263.
92. Gattone VH 2nd, Cowley BD Jr, Barash BD, Nagao S, Takahashi H, Yamaguchi T, et al. Methylprednisolone retards the progression of inherited polycystic kidney disease in rodents. Am J Kidney Dis. 1995;25(2):302–13. PubMed PMID: 7847359.
93. Zhang T, Wang L, Xiong X, Mao Z, Wang L, Mei C. Mycophenolate mofetil versus rapamycin in Han: SPRD rats with polycystic kidney disease. Biol Res. 2009;42(4):437–44. Epub 2010/02/09. doi: /S0716-97602009000400005. PubMed PMID: 20140299.
94. Sankaran D, Bankovic-Calic N, Ogborn MR, Crow G, Aukema HM. Selective COX-2 inhibition markedly slows disease progression and attenuates altered prostanoid production in Han:SPRD-cy rats with inherited kidney disease. Am J Physiol Renal Physiol. 2007;293(3):F821–30. Epub 2007/06/01. https://doi.org/10.1152/ajprenal.00257.2006. PubMed PMID: 17537981.
95. Kawai T, Masaki T, Doi S, Arakawa T, Yokoyama Y, Doi T, et al. PPAR-gamma agonist attenuates renal interstitial fibrosis and inflammation through reduction of TGF-beta. Lab Inv; J Tech Methods Pathol. 2009;89(1):47–58. Epub 2008/11/13. https://doi.org/10.1038/labinvest.2008.104. PubMed PMID: 19002105.
96. Perico N, Zoja C, Corna D, Rottoli D, Gaspari F, Haskell L, et al. V1/V2 vasopressin receptor antagonism potentiates the renoprotection of renin-angiotensin system inhibition in rats with renal mass reduction. Kidney Int. 2009;76(9):960–7. Epub 2009/07/25. https://doi.org/10.1038/ki.2009.267. PubMed PMID: 19625993.
97. Wang X, Gattone V 2nd, Harris PC, Torres VE. Effectiveness of vasopressin V2 receptor antagonists OPC-31260 and OPC-41061 on polycystic kidney disease development in the PCK rat. J Am Soc Nephrol. 2005;16(4):846–51. PubMed PMID: 15728778.
98. Rossetti S, Chauveau D, Kubly V, Slezak JM, Saggar-Malik AK, Pei Y, et al. Association of mutation position in polycystic kidney disease 1 (PKD1) gene and development of a vascular phenotype. Lancet. 2003;361(9376):2196–201. PubMed PMID: 12842373.
99. Antiga L, Piccinelli M, Fasolini G, Ene-Iordache B, Ondei P, Bruno S, et al. Computed tomography evaluation of autosomal dominant polycystic kidney disease progression: a progress report. Clin J Am Soc Nephrol: CJASN. 2006;1(4):754–60. Epub 2007/08/21. https://doi.org/10.2215/CJN.02251205. PubMed PMID: 17699283.
100. Wilson PD, Norman JT, Kuo NT, Burrow CR. Abnormalities in extracellular matrix regulation in autosomal dominant polycystic kidney disease. Contrib Nephrol. 1996;118:126–34. Epub 1996/01/01. PubMed PMID: 8744049.
101. Wilson PD, Hreniuk D, Gabow PA. Abnormal extracellular matrix and excessive growth of human adult polycystic kidney disease epithelia. J Cell Physiol. 1992;150(2):360–9. Epub 1992/02/01. https://doi.org/10.1002/jcp.1041500220. PubMed PMID: 1734038.
102. Wilson PD, Sherwood AC. Tubulocystic epithelium. Kidney Int. 1991;39(3):450–63. Epub 1991/03/01. PubMed PMID: 1648146.
103. Wilson PD, Geng L, Li X, Burrow CR. The PKD1 gene product, "polycystin-1," is a tyrosine-phosphorylated protein that colocalizes with alpha2beta1-integrin in focal clusters in adherent renal epithelia. Lab Inv; J Tech Methods Pathol. 1999;79(10):1311–23. Epub 1999/10/26. PubMed PMID: 10532593.
104. Wilson PD, Burrow CR. Cystic diseases of the kidney: role of adhesion molecules in normal and abnormal tubulogenesis. Exp Nephrol. 1999;7(2):114–24. Epub 1999/04/24. doi: 20592. PubMed PMID: 10213865.
105. Norman J. Fibrosis and progression of autosomal dominant polycystic kidney disease (ADPKD). Biochim Biophys Acta. 2011;1812(10):1327–36. Epub 2011/07/13. https://doi.org/10.1016/j.bbadis.2011.06.012. PubMed PMID: 21745567; PubMed Central PMCID: PMC3166379.
106. Liu D, Wang CJ, Judge DP, Halushka MK, Ni J, Habashi JP, et al. A Pkd1-Fbn1 genetic interaction implicates TGF-beta signaling in the pathogenesis of vascular complications in autosomal dominant polycystic kidney disease. J Am Soc Nephrol. 2014;25(1):81–91. Epub 2013/09/28. https://doi.org/10.1681/ASN.2012050486. PubMed PMID: 24071006; PubMed Central PMCID: PMC3871766.
107. Hassane S, Leonhard WN, van der Wal A, Hawinkels LJ, Lantinga-van Leeuwen IS, ten Dijke P, et al. Elevated TGFbeta-Smad signalling in experimental Pkd1 models and human patients with polycystic kidney disease. J Pathol. 2010;222(1):21–31. Epub 2010/06/16. https://doi.org/10.1002/path.2734. PubMed PMID: 20549648.

108. Mangos S, Lam PY, Zhao A, Liu Y, Mudumana S, Vasilyev A, et al. The ADPKD genes pkdla/b and pkd2 regulate extracellular matrix formation. Dis Model Mech. 2010;3(5–6):354–65. Epub 2010/03/26. https://doi.org/10.1242/dmm.003194. PubMed PMID: 20335443; PubMed Central PMCID: PMC2860853.
109. Du J, Wilson PD. Abnormal polarization of EGF receptors and autocrine stimulation of cyst epithelial growth in human ADPKD. Am J Phys. 1995;269(2 Pt 1):C487–95. Epub 1995/08/01. PubMed PMID: 7653531.
110. Kuo NT, Norman JT, Wilson PD. Acidic FGF regulation of hyperproliferation of fibroblasts in human autosomal dominant polycystic kidney disease. Biochem Mol Med. 1997;61(2):178–91. Epub 1997/08/01. PubMed PMID: 9259983.
111. Horie S, Higashihara E, Nutahara K, Mikami Y, Okubo A, Kano M, et al. Mediation of renal cyst formation by hepatocyte growth factor. Lancet. 1994;344(8925):789–91. Epub 1994/09/17. PubMed PMID: 7916076.
112. Hu MC, Piscione TD, Rosenblum ND. Elevated SMAD1/beta-catenin molecular complexes and renal medullary cystic dysplasia in ALK3 transgenic mice. Development. 2003;130(12):2753–66. Epub 2003/05/09. PubMed PMID: 12736218.
113. Jena N, Martin-Seisdedos C, McCue P, Croce CM. BMP7 null mutation in mice: developmental defects in skeleton, kidney, and eye. Exp Cell Res. 1997;230(1):28–37. Epub 1997/01/10. PubMed PMID: 9013703.
114. Sato M, Morrissey J, Klahr S. Bone morphogenetic protein-7 (BMP-7) delays cyst formation in a mouse model of polycystic kidney disease. J Am Soc Nehrol. 2004;15:659A.
115. Leonhard W, Kunnen S, Bouazzaoui F, Veraar K, Breuning M, De Heer E, et al. Soluble activin type IIB receptor treatment effectively blocks cyst formation in a mouse model for ADPKD. J Am Soc Nehrol. 2014;25:772A.
116. Eddy AA. Molecular insights into renal interstitial fibrosis. J Am Soc Nephrol. 1996;7(12):2495–508. Epub 1996/12/01. PubMed PMID: 8989727.
117. Rankin CA, Suzuki K, Itoh Y, Ziemer DM, Grantham JJ, Calvet JP, et al. Matrix metalloproteinases and TIMPS in cultured C57BL/6J-cpk kidney tubules. Kidney Int. 1996;50(3):835–44. Epub 1996/09/01. PubMed PMID: 8872958.
118. Schieren G, Rumberger B, Klein M, Kreutz C, Wilpert J, Geyer M, et al. Gene profiling of polycystic kidneys. Nephrol Dial Transplant. 2006;21(7):1816–24. PubMed PMID: 16520345.
119. Nakamura T, Ushiyama C, Suzuki S, Ebihara I, Shimada N, Koide H. Elevation of serum levels of metalloproteinase-1, tissue inhibitor of metalloproteinase-1 and type IV collagen, and plasma levels of metalloproteinase-9 in polycystic kidney disease. Am J Nephrol. 2000;20(1):32–6. Epub 2000/01/25. doi: 13552. PubMed PMID: 10644865.
120. Snelgrove RJ, Jackson PL, Hardison MT, Noerager BD, Kinloch A, Gaggar A, et al. A critical role for LTA4H in limiting chronic pulmonary neutrophilic inflammation. Science. 2010;330(6000):90–4. Epub 2010/09/04. https://doi.org/10.1126/science.1190594. PubMed PMID: 20813919; PubMed Central PMCID: PMC3072752.
121. Geiger B, Bershadsky A, Pankov R, Yamada KM. Transmembrane crosstalk between the extracellular matrix – cytoskeleton crosstalk. Nat Rev Mol Cell Biol. 2001;2(11):793–805. Epub 2001/11/21. https://doi.org/10.1038/35099066. PubMed PMID: 11715046.
122. Ehrhardt A, Ehrhardt GR, Guo X, Schrader JW. Ras and relatives – job sharing and networking keep an old family together. Exp Hematol. 2002;30(10):1089–106. Epub 2002/10/18. PubMed PMID: 12384139.
123. Wozniak MA, Modzelewska K, Kwong L, Keely PJ. Focal adhesion regulation of cell behavior. Biochim Biophys Acta. 2004;1692(2–3):103–19. Epub 2004/07/13. https://doi.org/10.1016/j.bbamcr.2004.04.007. PubMed PMID: 15246682.
124. Zeltner R, Hilgers KF, Schmieder RE, Porst M, Schulze BD, Hartner A. A promoter polymorphism of the alpha 8 integrin gene and the progression of autosomal-dominant polycystic kidney disease. Nephron Clin Pract. 2008;108(3):c169–75. Epub 2008/02/16. https://doi.org/10.1159/000116887. PubMed PMID: 18277079.
125. Wallace DP, Quante MT, Reif GA, Nivens E, Ahmed F, Hempson SJ, et al. Periostin induces proliferation of human autosomal dominant polycystic kidney cells through alphaV-integrin receptor. Am J Physiol Renal Physiol. 2008;295(5):F1463–71. Epub 2008/08/30. https://doi.org/10.1152/ajprenal.90266.2008. PubMed PMID: 18753297; PubMed Central PMCID: PMC2584901.
126. Joly D, Morel V, Hummel A, Ruello A, Nusbaum P, Patey N, et al. Beta4 integrin and laminin 5 are aberrantly expressed in polycystic kidney disease: role in increased cell adhesion and migration. Am J Pathol. 2003;163(5):1791–800. Epub 2003/10/28. PubMed PMID: 14578180; PubMed Central PMCID: PMC1892423.
127. Wu W, Kitamura S, Truong DM, Rieg T, Vallon V, Sakurai H, et al. Beta1-integrin is required for kidney collecting duct morphogenesis and maintenance of renal function. Am J Physiol Renal Physiol. 2009;297(1):F210–7. Epub 2009/05/15. https://doi.org/10.1152/ajprenal.90260.2008. PubMed PMID: 19439520; PubMed Central PMCID: PMC2711709.
128. McGlashan SR, Jensen CG, Poole CA. Localization of extracellular matrix receptors on the chondrocyte primary cilium. J Histochem Cytochem. 2006;54(9):1005–14. Epub 2006/05/03. https://doi.org/10.1369/jhc.5A6866.2006. PubMed PMID: 16651393.
129. Qi W, Chen X, Poronnik P, Pollock CA. The renal cortical fibroblast in renal tubulointerstitial fibro-

sis. Int J Biochem Cell Biol. 2006;38(1):1–5. Epub 2005/10/19. https://doi.org/10.1016/j.biocel.2005.09.005. PubMed PMID: 16230044.
130. Desmouliere A, Geinoz A, Gabbiani F, Gabbiani G. Transforming growth factor-beta 1 induces alpha-smooth muscle actin expression in granulation tissue myofibroblasts and in quiescent and growing cultured fibroblasts. J Cell Biol. 1993;122(1):103–11. Epub 1993/07/01. PubMed PMID: 8314838; PubMed Central PMCID: PMC2119614.
131. Follonier Castella L, Gabbiani G, McCulloch CA, Hinz B. Regulation of myofibroblast activities: calcium pulls some strings behind the scene. Exp Cell Res. 2010;316(15):2390–401. Epub 2010/05/11. https://doi.org/10.1016/j.yexcr.2010.04.033. PubMed PMID: 20451515.
132. Wada T, Sakai N, Sakai Y, Matsushima K, Kaneko S, Furuichi K. Involvement of bone-marrow-derived cells in kidney fibrosis. Clin Exp Nephrol. 2011;15(1):8–13. Epub 2010/12/15. https://doi.org/10.1007/s10157-010-0372-2. PubMed PMID: 21152947.
133. Nishio S, Hatano M, Nagata M, Horie S, Koike T, Tokuhisa T, et al. Pkd1 regulates immortalized proliferation of renal tubular epithelial cells through p53 induction and JNK activation. J Clin Invest. 2005;115(4):910–8. Epub 2005/03/12. https://doi.org/10.1172/JCI22850. PubMed PMID: 15761494; PubMed Central PMCID: PMC1059447.
134. Niedermeier M, Reich B, Rodriguez Gomez M, Denzel A, Schmidbauer K, Gobel N, et al. CD4+ T cells control the differentiation of Gr1+ monocytes into fibrocytes. Proc Natl Acad Sci U S A. 2009;106(42):17892–7. Epub 2009/10/10. https://doi.org/10.1073/pnas.0906070106. PubMed PMID: 19815530; PubMed Central PMCID: PMC2764893.
135. Anders HJ, Ryu M. Renal microenvironments and macrophage phenotypes determine progression or resolution of renal inflammation and fibrosis. Kidney Int. 2011;80(9):915–25. Epub 2011/08/05. https://doi.org/10.1038/ki.2011.217. PubMed PMID: 21814171.
136. Vernon MA, Mylonas KJ, Hughes J. Macrophages and renal fibrosis. Semin Nephrol. 2010;30(3):302–17. Epub 2010/07/14. https://doi.org/10.1016/j.semnephrol.2010.03.004. PubMed PMID: 20620674.
137. Semedo P, Donizetti-Oliveira C, Burgos-Silva M, Cenedeze MA, Avancini Costa Malheiros DM, Pacheco-Silva A, et al. Bone marrow mononuclear cells attenuate fibrosis development after severe acute kidney injury. Lab Investig. 2010;90(5):685–95. Epub 2010/03/24. https://doi.org/10.1038/labinvest.2010.45. PubMed PMID: 20308984.
138. Snelgrove SL, Kausman JY, Lo C, Lo C, Ooi JD, Coates PT, et al. Renal dendritic cells adopt a pro-inflammatory phenotype in obstructive uropathy to activate T cells but do not directly contribute to fibrosis. Am J Pathol. 2012;180(1):91–103. Epub 2011/11/15. https://doi.org/10.1016/j.ajpath.2011.09.039. PubMed PMID: 22079432.
139. Heymann F, Meyer-Schwesinger C, Hamilton-Williams EE, Hammerich L, Panzer U, Kaden S, et al. Kidney dendritic cell activation is required for progression of renal disease in a mouse model of glomerular injury. J Clin Invest. 2009;119(5):1286–97. Epub 2009/04/22. https://doi.org/10.1172/JCI38399. PubMed PMID: 19381017; PubMed Central PMCID: PMC2673875.
140. Kim DH, Moon SO, Jung YJ, Lee AS, Kang KP, Lee TH, et al. Mast cells decrease renal fibrosis in unilateral ureteral obstruction. Kidney Int. 2009;75(10):1031–8. Epub 2009/02/27. https://doi.org/10.1038/ki.2009.1. PubMed PMID: 19242503.
141. Kriz W, Kaissling B, Le Hir M. Epithelial-mesenchymal transition (EMT) in kidney fibrosis: fact or fantasy? J Clin Invest. 2011;121(2):468–74. Epub 2011/03/04. PubMed PMID: 21370523; PubMed Central PMCID: PMC3026733.
142. Kistler AD, Mischak H, Poster D, Dakna M, Wuthrich RP, Serra AL. Identification of a unique urinary biomarker profile in patients with autosomal dominant polycystic kidney disease. Kidney Int. 2009;76(1):89–96. Epub 2009/04/03. https://doi.org/10.1038/ki.2009.93. PubMed PMID: 19340089.
143. Kistler AD, Serra AL, Siwy J, Poster D, Krauer F, Torres VE, et al. Urinary proteomic biomarkers for diagnosis and risk stratification of autosomal dominant polycystic kidney disease: a multicentric study. PLoS One. 2013;8(1):e53016. Epub 2013/01/18. https://doi.org/10.1371/journal.pone.0053016. PubMed PMID: 23326375; PubMed Central PMCID: PMC3542378.

Part III

ADPKD: Clinical Features

Imaging-Based Diagnosis of Autosomal Dominant Polycystic Kidney Disease

7

Young-Hwan Hwang, Moumita Barua, Anna McNaught, Korosh Khalili, and York Pei

Introduction

Autosomal dominant polycystic kidney disease (ADPKD) is the most common Mendelian genetic kidney disease, affecting 1 in 500–1000 births worldwide [1]. Focal development of an increasing number of renal cysts with age is a hallmark of ADPKD, leading to the distortion of normal kidney architecture and, ultimately, end-stage renal disease (ESRD) in a majority of patients [2]. Mutations of two genes, *PKD1* and *PKD2*, have been, respectively, implicated for the disease in 85% and 15% of linkage-characterized European families [3]. However, a more recent population-based study has reported a higher prevalence of PKD2 of 26% [4]. Disease severity and progression is highly variable in ADPKD in part due to strong effects from the gene locus and alleles [5–11]. Adjusted for age, patients with PKD1 have more renal cysts, larger kidneys, and earlier onset of ESRD than patients with PKD2 (mean age at ESRD: 53.4 vs. 72.7 years, respectively) [7, 8]. More recent studies have further demonstrated a significant allelic effect in PKD1 with milder renal disease associated with non-truncating mutations and severe disease, with truncating mutations [9–11]. Marked renal disease variability within families has been well documented in ADPKD and suggests a modifier effect from genetic and environmental factors [12, 13].

Imaging-based testing is commonly performed for presymptomatic screening or clinical diagnosis of ADPKD. Conventional ultrasound, which is inexpensive and widely available, is the most common modality used for presymptomatic screening of ADPKD. As simple cysts occur with increasing age in the general [14] and hospital patient [15] population, age-dependent ultrasound diagnostic criteria have been established for PKD1 [16] and subsequently refined and extended for evaluation of at-risk subjects of unknown gene type (a.k.a. "unified diagnostic criteria") [17]. More recently, highly sensitive and specific criteria based on magnetic resonance imaging (MRI) have also been derived for earlier diagnosis and exclusion of ADPKD in younger at-risk subjects [18]. In general, presymptomatic

Y.-H. Hwang, MD, PhD
Department of Medicine, Eulji General Hospital, Seoul, South Korea

Divisions of Nephrology and Genomic Medicine, University Health Network and University of Toronto, Toronto, ON, Canada

M. Barua, MD · Y. Pei, MD (✉)
Divisions of Nephrology and Genomic Medicine, University Health Network and University of Toronto, Toronto, ON, Canada
e-mail: Moumita.Barua@uhn.ca; york.pei@uhn.ca

A. McNaught, MD · K. Khalili, MD
Department of Medical Imaging, University Health Network and University of Toronto, Toronto, ON, Canada
e-mail: Anna.Mcnaught@health.nsw.gov.au; Korosh.Khalili@uhn.ca

B. D. Cowley, Jr., J. J. Bissler (eds.), *Polycystic Kidney Disease*,
https://doi.org/10.1007/978-1-4939-7784-0_7

screening of at-risk children (under 18 years of age) cannot be recommended at this time based on the potential risks including adverse psychological consequences and denial of future insurance coverage. Additionally, there is currently no evidence that clinical management in this setting would improve outcomes. The possible implications of all diagnostic screening should be discussed beforehand, and the results clearly explained to the test subjects. Blood pressure assessment should be performed routinely in at-risk subjects of all age groups whether or not they undergo the screening.

It is important to note that the diagnostic criteria derived for US and MRI are applicable only to test subjects with a definitive family history of ADPKD who are born with a 50% risk of disease. By contrast, the pretest probability of subjects without a positive family history is that of the population risk (i.e., 1 in 500–1000); thus, the above criteria may not be valid. Moreover, the possibility of other genetic and nongenetic causes of PKD needs to be considered in the latter setting [2]. In subjects without a positive family history, it is useful to screen their parents and older first-degree relatives with ultrasound as mild disease associated with a *PKD2* or non-truncating *PKD1* mutation may not be apparent, especially in small families [2]. If one or both parents are deceased, review of their medical record for prior renal imaging results may be helpful. The documentation of at least one affected first-degree relative with bilaterally enlarged kidneys and numerous cysts is sufficient evidence to support the use of the imaging-based diagnostic criteria. On the other hand, the presence of several cysts without kidney enlargement in an elderly relative may be due to simple cysts and should not be considered as sufficient evidence for a positive family history.

Diagnosis of ADPKD by Conventional Ultrasound

The diagnosis of ADPKD is generally straightforward in patients with symptomatic disease and a positive family history. For presymptomatic screening of at-risk subjects, age-dependent criteria based on conventional ultrasound have been derived for PKD1 [16]. However, the utility of these criteria is limited by the unknown gene type of most test subjects in the clinical setting and the negative impact on diagnostic performance by the milder cases associated with PKD2. To overcome these limitations, Pei et al. derived age-dependent diagnostic criteria from a cohort of 948 at-risk subjects by comparing their molecular genetic results (for the presence or absence of disease) and ultrasound findings, using a simulated case mix of 85–15% for PKD1 and PKD2, respectively [17]. Based on the "unified criteria" derived from this study (Table 7.1), the presence of "a total of three or more renal cysts" for at-risk subjects aged 15–39 years and "two cysts or more in each kidney" for at-risk subjects aged 40–59 years can be considered as sufficient for diagnosis. Conversely, the "absence of any renal cyst" can be considered sufficient for disease exclusion only in at-risk subjects aged 40 years or older. It should be noted that a resolution of approximately 1 cm or more is required for conventional ultrasound to detect most of the renal cysts. Thus, the validity of the unified criteria should not be extrapolated to high-resolution ultrasound using modern scanners, which has imaging resolution enabling routine detection of very small renal cysts of 2–3 mm. It is also clear that reduced diagnostic sensitivity (e.g., ~81% for unknown gene type) is a limitation of conventional ultrasound rendering early diagnosis of at-risk subjects with milder disease suboptimal. A corollary is that the "absence of any renal cyst" cannot be used as definitive evidence for disease exclusion in younger at-risk subjects of unknown gene type, where their negative predictive values are ~91% and 98%, under 30 and between 30 and 39 years of age, respectively.

Diagnosis of ADPKD by MRI and High-Resolution Ultrasound

Given that younger subjects at risk for ADPKD are increasingly being evaluated as potential living kidney donors [19, 20], there is a need to

Table 7.1 Criteria for diagnosis and exclusion of ADPKD using conventional ultrasound

Age (years)	Criterion	PKD1	PKD2	Unknown gene type
Performance of criteria for diagnostic confirmation				
15–29	A total of three or more cysts[a]	PPV = 100%	PPV = 100%	PPV = 100%
		SEN = 94.3%	SEN = 69.5%	SEN = 81.7%
30–39	A total of three or more cysts[a]	PPV = 100%	PPV = 100%	PPV = 100%
		SEN = 96.6%	SEN = 94.9%	SEN = 95.5%
40–59	≥2 cysts in each kidney	PPV = 100%	PPV = 100%	PPV = 100%
		SEN = 92.6%	SEN = 88.8%	SEN = 90%
Performance of criteria for disease exclusion				
15–29	No renal cyst	NPV = 99.1%	NPV = 83.5%	NPV = 90.8%
		SPEC = 97.6%	SPEC = 96.6%	SPEC = 97.1%
30–39	No renal cyst	NPV = 100%	NPV = 96.8%	NPV = 98.3%
		SPEC = 96%	SPEC = 93.8%	SPEC = 94.8%
40–59	No renal cyst	NPV = 100%	NPV = 100%	NPV = 100%
		SPEC = 93.9%	SPEC = 93.7%	SPEC = 93.9%

[a]Unilateral or bilateral

develop highly sensitive and specific tests for disease exclusion. While molecular diagnostics may be used here for disease exclusion, it is expensive and time-consuming and may not provide a definitive diagnosis in up to one third of cases [21]. With increased resolution for detecting very small cysts by magnetic resonance imaging (MRI) and contrast-enhanced computed tomography (CT), many transplant centers have routinely included one of these imaging modalities in their evaluation of subjects at risk of ADPKD. However, until recently, validated diagnostic criteria for these modalities were lacking [19, 20]. Thus, Huang et al. empirically proposed that CT or MRI be used for screening in this setting, and if there are at least three unilateral or bilateral renal cysts, that the kidney donation be deferred pending the results of molecular genetic testing [19]. On the other hand, Niaudet proposes that CT or MRI be used for detection of small renal cysts in at-risk subjects under 30 years of age and, if the scan is negative, molecular genetic testing be considered for disease exclusion [20].

With improved resolution to detect smaller cysts, there is a general concern that MRI or CT may also detect more simple renal cysts. However, until recently, there was no data on the prevalence of simple renal cysts detected by these imaging modalities in the heathy general population. Instead, a widely quoted study by Nascimento et al. [15] provides a retrospective survey of the prevalence of renal cysts by MRI in 528 patients with various non-specified medical conditions from a large university hospital in the United States. In this study, 31% (i.e., 11/35) and 51% (i.e., 97/190) of the patients aged 18–29 years and 30–44 years, respectively, had at least one renal cyst, and 11% (i.e., 4/35) and 12% (i.e., 23/190) of the patients from the two respective age strata had a total of three or more renal cysts. However, chronic renal disease (including polycystic kidney disease), if not manifested as renal atrophy, was not excluded in the study. Furthermore, molecular genetic analysis was not employed to ascertain whether those patients with renal cysts had ADPKD. Thus, the prevalence estimates of renal cysts provided by this study should not be taken to reflect those from a healthy general population.

The Toronto Radiological Imaging Study of Polycystic kidney disease (TRISP) has recently shown that MRI and high-resolution ultrasound provide improved performance for early diagnosis and exclusion of ADPKD compared to conventional ultrasound [18]. In this study, we prospectively enrolled 126 subjects at risk for ADPKD aged 16–40 years to undergo renal MRI and high-resolution ultrasound as well as comprehensive mutation screening of *PKD1* and *PKD2* (to define the disease status). Concurrently, 46 age-matched healthy controls without a family history of ADPKD also underwent the same imaging protocol to provide specificity data. Using these imaging modalities, we were able to detect very small renal cysts down to 3 mm in diameter. Despite increased sensitivity for detecting very small cysts by MRI, we only found 1/82 unaffected subject aged 16–40 years with more than three renal cysts. Thus, simple renal cysts in this healthy population remain few in number despite enhanced resolution for detecting very small cysts. By contrast, all but one (i.e., 72/73) of our genetically affected subjects had a total of more than 20 renal cysts (*left panel*, Fig. 7.1). These two features together enable MRI to provide highly discriminant diagnostics for ADPKD. Thus, the presence of "a total of more than 10 renal cysts" (with both positive predictive value and sensitivity of 100%) can be considered as sufficient for diagnosis in a subject at risk of ADPKD. Conversely, "less than a total of 10 renal cysts" (with both negative predictive value and specificity of 100%) can be considered as sufficient for disease exclusion. For evaluation of living kidney donors, among whom the clinical agenda is disease exclusion with high certainty, we recommend using "less than a total of 5 renal cysts" (with negative predictive value of 100% and specificity of 98.3%) as a more stringent criterion. Pending future studies demonstrating diagnostic equivalence between the two modalities, we do not recommend extrapolating the MRI-specific criteria to contrast-enhanced CT.

Overall, we found improved diagnostic performance by high-resolution ultrasound compared to conventional ultrasound [18]. Specifically, we noted a significant increase in sensitivity with a small decrease in specificity across all the criteria tested, likely due to increased imaging resolution in detecting cysts as small as 3 mm with the modern scanners and experienced operators attuned to detection of small cysts. Using the unified criterion of "a total of three or more renal cysts" in at-risk subjects under 30 years of age, we found a significant increase in sensitivity (i.e., 97.3% from 81.7%) with a small decrease in positive predictive value (i.e., 100–97.3%). To minimize false-positive cases with high-resolution ultrasound, a more stringent criterion such as "two or more cysts in

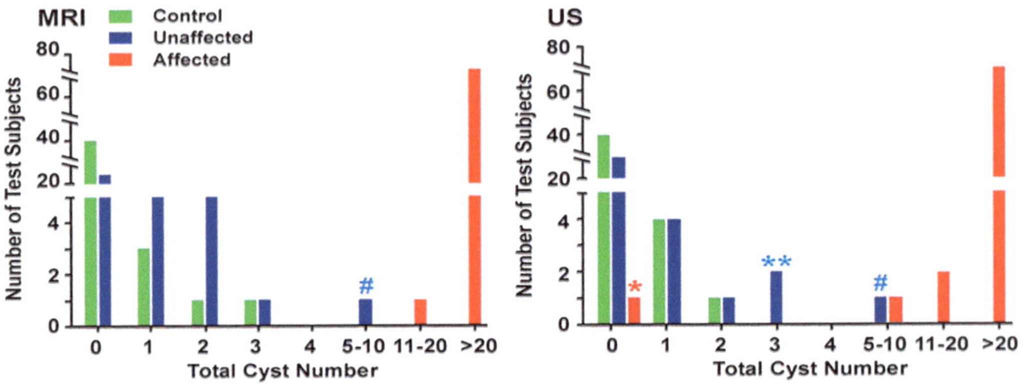

Fig. 7.1 *Distribution of total renal cyst counts by disease status: MRI (left panel) versus high-resolution US (right panel).* Both MRI and HR-US provided highly discriminant diagnostics for ADPKD; however, HR-US is both operator- and center-dependent and may be affected by the body habitus of the test subject (Adapted from Pei et al. JASN; [18]). *TOR190.1 is a genetically affected subject with a BMI of 35.6 kg/m^2 who had more than 20 renal cysts by MRI but no cyst detectable by a suboptimal US. #TOR31.2 is a subject with six renal cysts on US and ten renal cysts on MRI; he did not carry the familial *PKD2* mutation and was considered as unaffected. **TOR404.1 and TOR208.5 were both unaffected but had three renal cysts by US

each kidney" (with positive predictive value of 100%) should be used. Conversely, the "absence of any renal cyst" by high-resolution ultrasound may be considered sufficient for disease exclusion in at-risk subjects aged 30–40 years, but not younger. An important caveat is that a suboptimal scan (e.g., due to body habitus) should be interpreted as indeterminate, and this point was well illustrated by patient TOR190.1 (*right panel*, Fig. 7.1). Another limitation of ultrasound is that its diagnostic performance is both operator- and center-dependent, reflecting differences such as imaging resolution of the scanners and experience of the technicians/radiologists. Thus, current availability of ultrasound scanners with different imaging resolution has important implication for diagnostic testing. Specifically, the diagnostic criteria we derived here should be applicable to experienced centers using high-resolution ultrasound; otherwise, the unified criteria [17] should be used for centers that utilize conventional ultrasound. While conventional ultrasound will continue to be the first-line test for presymptomatic screening of ADPKD, MRI or high-resolution ultrasound will be useful for diagnostic clarification in cases with equivocal results and for disease exclusion in at-risk subjects being evaluated as potential kidney donors. Moreover, MRI also provides an assessment of renal cystic burden and disease severity in affected subjects (Fig. 7.2).

Diagnosis of ADPKD Without a Positive Family History

The absence of a positive family history in 15–28% of patients with suspected ADPKD poses a diagnostic challenge [2, 22, 23]. This problem is well illustrated by our findings in the *T*oronto *G*enetic *E*pidemiology *S*tudy of *P*KD (TGESP) in which 28% (58/209) of our probands

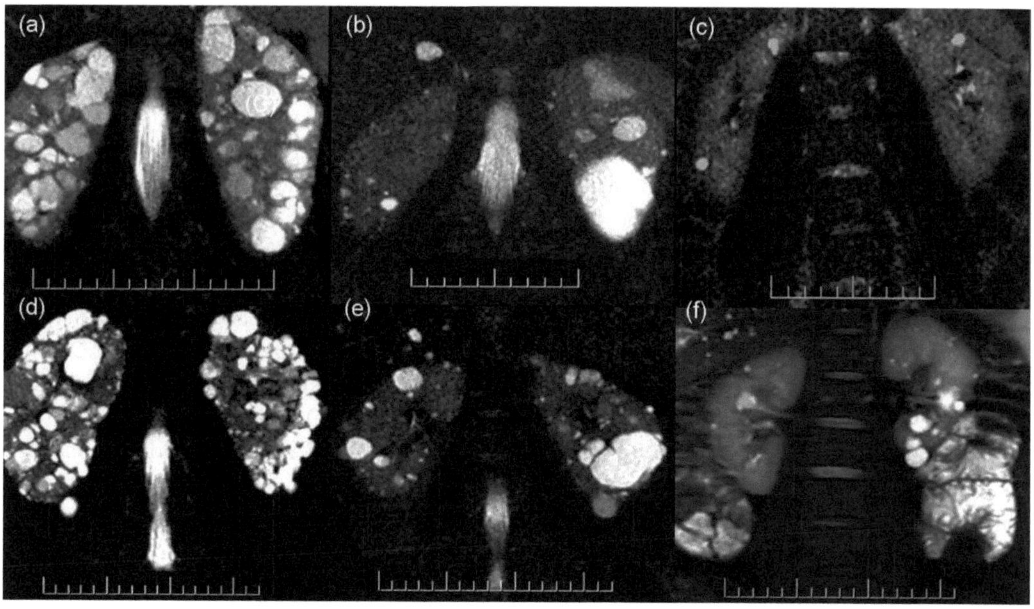

Fig. 7.2 *T2-weighted MRI images showing a spectrum of autosomal dominant polycystic kidney disease.* (**a**) 26-year-old female with a protein-truncating *PKD1* mutation (TKV = 890 ml), (**b**) 22-year-old female with a protein-truncating *PKD2* mutation (TKV = 610 ml), (**c**) 26-year-old male with a hypomorphic *PKD1* mutation (TKV = 310 ml), (**d**) 42-year-old male with protein-truncating PKD 1 mutation (TKV = 1280 ml), (**e**) 40-year-old male with a complete *PKD2* deletion (TKV = 470 ml), and (**f**) 43-year-old male with a hypomorphic *PKD1* mutation (TKV = 470 ml). Each small unit of the ruler denotes 1 cm

did not report a family history of ADPKD [22]. In this subgroup of patients, we reviewed their parental medical records and screened all available parents by renal imaging. We found that 15.3% (32/209) of them had de novo PKD, 2% (4/209) had a positive family history in retrospect due to mild disease from non-truncating *PKD1* mutations in one of their parents, and 10.5% (22/209) had an indeterminate family history due to missing parental information. Of interest, no pathogenic *PKD1* and *PKD2* mutation could be identified in ~16% (34/209) of our patients with atypical (i.e. asymmetric, focal, or unilateral) polycystic kidney disease on renal imaging. In one family with both an affected mother (proband) and daughter, we were able to prove that the mother was a somatic mosaic harboring a frameshift *PKD1* mutation. Somatic mosaicism of a dominantly inherited disease such as ADPKD results from a pathogenic somatic mutation affecting one of the pluripotent progenitor cells during early embryo development [24]. The hallmark of somatic mosaicism is the presence of two distinct cell populations (i.e., one with and one without the pathogenic mutation) in the affected subject whose disease is typically focal, milder, and variably expressed due to dilution of the mutant gene dosage at one or more disease tissues [25]. This diagnosis should be considered in patients with asymmetric polycystic kidney disease of de novo onset (see molecular genetic testing).

In the absence of a family history of ADPKD, other causes of renal cystic diseases need to be considered in the differential diagnosis (Table 7.2). Autosomal dominant polycystic liver disease (ADPLD) [MIM 174050] is caused by mutations in at least two genes that are distinct from *PKD1* and *PKD2* [26]. In the classical form, ADPLD presents as a late-onset disease with liver cysts. However, patients with ADPLD may have a few renal cysts which can be confused as mild ADPKD. By contrast, patients with autosomal recessive polycystic kidney disease (ARPKD) [MIM 263200] can present with enlarged echogenic kidneys in the prenatal period as an incidental finding detected by screening ultrasound. The presence of oligohydramnios and respiratory failure at the perinatal period or congenital hepatic fibrosis and renal failure during childhood heralds more severe disease typically associated with two protein-truncating mutations [27]. Two other syndromic forms of PKD due to tuberous sclerosis complex (TSC) [MIM 191100] [28] and Von Hippel-Lindau (VHL) syndrome [MIM 193300] [29] should be easily recognized by their extrarenal clinical features (Table 7.2). However, when present atypically they can mimic ADPKD. Of note, the characteristic renal angiomyolipomas or skin lesions may be absent in up to 30% of patients with mild disease, some of whom may harbor TSC somatic mosaicism [28]. Glomerulocystic kidney disease [MIM 137920] due to hepatocyte nuclear factor 1-beta (*HNF-1B*) gene mutations can mimic ADPKD. However, the association of renal cysts with urogenital abnormalities, maturity onset diabetes mellitus, as well as chronic renal insufficiency that is discordant with the cystic disease burden (i.e., renal insufficiency without enlarged cystic kidneys) should raise a suspicion for this disorder [30]. Autosomal dominant medullary cystic kidney disease [OMIM 174000 and 603,860] typically presents as chronic renal insufficiency with few or no renal cysts and may be associated with hyperuricemia and gout [31, 32]. Other non-syndromic causes of PKD including simple renal cysts, acquired renal cystic disease, medullary sponge kidney [33], and somatic mosaicism of ADPKD should also be considered in patients without a family history of ADPKD. Examples of both syndromic and non-syndromic forms of PKD are shown in Fig. 7.3.

An Integrated Approach for Diagnosis of Renal Cysts

We present in Fig. 7.4 an integrated approach for the evaluation of patients with renal cysts. The first step in the evaluation is a detailed

Table 7.2 Differential diagnosis for renal cysts without a family history of ADPKD

Cystic disorder	Inheritance	Prevalence	Renal findings	Distinguishing extrarenal findings
Syndromic				
Polycystic liver disease	AD; often unrecognized	Unknown	Few renal cysts	Asymptomatic liver cysts; rarely presents with severe PLD predominantly in women
Autosomal recessive polycystic kidney disease (ARPKD)	AR	~1/20,000	Echogenic kidneys with renal cysts	Oligohydramnios and pulmonary hypoplasia in utero, congenital hepatic fibrosis and ESRD in severe cases. Patients with one non-truncating *PKHD1* mutation may have mild renal disease
Tuberous sclerosis complex (TSC)	AD; de novo onset in 2/3 of cases	~1/10,000	Renal angiomyolipomas and cysts; contiguous deletion syndrome of *PKD1* and *TSC2* causes severe PKD with ESRD by teenage years	Skin lesions (facial angiofibromas, periungual fibroma, hypomelanotic macules, shagreen patch); retinal hamartomas; cortical tuber, subependymal giant cell astrocytoma, seizures, mental retardation and autism-spectrum symptoms; lymphangioleiomyomatosis. Patients with somatic mosaicism or hypomorphic mutations have mild and atypical disease
Von Hippel-Lindau (VHL) syndrome	AD; de novo onset in ~20% of cases	~1/50,000	Renal cysts and renal cell carcinomas	Cerebellar, spinal and retinal hemangioblastoma; pancreatic cysts and neuroendocrine tumors; pheochromocytoma
Glomerulocystic kidney disease	AD	Rare	Renal cysts associated with echogenic kidneys, renal hypoplasia, or dysplasia	Mature-onset diabetes of the young (MODY); genital tract abnormalities such as epididymal cysts, atresia of vas deferens, and bicornuate uterus
Medullary cystic kidney disease (MCKD)	AD	Rare	Chronic interstitial disease. Rarely, medullary cysts. Normal or small kidneys	Hyperuricemia and gout
Non-syndromic				
Simple cysts	Nongenetic	Common	Cysts increase in number and size with age	None
Acquired cystic kidney disease (ACKD)	Nongenetic	Common	Associated with CKD or ESRD. Multiple cysts with normal or small kidneys	None
Medullary sponge kidney (MSK)	AD with reduced penetrance	~1/5000	Nephrocalcinosis; kidney stones; "brush" or linear striations on CT urogram	None
Somatic mosaicism	Potentially	Unknown	Asymmetric or mild PKD of de novo onset	None

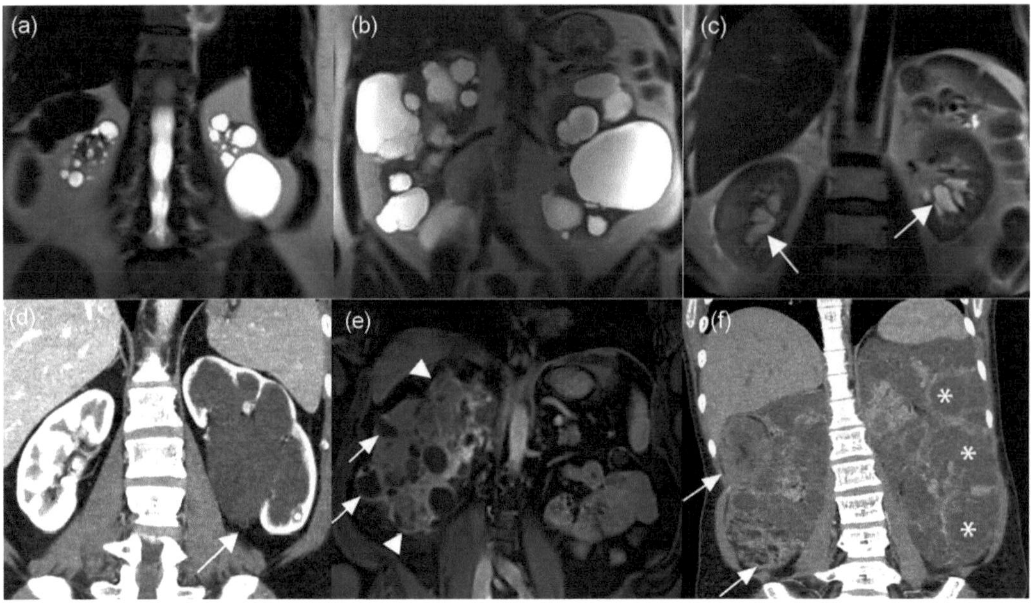

Fig. 7.3 *Examples of other cystic disorders.* (**a**) Acquired cystic kidney disease in a 63-year-old female with end-stage renal failure due to diabetés mellitus, (**b**) simple renal cysts in a 61-year-old-male with normal eGFR and negative *PKD1* and *PKD2* mutation screen, (**c**) parapelvic cysts (arrows) in a 64-year-old-male, (**d**) unilateral ureteropelvic junction (UPJ) obstruction in a 44-year-old-male with markedly distended left renal collecting system and abrupt transition at UPJ (arrow), (**e**) multiple renal cysts (arrows) and renal cell carcinomas (RCCs) (arrowheads) in a 44-year-old male with Von-Hippel Lindau disease and a previous left nephrectomy for RCC, and (**f**) kidney enlargement from numerous cysts (asterisks) and angiomyolipomas (arrows) in a 32-year-old female with tuberous sclerosis complex. All figures are T2-weighted MRI images except for panels (**d**) and (**f**) which are from contrast-enhanced CT scans

family history including renal disease severity (i.e., age at ESRD) in older affected family members. For at-risk subjects with a definitive family history of ADPKD, the unified criteria based on conventional ultrasound can be used for both diagnosis and disease exclusion (Table 7.1). Specifically, the presence of "a total of three or more renal cysts" for at-risk subjects aged 15–39 years and "two cysts or more in each kidney" for at-risk subjects aged 40–59 years can be considered as sufficient for diagnosis. Conversely, the "absence of any renal cyst" can be considered sufficient for disease exclusion only in at-risk subjects aged 40 years or older. In addition, the absence of any renal cyst by 30 years of age ("Ravine criterion") can be used for disease exclusion in at-risk subjects from families with one or more affected member who developed ESRD before 50 years of age or known truncating *PKD1* mutations [4]. In at-risk subjects with equivocal results, MRI may be used for further diagnostic clarification [18]. Specifically, the presence of "a total of more than 10 renal cysts" can be considered as sufficient for diagnosis and "less than a total of 5 renal cysts" for disease exclusion with high stringency. In patients without an apparent family history of ADPKD, review of medical record or ultrasound screening of other older first-degree relatives may uncover one or more affected but undiagnosed members with mild disease due to *PKD2* or non-truncating *PKD1* mutations. In the absence of a definitive family history of ADPKD, the differential diagnosis will need to broaden to include other syndromic and non-syndromic causes of renal cysts (Table 7.2) with molecular genetic testing often indicated for diagnostic clarification.

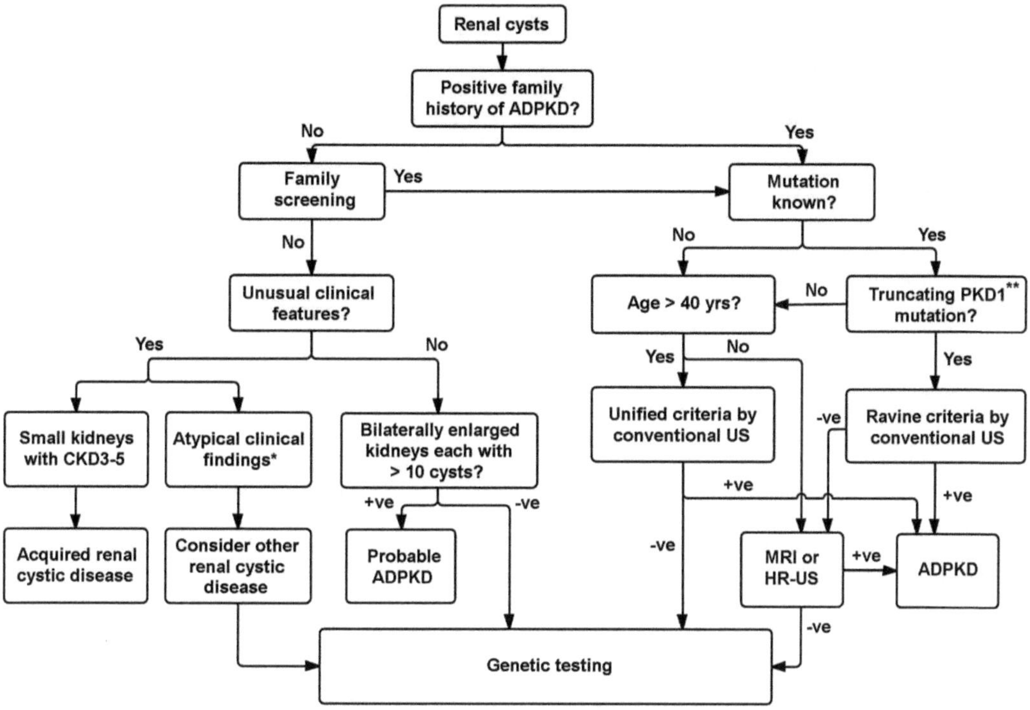

Fig. 7.4 *An integrated approach for evaluation of renal cysts detected by conventional ultrasound (US).* The documentation of a positive family history is a critical step allowing the use of age-dependent imaging-based criteria for both diagnosis and exclusion of ADPKD. In the absence of a family history, the differential diagnosis needs to include other syndromic and non-syndromic causes of renal cysts. *See Table 7.2 for differential diagnosis of atypical polycystic kidney disease; **at-risk subjects from families with known protein-truncating *PKD1* mutations may use the Ravine criteria for earlier disease exclusion; MRI magnetic resonance imaging, HR-US high-resolution ultrasound

References

1. Harris PC, Torres V. Polycystic kidney disease. Annu Rev Med. 2009;60:321–37.
2. Pei Y, Watnick T. Diagnosis and screening of autosomal dominant polycystic kidney disease. Adv Chronic Kidney Dis. 2010;17:140–52.
3. Peters D, Sandkuijl L. Genetic heterogeneity of polycystic kidney disease in Europe. Contrib Nephrol. 1992;97:128–39.
4. Barua M, Cil O, Paterson AD, Wang KW, et al. Family history of renal disease severity predicts the mutated gene in ADPKD. J Am Soc Nephrol. 2009; 20:1833–8.
5. Dicks E, Ravani P, Langman D, et al. Incident renal events and risk factors in autosomal dominant polycystic kidney disease: a population and family-based cohort followed for 22 years. Clin J Am Soc Nephrol. 2006;1:710–7.
6. Magistroni R, He N, Wang KR, et al. Genotype-renal function correlation in type 2 autosomal dominant polycystic kidney disease. J Am Soc Nephrol. 2003;14:1164–74.
7. Hateboer N, Dijk MA V, Bogdanova N, et al. Comparison of phenotypes of polycystic kidney disease types 1 and 2. European PKD1-PKD2 Study Group. Lancet. 1999;353:103–7.
8. Harris PC, Bae KT, Rossetti S, et al. Cyst number but not the rate of cystic growth is associated with the mutated gene in autosomal dominant polycystic kidney disease. J Am Soc Nephrol. 2006;17:3013–9.
9. Rossetti S, Kubly VJ, Consugar MB, et al. Incomplete penetrant *PKD1* alleles suggest a role for gene dosage in cyst initiation in polycystic kidney disease. Kidney Int. 2009;75:848–55.
10. Pei Y, Lan Z, Wang KR, et al. Attenuated renal disease severity associated with a missense PKD1 mutation. Kidney Int. 2012;81:412–7.
11. Cornec-Le Gall E, Audrezet M-P, Chen JM, et al. Type of PKD1 mutation influences renal outcome in ADPKD. J Am Soc Nephrol. 2013;24:1006–13.
12. Paterson AD, Magistroni R, He N, et al. Progressive loss of renal function is a heritable trait in type 1

autosomal dominant polycystic kidney disease. J Am Soc Nephrol. 2005;16:755–62.
13. Liu Q-X, Shi S, Senthilnathan S, et al. Genetic variation of DKK3 may modify renal disease severity in PKD1. J Am Soc Nephrol. 2010;21:1510–20.
14. Carrim ZI, Murchison JT. The prevalence of simple renal and hepatic cysts detected by spiral computed tomography. Clin Radiol. 2003;58:626–9.
15. Nascimento AB, Mitchell DG, Zhang XM, et al. Rapid MR imaging detection of renal cysts: age-based standards. Radiology. 2001;221:628–32.
16. Ravine D, Gibson RN, Walker RG, et al. Evaluation of ultrasonographic diagnostic criteria for autosomal dominant polycystic kidney disease 1. Lancet. 1994;343:824–7.
17. Pei Y, Obaji J, Dupuis A, et al. Unified criteria for ultrasonographic diagnosis of ADPKD. J Am Soc Nephrol. 2009;20:205–12.
18. Pei Y, Hwang YH, Conklin J, et al. Imaging-based diagnosis of autosomal dominant polycystic kidney disease. J Am Soc Nephrol. 2015;26:746–53.
19. Huang E, Samaniego-Picota M, McCune T, et al. DNA testing for live kidney donors at risk for autosomal dominant polycystic kidney disease. Transplantation. 2009;87:133–7.
20. Niaudet P. Living donor kidney transplantation in patients with hereditary nephropathies. Nat Rev Nephrol. 2010;6:736–43.
21. Rossetti S, Consugar M, Chapman A, et al. Comprehensive molecular diagnostics in autosomal dominant polycystic kidney disease. J Am Soc Nephrol. 2007;18:2143–60.
22. Iliuta I-A, Kalatharan V, Wang KR, et al. Polycystic kidney disease without an apparent family history. J Am Soc Nephrol. 2017;28:2768–76.
23. Reed B, McFann K, Kimberling WJ, et al. Presence of de novo mutations in autosomal dominant polycystic kidney disease patients without family history. Am J Kidney Dis. 2008;52:1042–50.
24. Youssoufian H, Pyeritz R. Mechanisms and consequences of somatic mosaicism in humans. Nat Rev Genet. 2002;3:748–58.
25. Gottlieb B, Beitel L, Trifiro M. Somatic mosaicism and variability expressivity. Trends Genet. 2001;17:79–82.
26. Gevers TJ, Drenth JP. Diagnosis and management of polycystic liver disease. Nat Rev Gastroenterol Hepatol. 2013;10:101–8.
27. Adeva M, El-Youssef M, Rossetti S, et al. Clinical and molecular characterization defines a broadened spectrum of autosomal recessive polycystic kidney disease. Medicine (Baltimore). 2006;85:1–21.
28. Curatolo P, Bombardieri R, Jozwiak S. Tuberous sclerosis. Lancet. 2008;372:657–68.
29. Lonser RR, Glenn GM, Walther M, et al. von Hippel-Lindau disease. Lancet. 2003;361:2059–67.
30. Ulinski T, Lescure S, Beaufils S, et al. Renal phenotypes related to HNF1B mutations in a pediatric cohort. J Am Soc Nephrol. 2006;17:497–503.
31. Heidet L, Decramer S, Pawtowski A, et al. Spectrum of HNF1B mutations in a large cohort of patients who harbor renal disease. Clin J Am Soc Nephrol. 2010;5:1079–90.
32. Ekici A, Hackenbeck T, Moriniere V, et al. Renal fibrosis is the common feature of autosomal dominant tubulointerstitial kidney diseases caused by mutations in mucin 1 or uromodulin. Kidney Int. 2014;86:589–99.
33. Fabris A, Lupo A, Ferraro P, et al. Familial clustering of medullary sponge kidney is autosomal dominant with reduced pnentrance and variable expressivity. Kidney Int. 2013;83:272–7.

8 Renal Structural Involvement in Autosomal Dominant Polycystic Kidney Disease: Cyst Growth and Total Kidney Volume – Lessons from the Consortium for Radiologic Imaging of Polycystic Kidney Disease (CRISP)

Frederic Rahbari-Oskoui, Harpreet Bhutani, Olubunmi Williams, Ankush Mittal, and Arlene Chapman

Epidemiology

ADPKD is the most common hereditary kidney disease, characterized by progressive kidney cyst growth and enlargement over decades, ultimately leading to loss of kidney function and end-stage renal disease (ESRD) [1]. ADPKD is the fourth most common cause of renal failure in the United States with approximately 200,000 individuals diagnosed. There are two identified genes, *PKD1* and *PKD2*, which code for the proteins polycystin-1 and polycystin-2, and mutations in these genes account for approximately 85% and 15% of all diagnosed cases, respectively. Patients with *PKD2* disease have a less severe phenotype with a later age of onset of ESRD (mean age 74.0 versus 54.3 years *PKD2* vs. *PKD1*), later onset of hypertension, and a greater life expectancy [2, 3].

ADPKD is a systemic disorder and includes both renal and extrarenal manifestations such as hypertension, kidney pain, hematuria, cyst hemorrhage and infection, urinary tract infections, nephrolithiasis, liver and pancreatic cysts, abdominal hernias, valvular heart disease, left ventricular hypertrophy, biventricular diastolic dysfunction, and intracerebral aneurysms [1]. Clinical and genetic characteristics that associate with an earlier age of onset of ESRD include the *PKD1* genotype, male gender, proteinuria, gross hematuria before the age of 30, hypertension before the age of 35, and a history of three or more pregnancies [4]. All of these characteristics, as well as pain, are directly related to the degree of cystic involvement as measured by total kidney volume (TKV).

The characteristically increased TKV found in ADPKD differentiates this disease from other renal cystic diseases. ADPKD is characterized by unrelenting progression, a gradual but insistent nature of increase, and the appearance of

Disclosures: Arlene Chapman consultant to Otsuka, Pfizer, and Sanofi.

F. Rahbari-Oskoui, MD, MS · H. Bhutani, MD
O. Williams, MD, MPH · A. Mittal, BS
A. Chapman, MD (✉)
Department of Medicine,
Emory University School of Medicine,
Atlanta, GA, USA
e-mail: frahbar@emory.edu;
olubunmi.williams@emory.edu;
Achapman1@bsd.uchicago.edu

B. D. Cowley, Jr., J. J. Bissler (eds.), *Polycystic Kidney Disease*,
https://doi.org/10.1007/978-1-4939-7784-0_8

enlarged cysts throughout both the medulla and cortex. Although other hereditary cystic disorders carry similar manifestations, increased TKV is not a universal finding. The increase in TKV in ADPKD can be seen in utero or during childhood, is predominant in adult life, and does not reverse [5]. Acquired cystic kidney disease, the most common non-hereditary cystic disease of the kidney, observed in patients with advanced renal disease, typically presents with multiple small- to moderate-sized renal cysts, an echogenic cortex, and small- to normal-sized kidneys. Other cystic disease of the kidneys, such as medullary cystic kidney disease, juvenile nephronophthisis, glomerulocystic kidney disease, and von Hippel-Lindau syndrome, are typically not associated with increased TKV [6], and cyst distribution is often limited to the medulla or the cortex, typically without extremely large cysts [7].

Pathogenesis of Cyst Formation in ADPKD

Cysts in ADPKD arise from the nephrons and can arise from any nephron segment, as well as the glomerulus; however cysts occur in only 5% of all nephrons due to a required "second hit" or somatic mutation that results in focal, clonal proliferation [8–10]. Cysts form as focal, segmental dilatations of the tubule that ultimately disconnect from the parent tubule (typically once the cyst reaches a diameter of 2 mm or greater) and continue to grow through autonomous proliferation and fluid secretion [8, 11]. The process of cystogenesis can start in utero with an initial growth rate reaching 2400%/year, arising from 100 μm tubules and growing to 5 mm or 5000 μm size by birth. This level of cyst expansion is undetectable by clinical imaging techniques, and increased kidney size with echogenicity is often the only ultrasound (US) finding [12]. The growth rate of cysts measured by magnetic resonance imaging and US is approximately 17%/year during childhood. [13]. The process of continual cyst growth and expansion commonly results in an impressive TKV of approximately 1 L by the age of 30 or a weight of 5 kg/kidney once closer to ESRD. This is dramatic in contrast with a normal kidney weight of 0.15 kg.

The polycystins are essential to maintain a fully differentiated tubular epithelium. Reduction in one of these proteins below a critical threshold results in an increased rate of proliferation and apoptosis, expression of a secretory phenotype, inability to maintain planar cell polarity, and remodeling of the extracellular matrix [14]. Polycystins 1 and 2 are two transmembrane proteins that form a single functional complex [15–18]. Polycystin-2 is a nonselective cation channel capable of transporting calcium (Ca^2+) into the cell by interacting with the transient receptor potential channel 1 (TRPC1) [19, 20]. Polycystin-1 is a receptor for an unidentified ligand. The polycystins are located together in the primary cilium [21, 22], a hairlike organelle projecting from the apical surface of tubular epithelial cells into the lumen. The polycystin complex contributes to ciliary function as a mechanosensor, detecting changes in urinary flow. Calcium influx secondary to activation of the calcium channel via polycystin-2 in turn induces release of calcium from intracellular stores within the endoplasmic reticulum. [23]. In the setting of decreased availability of functional polycystins, reduced intracellular concentrations of calcium and increased intracellular concentrations of cyclic AMP (cAMP) are present which lead to alterations in epithelial cell signaling and increased cellular proliferation [24, 25]. Decreased polycystin levels also lead to aberrant apical secretion of chloride. The progressive chloride accumulation within the cyst lumen drives sodium and water secretion following transepithelial potential and osmotic gradients [14] ultimately resulting in cyst expansion.

Natural History of ADPKD: Kidney Cyst Burden and Decline in Kidney Function

Renal cyst growth and kidney enlargement are cardinal features of ADPKD. In the first systematic and extensive review of 284 patients with ADPKD in 1955, Dalgaard identified the value

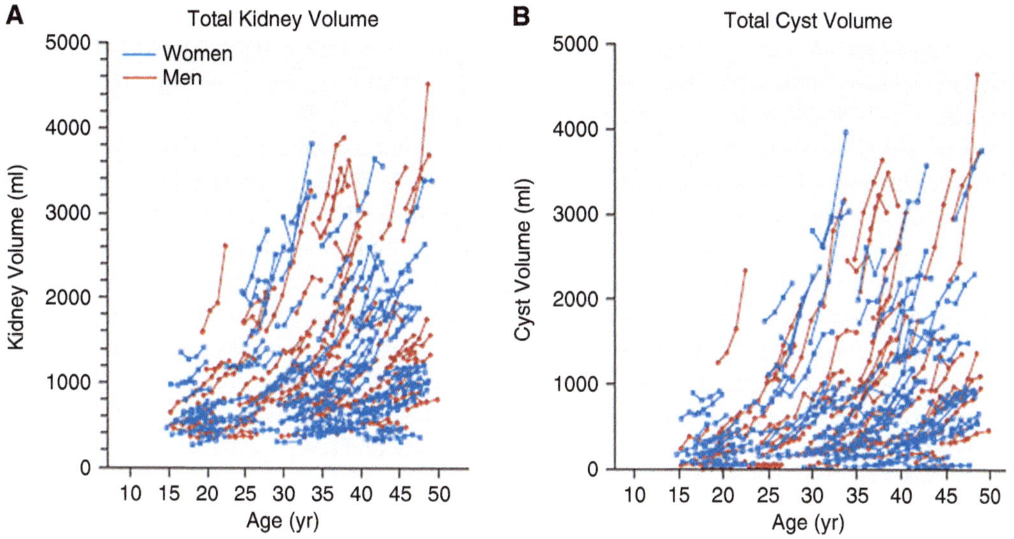

Fig. 8.1 Total kidney volume (**a**) and total cyst volume (**b**) in relation to age in women (in blue) and men (in red). The lines connecting the four measurements for each patient in the 3 years of follow-up exhibit an exponential growth process (From Grantham et al. [40]. Copyright © Massachusetts Medical Society (2006). Reprinted with permission from the Massachusetts Medical Society)

of renomegaly on physical examination in diagnosing ADPKD and clarified that in some cases, renomegaly would be absent or unilateral, making a diagnosis of ADPKD more difficult [26]. In an early study of 38 patients with ADPKD where serial determinations of glomerular filtration rate, PAH clearance, and reciprocal serum creatinine were performed, renal function remained preserved for decades and ultimately decreased rapidly at a later stage. Franz and Reubi postulated that a complex nonlinear relationship exists between renal function, age, and the slow but constant growth of kidney cysts [27]. More contemporary large longitudinal studies of ADPKD demonstrate that GFR remains stable for decades despite significant increases in TKV. In fact, hyperfiltration has been reported in a number of studies [28–30]. While hyperfiltration of the remaining non-cystic nephrons allows GFR to be maintained within the normal range, this is falsely reassuring, particularly as TKV continues to increase and renal fibrosis is already present [31] (Fig. 8.1). In ADPKD, once GFR begins to decline (typically in the 5th decade of life) progression to renal failure is rapid and relatively uniform, with an average rate of decline of 4.4–5.9 mL/min/year, more predictable and faster than other progressive chronic kidney diseases [32].

Imaging Studies to Measure Total Kidney Volume (TKV)

Over the past three decades, different imaging modalities have been used to establish the importance of increases in TKV in ADPKD. US imaging was used at the University of Colorado to measure TKV using the ellipsoid formula in a 16-year longitudinal cohort of 241 patients. Sequential US-based TKV measurements were performed along with measurements of serum creatinine at a mean interval of 7.8 (±3.1) years. The mean increase in single TKV was 46 (±55) cm^3/year and correlated ($r = -0.53$) with a mean decline in GFR of 2.4 (±2.8) mL/min/1.73m^2/year. Men had greater kidney growth, more severe hypertension, and a faster decline in GFR than women of similar age. Multiple linear regression models showed a significant relationship between rate of change in GFR and TKV, rate of change in TKV, proteinuria, and age of initiation of ESRD [33].

Similarly, several studies reported CT-based TKV and cyst volume measurements in ADPKD. An early study from Denmark in 1983 evaluated 43 ADPKD patients with creatinine clearance levels between 8 and 130 ml/min. CT-based measures of TKV were 70% larger in patients with severely decreased renal function vs. patients with preserved kidney function (2053 ± 698 vs. 1212 ± 411 mls) [34]. Sise et al. analyzed two contrast-enhanced CTs more than 3 years apart in ten ADPKD patients with serum creatinine levels <1.6 mg/dl. The rate of TKV increase was 53.9 (±10.4) mL/year/kidney ($p < 0.001$), and 50% of the patients who reached dialysis within the following 11.2 years had a total cyst volume/kidney volume ratio of >0.43 [35]. Torres and colleagues used fast electron-beam CT weekly on three occasions 1 week apart in nine patients with serum creatinine levels of <1.3 mg/dl and were able to obtain follow up imaging 8 years later. They demonstrated high reproducibility and reliability of initial TKV measures with an average coefficient of variation for TKV, cyst volume, % cystic volume, and renal parenchymal volume of 3.4%, 7.2%, 5.3%, and 5.6%, respectively. Spearman rank correlation coefficients between slope of GFR and TKV and cyst volume were −0.48 and −0.78, respectively [36].

Even though these studies established the utility of CT imaging in ADPKD, the use of CT for longitudinal TKV measures is limited due to the risk associated with ionizing radiation and iodinated contrast exposures. Increased availability of magnetic resonance (MR) imaging in the 1990s has provided an alternative to CT imaging.

Total Kidney Volume by Magnetic Resonance Imaging (MRI) and the Consortium for Radiologic Imaging Studies of Polycystic Kidney Disease (CRISP)

Magnetic resonance imaging (MRI) relies on detecting a radio-frequency signal emitted by excited hydrogen atoms in the body (present in any tissue containing water molecules) using energy from an oscillating magnetic field applied at the appropriate resonant frequency. MRI has been used in rodent and human models of polycystic kidney disease to measure TKV and total cyst volume (TCV).

The first systematic assessment of MR-based TKV came from the National Institutes of Health (NIH)-funded Consortium for Radiologic Imaging Studies of Polycystic Kidney Disease (CRISP), which developed reliable and sensitive imaging modalities for assessment of kidney disease progression in ADPKD [37]. Before initiating the CRISP protocol, several steps were undertaken to establish the accuracy and reproducibility of TKV measurements.

MR-based phantom models were developed and tested to establish the accuracy and validity of TKV measures by MR [38]. In one model, a kidney-shaped mold of agarose (representing renal parenchyma) containing grapes (mimicking cysts) and olive oil (representing fat) was frozen and measured in two different 1.5 Tesla MRI machines. True individual grape and total phantom volumes were measured by volume of fluid displacement. An additional geometric phantom made of solidified agarose containing four water-filled balloons (5, 10, 20, 30 mls) was constructed to evaluate accuracy of cyst volume measurement across a broad range of volumes. Image segmentation and measurements were performed using stereology.

Measuring the whole simple phantom and the individual balloon volumes located within the phantom was accurate (mean coefficient of variation: 2.8% (2–5%)). The grape volume measurements were highly accurate (mean coefficient of variation 1.4% (0.1–3.1%)) and reliable (mean 1.8% (0.2–4.6%)). The accuracy and reliability of the second phantom for cyst/renal parenchyma were in close agreement (Siemens 149.8/396.9 cm^3, GE 147/383.3 cm^3 vs. fluid displacement methodology 150/385 cm^3).

Standardization of TKV acquisition methods was tested in a variety of ways [39]. Four small and large balloon phantoms were created and scanned at four different clinical centers using the methodology of Bae et al. [38]. To test reliability of MR-based TKV measures in humans, four patients (ages 21, 40, 48, and 58 with varying levels of kidney function) were scanned at each of the four participating centers for the CRISP consortium 2 weeks apart by Siemens, Phillips, or GE MR scanners. TKV was calculated from contiguous 3 mm, non-overlapping images by summing the products of the area measurements and the slice thickness (stereology method). A region-based thresholding method was used to calculate total cyst volume. A threshold was selected interactively by an analyst using T2-weighted images. Excellent reliability of measurement was found with reliability coefficients (interclass *r*) ranging between 0.961 and 0.998 for intra-reader and inter-reader variability. Both TKV and TCV were reproducible with repeat error for TKV and TCV ranging from 0.2% to 2.5% and 0.1% to 5.6% and mean difference between measurements of 1.3% and 4.0%, respectively.

CRISP participants were 15–46 years old with relatively intact renal function (24 h creatinine clearance >70 ml/min/1.73 m^2 or a Cockcroft-Gault estimate of creatinine clearance >70 ml/min or serum creatinine level of 1.6 mg/dl or less in men and 1.4 mg/dl or less in women). Two thirds of the study population had risk factors for progression to renal failure including the presence of hypertension before age of 35 or the presence of dipstick detectable proteinuria. Two hundred forty-one ADPKD individuals were enrolled and underwent non-radiolabeled iothalamate clearance, comprehensive clinical evaluation, blood pressure measurements, 24-h urinary albumin and electrolyte excretion, and MR renal imaging for TKV and renal blood flow annually. All measures were obtained annually for the first 3 years and alternate years thereafter [37].

The distribution of TKV in the CRISP population was widely skewed consistent with the known high variability of disease severity in ADPKD. TCV measurements were more variable than TKV measurements but remained highly correlated with TKV ($r = 0.99$), indicating that renal cyst expansion accounts for the increase in TKV seen in ADPKD (Fig. 8.1). Change in left and right TKVs was highly correlated with the left consistently larger than the right, similar to healthy individuals [40].

The first 3-year follow-up of the CRISP cohort demonstrated an exponential increase in TKV and TCV. The baseline mean (±SD) TKV was 1060 (±642) ml and increased by 204 ± 246 ml over a 3-year period (68 ml/year) or an annual growth rate of 5.27 ± 3.92%. TCV increased 218 ± 263 ml during the same period. The vast majority of CRISP participants demonstrated detectable increases in TKV over a relatively short (12-month) period. Baseline TKV predicted the subsequent rate of increase in TKV, independent of age. Importantly, although GFR did not decrease significantly in the overall CRISP cohort during the first 3 years of observation, those with TKV greater than 1500 ml ($n = 51$) had an associated decline in GFR of 4.33 ± 8.07 ml/min/year, $P < 0.001$. Baseline TKV was greater in the 135 patients with a *PKD1* mutation than in the 28 patients with a *PKD2* mutation (994 vs. 678 mL, $p = 0.0003$). However the rate of increase in TKV were similar for patients in both groups (5.51 vs. 4.99%/year, p = NS). There was a gradual nonsignificant decline in renal function by non-radiolabeled iothalamate clearance (mean slope −1.5%/year; SD = 9.3%), by MDRD equation (mean −3.0%/year; SD = 7.0%), and by Cockcroft-Gault equation (mean −1.8%/year; SD 6.7%) [31].

MR measures with and without gadolinium were performed in CRISP participants until 2007. After a warning regarding the risk of nephrogenic systemic fibrosis related to gadolinium exposure was issued by the US Food and Drug Administration, gadolinium-enhanced imaging was discontinued. Comparison of MR measures of TKV with and without gadolinium showed that measurements were highly correlated ($r = 0.99$) and that gadolinium-enhanced MRI measured a higher TKV for small-, medium-, and larger-sized kidneys (average variation of 43.55, 48.31, and 26.15 mL (or 9.59%, 5.9%, and 1.98%), respectively [39].

The relationship of TKV with other known risk factors for progression to ESRD in ADPKD is also highlighted in the CRISP cohort. Genotype, gender, age, proteinuria, and hypertension, all risk factors for progression to renal failure, were associated with a larger TKV [31].

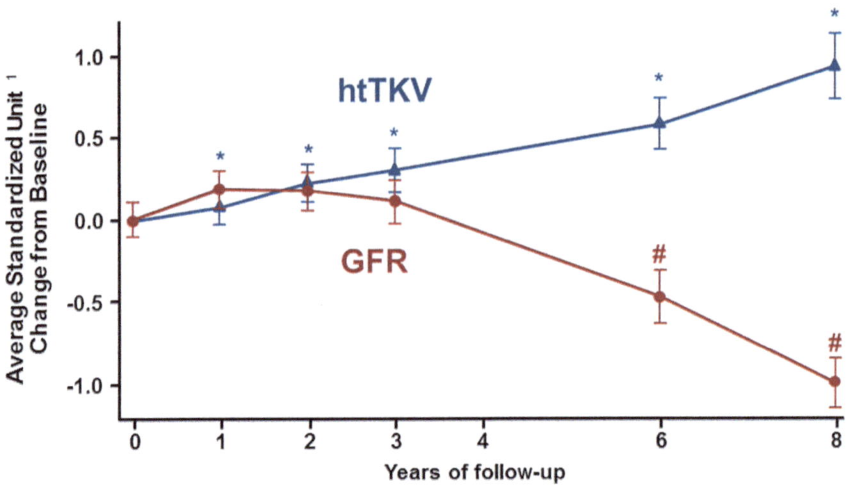

Fig. 8.2 Average standardized change in height adjusted total kidney volume (htTKV) and iothalamate GFR. HtTKV and iothalamate determinations at baseline and five subsequent visits until year 8 (n = 93 with complete data). $P < 0.01$ based on paired t-test comparing each year to baseline for htTKV (*) and GFR (#) (Republished with permission of the American Society of Nephrology from Chapman et al. [41]; permission conveyed through Copyright Clearance Center, Inc.)

The observed gender difference in TKV in CRISP was evaluated with regard to body size. Referencing baseline TKV to height, weight, body surface area, or BMI diminished the gender differences in TKV with height providing a male/female ratio of 1.037 similar to the differences seen in TKV. These data suggest that height-corrected TKV is a more suitable measure of cyst burden in ADPKD. GFR was referenced to body surface area following the conventional notation in nephrology and the values for height and body surface area followed a similar degree of adjustment (1.036 and 0.965, respectively).

With further longitudinal follow-up of 8 years in CRISP participants in CRISP II, additional insight was obtained regarding TKV progression and its relationship with the decline in kidney function. The mean rate of increase in TKV continued unchanged (5.2%/year), resulting in an 8-year increase of 55% from baseline [41]. Thirty-one percent of the CRISP participants reached CKD Stage 3 during this time. The negative correlation between htTKV and GFR at baseline increased at years 3 and 8 of follow-up (r = −0.22 baseline, −0.44 year 3 and −0.65 year 8) (Fig. 8.2). Prediction models established that a baseline htTKV of ≥600 cc/m (equivalent to a TKV of 1047 mls) strongly predicted the development of CKD Stage 3 within 8 years with a receiver-operating characteristic (ROC) value of 0.84. Each increase in baseline htTKV of 100 cc/m significantly predicted the development of CKD 3 with an odds ratio of 1.48. HtTKV was a stronger predictor than age, genotype, serum creatinine, blood urea nitrogen, urinary albumin, or urinary monocyte chemotactic protein-1 (MCP-1) for future CKD Stage 3.

The relationship between htTKV and complications in ADPKD (hypertension, renal pain, gross hematuria, nephrolithiasis, and urinary tract infections) was evaluated in the CRISP population. More than 50% had experienced at least one complication by the time of enrollment (mean age 33 years). TKV associated significantly with gross hematuria, pain, and hypertension but not nephrolithiasis or urinary tract infection. Each 100 ml increase in htTKV was associated with an increased likelihood of HTN (53%), gross hematuria (14%), and kidney pain (19%) [42].

These findings confirmed previous assessments in multiple ADPKD populations and provided direct evidence for the strong association between kidney size, symptoms, and complications in ADPKD. In a French pediatric study of

29 children screened prenatally and followed for 25 years, those with in utero or neonatal cysts had a higher frequency of symptoms (pain, urinary tract infection, hematuria) vs. those without any cysts at birth [43]. In adults with ADPKD, those with repeated episodes of gross hematuria, proteinuria, albuminuria, hypertension, renal pain, progressive renal insufficiency, and abdominal distention had significantly larger TKV than patients without those features [31, 33, 34, 44–49].

Other contemporary ADPKD populations have been studied utilizing MR imaging and report rates of TKV growth similar to the CRISP study (Table 8.1). The Suisse cohort of 100 European ADPKD individuals with relatively intact kidney function similar to CRISP followed for 2 years and imaged every 6 months demonstrated a TKV growth rate of 5.8%/year measured by MRI [50]. A Japanese cohort of 65 patients followed for 39 months demonstrated a significant inverse correlation between Log htTKV and eGFR with a correlation coefficient of $r = -0.6688$ ($p < 0.001$) [51]. Larger baseline TKV was associated with a steeper eGFR slope, supporting the observation that eGFR declines faster in patients with larger TKV [51]. Data from the participants in the placebo arms of the everolimus, sirolimus, and tolvaptan clinical trials also showed rates of TKV growth similar to the CRISP cohort [52–54].

The CRISP consortium continues to look for more efficient and automated ways of measuring TKV. CRISP TKV measurements were done by stereology (manually traced renal contours) and TCV by a thresholding method. A semiautomated method for the segmentation of individual renal cysts from MRI images has been compared to manual segmentation. The total number of cysts in each kidney measured with the two methods correlated well (intraclass correlation coefficient, ICC, of 0.99), with a very small relative bias (0.3% increase) with the semiautomated method. TCV measured using both methods also correlated well (ICC, 1.00), with a small relative bias of 9.0% decrease in the semiautomated method. These findings suggest that a reliable semiautomated quantitative measurements of TCV can be performed as an indicator of disease severity in early and moderate ADPKD [55]. Another Italian group has also developed and validated a similar automatic method with the same level of reliability [56].

Members of the CRISP consortium developed mathematical models that reliably estimate TKV at age 18 for each CRISP participant based on their baseline age and TKV assuming that TKV increases at a constant rate in an exponential fashion. When imputing cyst dosage or number at a given age, and employing different rates of TKV growth, reliable age-based TKV could be established. Importantly, although cyst dose, rate of cyst growth, and age of cyst development were all contributors to TKV in ADPKD, development of cysts at a later age contributed very little to the ultimate TKV attained. Computational modeling that integrated cyst surface area, cyst volume, and a rate of cyst growth similar to the rate measured in the CRISP study indicates that cysts that developed early in life are the main contributors to the TKV observed [57].

To translate the observations of CRISP back to the clinical management of ADPKD patients, the role of ultrasound (US)-measured TKV is worthy of discussion. CRISP participants underwent US measurement during the first year of participation in CRISP. US calculations of TKV were determined by using a modified ellipsoid formulae [$TKV = 4/3\ \pi \times ½$(anterior–posterior diameter) × ½(width) × ½(length)] by trained ultrasonographers and were compared to TKV measured by MR. The correlation coefficient of US vs. MRI TKV was 0.88 and US TKV underestimated MR-based TKV by up to as much as 25% [58]. Reproducibility or coefficient of variation was greater with US (21–35%) vs. MRI (2.1–2.5%). All patients with an US TKV less than 700 mls had an MRI TKV less than 1000 mls, and all patients with an US TKV greater than 1700 mls had an MRI TKV greater than 1000 mls. TKV increased 12 ± 36% by US and 4.2 ± 7.2% by MR in the first year of CRISP. These data indicate that US-based TKV is significantly less precise than MR and that over short periods of time of follow-up, US is unreliable regarding the change in TKV. However the correlation between renal

Table 8.1 Relationship between TKV and GFR in five cohorts of ADPKD patients

Cohort	Sample size	Follow-up (months)	Baseline TKV (mean ± SD)	Mean annual increase in TKV (in mls, %)	GFR (mean ± SD) mL/min/1.73 m^2	Annual decline in GFR (mL/min/1.73 m^2/year)	Age (mean ± SD years)	HTN (%)	Gender (male %)	Race White/Asian/others (%)
Japanese cohort [51]	64	40	1681 ± 1001	(109.5, 5.9%)	60.2 ± 27.38	1.02 (3.6)	47 ± 14.1	88	32.8	0/100/0
Sirolimus study- placebo group [52]	50	18	1003 ± 424 (median)	(66, 5.2%)	91 ± 17	2.33	32 ± 6	64	64	98/2/0
Tempo trial- placebo group [54]	484	36	1668 ± 873	(not reported, 5.5%)	82.14 ± 22.73	Not reported	39 ± 7	78.9	51.9	84/13/3
Everolimus trial-placebo group [53]	216	24	1911 ± 1153	(150, 7.88%)	56.0 ± 19.9	3.5	44.4 ± 10.5	88	53.7	100/0/0
CRISP-I cohort- 3-year FU [37–40]	241	36	1060 ± 642	(63.4, 5.27%)	98.2 ± 24.9	Not reported	33.8 ± 8.9	61.4	39.8	87/1/12

HTN Hypertension, *M* male, *F* female, *GFR* glomerular filtration rate, *TKV* total kidney volume length (commonly obtained in clinical practice) measured by US and MR and TKV measured by MR is particularly strong ($r = 0.97$). The agreement between US and MR renal length and US and MR TKV was strong until kidney length exceeded 16 cm (the maximal length of kidney typically obtained in a single US image). Additionally, US renal length predicted future CKD Stage 3 strongly (ROC = 0.91) equal to TKV [59].

Cyst Growth and Total Kidney Volume in Children with ADPKD

Data on cyst growth and disease progression is sparse in pediatric ADPKD patients. The assessment of TKV in children with ADPKD is hindered by normal renal growth in the healthy population. To date, there are only three studies on TKV in ADPKD children. One study from the University of Colorado examined longitudinal TKV and TCV measured by MR in ADPKD children [60]. Three hundred two MRIs from 77 children aged 4–21 were performed. ADPKD children demonstrated a 14% and 9%/year increase in hypertensive and normotensive children [60]. In this study, hypertension was defined as having blood pressures >75th percentile for age and gender.

In a small study from the Czech Republic, US and ambulatory blood pressure monitoring were performed in 62 ADPKD children (22 hypertensive and 40 normotensive) with normal renal function (mean age 12.3 ± 4.3 years). Mean TKV was significantly greater in hypertensive vs. normotensive children (2.7 ± 2.3 SDS versus 1.2 ± 2.5 SDS, $P < 0.01$) with similar anthropometric data and renal function. In addition, the mean number of cysts was significantly higher in hypertensive vs. normotensive individuals (35 ± 15 cysts versus 23 ± 14 cysts, $P < 0.01$). TKV correlated with daytime as well as with night-time systolic and diastolic BP ($r = 0.41$–0.47, $P < 0.01$). Correlations with renal length and the number of renal cysts were also significant ($r = 0.29$–0.43, $P < 0.05$ and 0.01, respectively). This study indicates that ADPKD children should have their BP checked regularly, especially those who show increased TKV or a high number of renal cysts on US [61].

The third study from Emory University identified accelerated cyst growth during adolescence. Twenty-nine adolescents and young adults with ADPKD and age and gender matched healthy controls less than 18 years of age underwent MR-based TKV and routine laboratory analyses. Data indicated an accelerated TKV and TCV growth curve with an inflection point at 12.5 and 12.7 years for TKV and TCV, respectively [62]. This study also demonstrated an association between TKV and increased systolic and diastolic blood pressures. These data taken together, suggest that it is important to monitor children at risk for ADPKD with regard to blood pressure. For those diagnosed with ADPKD, it is now possible to identify individuals at increased risk for faster disease progression to allow for more intensive monitoring and treatment options.

Conclusions

There is a significant body of evidence that now supports htTKV as a prognostic marker of disease severity in ADPKD. Many associated complications of ADPKD including hypertension, gross hematuria, pain, and renal insufficiency are inextricably linked to TKV. The establishment of TKV as an acceptable biomarker for clinical trial enrichment is currently under review by the US Food and Drug Administration. Future evaluations, including further follow-up in CRISP III, will help to evaluate TKV as a suitable primary endpoint for interventional trials in ADPKD.

References

1. Gabow P. Autosomal dominant polycystic kidney disease. N Engl J Med. 1993;329(5):332–42.
2. Hateboer N, et al. Comparison of phenotypes of polycystic kidney disease types 1 and 2. European PKD1-PKD2 Study Group. Lancet. 1999;353(9147):103–7.
3. Torra R, Darnell A, Nicolau C, Volpini V, Revert L, Estivill X. Linkage, clinical features, and prognosis of autosomal dominant polycystic kidney disease types 1 and 2. J Am Soc Nephrol. 1996;7(10):2142–51.
4. Fick GM, Gabow P. Natural history of autosomal dominant polycystic kidney disease. Annu Rev Med. 1994;45:23–9.
5. Gunay-Aygun M, Font-Montgomery E, Lukose L, Tuchman M, Graf J, Bryant JC, Kleta R, Garcia A, Edwards H, Piwnica-Worms K, Adams D, Bernardini I, Fischer RE, Krasnewich D, Oden N, Ling A, Quezado Z, Zak C, Daryanani KT, Turkbey B, Choyke P, Guay-Woodford LM, Gahl WA. Correlation of kidney function, volume and imaging findings, and PKHD1 mutations in 73 patients with autosomal recessive polycystic kidney disease. Clin J Am Soc Nephrol. 2010;5(6):972–84.
6. Rizk D, Chapman A. Cystic and inherited kidney diseases. Am J Kidney Dis. 2003;42(6):1305–17.
7. Bisceglia M, et al. Renal cystic diseases: a review. Adv Anat Pathol. 2006;13(1):26–56.
8. Baert L. Hereditary polycystic kidney disease (adult form): a microdissection study of two cases at an early stage of the disease. Kidney Int. 1978;13(6):519–25.
9. Heggo O. A microdissection study of cystic disease of the kidneys in adults. JPatholBact. 1966;91:311–5.
10. Grantham JJ, Geiser J, Evan AP. Cyst formation and growth in autosomal dominant polycystic kidney disease. Kidney Int. 1987;31(5):1145–52.
11. Cuppage FE, et al. Ultrastructure and function of cysts from human adult polycystic kidneys. Kidney Int. 1980;17(3):372–81.
12. Emmanuelli V, et al. Prenatal diagnosis of hyperechogenic kidneys: a study of 17 cases. J Gynecol Obstet Biol Reprod (Paris). 2010;39(8):637–46.
13. Grantham JJ, et al. Evidence of extraordinary growth in the progressive enlargement of renal cysts. Clin J Am Soc Nephrol. 2010;5(5):889–96.
14. Torres VE, Harris PC. Autosomal dominant polycystic kidney disease: the last 3 years. Kidney Int. 2009;76(2):149–68.
15. Hanaoka K, et al. Co-assembly of polycystin-1 and -2 produces unique cation-permeable currents. Nature. 2000;408(6815):990–4.
16. Qian F, et al. Cleavage of polycystin-1 requires the receptor for egg jelly domain and is disrupted by human autosomal-dominant polycystic kidney disease 1-associated mutations. Proc Natl Acad Sci U S A. 2002;99(26):16981–6.
17. Qian F, et al. PKD1 interacts with PKD2 through a probable coiled-coil domain. Nat Genet. 1997;16(2):179–83.
18. Chauvet V, et al. Mechanical stimuli induce cleavage and nuclear translocation of the polycystin-1 C terminus. J Clin Invest. 2004;114(10):1433–43.
19. Gonzalez-Perrett S, et al. Polycystin-2, the protein mutated in autosomal dominant polycystic kidney disease (ADPKD), is a Ca2+-permeable nonselective cation channel. Proc Natl Acad Sci U S A. 2001;98(3):1182–7.
20. Vassilev PM, et al. Polycystin-2 is a novel cation channel implicated in defective intracellular Ca(2+) homeostasis in polycystic kidney disease. Biochem Biophys Res Commun. 2001;282(1):341–50.
21. Pazour GJ, et al. Polycystin-2 localizes to kidney cilia and the ciliary level is elevated in orpk mice with polycystic kidney disease. Curr Biol. 2002;12(11):R378–80.
22. Yoder BK, Hou X, Guay-Woodford LM. The polycystic kidney disease proteins, polycystin-1, polycystin-2, polaris, and cystin, are co-localized in renal cilia. J Am Soc Nephrol. 2002;13(10):2508–16.
23. Nauli SM, et al. Polycystins 1 and 2 mediate mechanosensation in the primary cilium of kidney cells. Nat Genet. 2003;33(2):129–37.
24. Yamaguchi T, et al. Renal accumulation and excretion of cyclic adenosine monophosphate in a murine model of slowly progressive polycystic kidney disease. Am J Kidney Dis. 1997;30(5):703–9.
25. Hanaoka K, Guggino WB. cAMP regulates cell proliferation and cyst formation in autosomal polycystic kidney disease cells. J Am Soc Nephrol. 2000;11(7):1179–87.
26. Dalgaard OZ, Norby S. Autosomal dominant polycystic kidney disease in the 1980's. Clin Genet. 1989;36(5):320–5.
27. Franz KA, Reubi F. Rate of functional deterioration in polycystic kidney disease. Kidney Int. 1983;23(3):526–9.
28. Dimitrakov D, et al. Glomerular hyperfiltration and serum beta 2-microglobulin used as early markers in diagnosis of autosomal dominant polycystic kidney disease. Folia Med (Plovdiv). 1993;35(1–2):59–62.
29. Wong H, et al. Patients with autosomal dominant polycystic kidney disease hyperfiltrate early in their disease. Am J Kidney Dis. 2004;43(4):624–8.
30. Helal I, et al. Glomerular hyperfiltration and renal progression in children with autosomal dominant polycystic kidney disease. Clin J Am Soc Nephrol. 2011;6(10):2439–43.
31. Grantham JJ, Chapman AB, Torres VE. Volume progression in autosomal dominant polycystic kidney disease: the major factor determining clinical outcomes. Clin J Am Soc Nephrol. 2006;1(1):148–57.
32. Klahr S, Breyer J, Beck GJ, Dennis VW, Hartman JA, Roth D, Steinman TI, Wang SR, Yamamoto ME. Dietary protein restriction, blood pressure control, and the progression of polycystic kidney disease. Modification of Diet in Renal Disease Study Group. J Am Soc Nephrol. 1995;5(12):2037–47.

33. Fick-Brosnahan GM, et al. Relationship between renal volume growth and renal function in autosomal dominant polycystic kidney disease: a longitudinal study. Am J Kidney Dis. 2002;39(6):1127–34.
34. Thomsen HS, et al. Volume of polycystic kidneys during reduction of renal function. Urol Radiol. 1981;3(2):85–9.
35. Sise C, et al. Volumetric determination of progression in autosomal dominant polycystic kidney disease by computed tomography. Kidney Int. 2000;58(6):2492–501.
36. King BF, et al. Quantification and longitudinal trends of kidney, renal cyst, and renal parenchyma volumes in autosomal dominant polycystic kidney disease. J Am Soc Nephrol. 2000;11(8):1505–11.
37. Chapman AB, et al. Renal structure in early autosomal-dominant polycystic kidney disease (ADPKD): The Consortium for Radiologic Imaging Studies of Polycystic Kidney Disease (CRISP) cohort. Kidney Int. 2003;64(3):1035–45.
38. Bae KT, Commean PK, Lee J. Volumetric measurement of renal cysts and parenchyma using MRI: phantoms and patients with polycystic kidney disease. J Comput Assist Tomogr. 2000;24(4):614–9.
39. Bae KT, et al. MRI-based kidney volume measurements in ADPKD: reliability and effect of gadolinium enhancement. Clin J Am Soc Nephrol. 2009;4(4):719–25.
40. Grantham JJ, et al. Volume progression in polycystic kidney disease. N Engl J Med. 2006;354(20):2122–30.
41. Chapman AB, et al. Kidney volume and functional outcomes in autosomal dominant polycystic kidney disease. Clin J Am Soc Nephrol. 2012;7(3):479–86.
42. Rahbari-Oskoui FF, et al. Relationship between renal complications and total kidney volume in autosomal dominant polycystic kidney disease from the Consortium for Radiologic Imaging of Polycystic Kidney Disease (CRISP) Cohort. J Am Soc Nephrol 2013;24:687A.
43. Boyer O, et al. Prognosis of autosomal dominant polycystic kidney disease diagnosed in utero or at birth. Pediatr Nephrol. 2007;22(3):380–8.
44. Johnson AM, Gabow P. Identification of patients with autosomal dominant polycystic kidney disease at highest risk for end-stage renal disease. J Am Soc Nephrol. 1997;8:1560–7.
45. Gabow PA, Duley I, Johnson AM. Clinical profiles of gross hematuria in autosomal dominant polycystic kidney disease. Am J Kidney Dis. 1992;20(2):140–3.
46. Gabow PA, et al. Factors affecting the progression of renal disease in autosomal-dominant polycystic kidney disease. Kidney Int. 1992;41(5):1311–9.
47. Sharp C, Johnson A, Gabow P. Factors relating to urinary protein excretion in children with autosomal dominant polycystic kidney disease. J Am Soc Nephrol. 1998;9:1908–14.
48. Chapman AB, Schrier RW. Pathogenesis of hypertension in autosomal dominant polycystic kidney disease. Semin Nephrol. 1991;11(6):653–60.
49. Fick GM, et al. The spectrum of autosomal dominant polycystic kidney disease in children. J Am Soc Nephrol. 1994;4(9):1654–60.
50. Kistler AD, et al. Increases in kidney volume in autosomal dominant polycystic kidney disease can be detected within 6 months. Kidney Int. 2009;75(2):235–41.
51. Higashihara E, et al. Kidney volume and function in autosomal dominant polycystic kidney disease. Clin Exp Nephrol. 2014;18(1):157–65.
52. Serra AL, et al. Sirolimus and kidney growth in autosomal dominant polycystic kidney disease. N Engl J Med. 2010;363(9):820–9.
53. Walz G, et al. Everolimus in patients with autosomal dominant polycystic kidney disease. N Engl J Med. 2010;363(9):830–40.
54. Torres VE, et al. Tolvaptan in patients with autosomal dominant polycystic kidney disease. N Engl J Med. 2012;367(25):2407–18.
55. Bae K, et al. Segmentation of individual renal cysts from MR images in patients with autosomal dominant polycystic kidney disease. Clin J Am Soc Nephrol. 2013;8(7):1089–97.
56. Mignani R, et al. Assessment of kidney volume in polycystic kidney disease using magnetic resonance imaging without contrast medium. Am J Nephrol. 2011;33(2):176–84.
57. Grantham JJ, et al. Determinants of renal volume in autosomal-dominant polycystic kidney disease. Kidney Int. 2008;73(1):108–16.
58. O'Neill WC, et al. Sonographic assessment of the severity and progression of autosomal dominant polycystic kidney disease: the Consortium of Renal Imaging Studies in Polycystic Kidney Disease (CRISP). Am J Kidney Dis. 2005;46(6):1058–64.
59. Chapman AB, S.V., Rahbari-Oskoui FF, Bhutani HS, Grantham JJ, Torres VE, Bae KT, Landslittel, O'Neill WC for the CRISP Investigators. Kidney length measured by ultrasound (US) predicts development of chronic kidney disease (CKD) stage 3 in autosomal dominant polycystic kidney disease (ADPKD): findings from the Consortium for the Radiographic Imaging Studies of Polycystic Kidney Disease (CRISP) cohort. J Am Soc Nephrol 2013;24:687A.
60. Cadnapaphornchai MA, et al. Magnetic resonance imaging of kidney and cyst volume in children with ADPKD. Clin J Am Soc Nephrol. 2011;6(2):369–76.
61. Seeman T, Dusek J, Vondrichová H, Kyncl M, John U, Misselwitz J, Janda J. Ambulatory blood pressure correlates with renal volume and number of renal cysts in children with autosomal dominant polycystic kidney disease. Blood Press Monit. 2003;8(3):107–10.
62. Risk D, Rahbari-Oskoui F; Chapman AB. Adolescence is a time of accelerated renal growth in ADPKD. J Am Soc Nephrol 2007;18:368A.

Renal Complications: Pain, Infection, and Nephrolithiasis

9

Cristian Riella, Peter G. Czarnecki, and Theodore I. Steinman

Introduction

While the predominant academic interest in polycystic kidney disease is related to the genetics, pathophysiology, clinical pathology, and therapeutic trials, clinicians and patients predominantly struggle with the management of symptoms and comorbid conditions [1]. Cyst-related pain and infection, as well as nephrolithiasis, represent a significant cause of morbidity inherent to the nature of PKD and require specific attention by the treating physician. Notably, more than 60% of patients with ADPKD are affected by abdominal and flank pain, acute or chronic, in their lifetime [2], arising from kidney, liver, or, less often, pancreatic cysts, independent of the actual cystic burden or clinical stage of chronic renal insufficiency. Moreover, in almost half of the patients with ADPKD, pain is a chronic complaint before the diagnosis of ADPKD is even made and represents the most common symptom that leads to the diagnosis. Along with pain, the high lifetime prevalence of cyst infection (30–50%) or nephrolithiasis (20–30%) requires clinicians treating PKD patients to be familiar with the fundamental clinico-pathologic aspects of these important complications. This chapter will outline the etiology and pathogenesis of pain in PKD; review pain in the context of specific clinical scenarios including cyst rupture, infection, and nephrolithiasis; and present differential diagnostic and therapeutic approaches. Further, the authors will provide an outlook on invasive and surgical therapeutic modalities, including videothoracoscopic kidney denervation.

C. Riella, MD
Beth Israel Deaconess Medical Center, Harvard Medical School, Boston, MA, USA
e-mail: criella@bidmc.harvard.edu

P. G. Czarnecki, MD
Brigham & Women's Hospital, Harvard Medical School, Boston, MA, USA
e-mail: pczarnecki@partners.org

T. I. Steinman, MD (✉)
Beth Israel Deaconess Medical Center and Brigham & Women's Hospital, Harvard Medical School, Boston, MA, USA
e-mail: tsteinma@bidmc.harvard.edu

Innervation of Kidneys and Ureters (Fig. 9.1)

The genitourinary tract is densely innervated by efferent nerves from the sympathetic and parasympathetic division of the autonomic nervous system. Afferent sensory nerve fibers mediate visceral sensory perception and travel along the sympathetic fibers.

The general principles of the autonomic nervous system organization apply to the kidney as

B. D. Cowley, Jr., J. J. Bissler (eds.), *Polycystic Kidney Disease*,
https://doi.org/10.1007/978-1-4939-7784-0_9

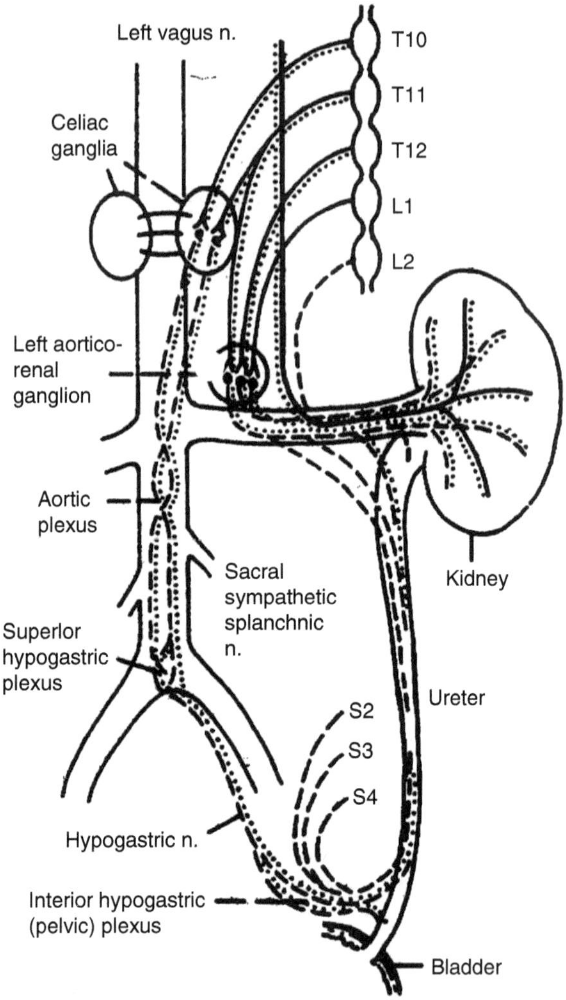

Fig. 9.1 Nerve supply to the kidney, ureter, and bladder (From Ansell et al. [86]. Reproduced with permission from Wolters Kluwer)

well [3]: Axons of preganglionic sympathetic fibers innervating the genitourinary tract originate from their cell bodies in segments T10 through L1 of the intermediolateral column (the lateral horn) of the spinal cord. After entering the anterior rami of the spinal nerves, they quickly separate out through the white rami communicantes to the paravertebral ganglia. Fibers coming from T10 to T11 travel with the lesser splanchnic nerves to the celiac and aorticorenal plexus; fibers from T12 and L1 run with the least splanchnic nerve to synapse with the postganglionic neurons at the level of the renal plexus. Their axons travel along the arteries to provide adrenergic innervation to the vascular smooth muscle cells of interlobar and arcuate arteries, juxtaglomerular afferent arterioles, as well as collecting system smooth muscle cells in the renal calyces and the pelvis.

Vagal and sacral nerves are responsible for the parasympathetic innervation. Long preganglionic fibers of the vagus nerve travel through the renal plexus along the vessels to reach the cell bodies of the short postganglionic fibers within the smooth musculature of the renal pelvis and superior ureter. While the role of parasympathetic innervation in the kidney is unclear, it does have a pacemaker function in the collecting system and mediates peristaltic activity along the ureter. The inferior part of the ureter receives additional parasympathetic innervation through the sacral outflow from S2 to S4 via the pelvic splanchnic nerves and the inferior hypogastric plexus.

Sensory input from the kidneys comes from afferent fibers originating from the parenchyma, the capsule, and the collecting system. Afferents from the kidney parenchyma are mainly unmyelinated C fibers, while afferents originating from the pelvis and calyces are thinly myelinated A-delta fibers. These travel together with the sympathetic efferent axons via the prevertebral plexus, the sympathetic trunk, the white rami communicantes, and anterior rami to the dorsal root ganglia T10–L1, where the cell bodies of these pseudo-unipolar neurons are situated. From here, the central processes reach the dorsal horn of the spinal cord. Similarly, afferents from the ureter travel along the pelvic splanchnic nerve to the dorsal root ganglia of S2–S4. Notably, the dorsal root ganglia neurons also receive sensory input from their respective dermatomes and synapse at the same second-order neurons in the dorsal horn of the spinal cord as the visceral sensory fibers from the genitourinary tract. In the context of inflammation along the genitourinary tract or distention of the renal capsule, the central nervous system cannot clearly discern whether the pain is coming from the body wall or from the viscera, and the perceived pain sensation is referred to areas such as the costovertebral angle, flank, inguinal region, scrotum, labia majora, or anterior thigh.

Acute Pain Syndromes

Parenchymal or cyst infection, cyst rupture or hemorrhage, and nephrolithiasis are the most common causes of acute abdominal pain in patients with PKD. Detailed evaluation outlined below will help in differentiating between the causes of the acute pain and defining the treatment approach accordingly.

Renal Parenchymal and Cyst Infections

Urinary tract infections are frequently noted in the ADPKD population, affecting women more commonly than men [4, 5]. Similar to the pattern noted in the general population, the predominance of gram-negative enteric pathogens suggests that the route of infection is ascending from the urethra and bladder [6–8].

Clinico-pathologically, upper urinary tract infections in ADPKD patients can be separated into two distinct categories – parenchymal (pyelonephritis) and isolated cyst infection [7]. The clinical course and response to therapy in patients with parenchymal infection is comparable to acute pyelonephritis in the general population. The typical presentation includes diffuse pain on the affected side and fever. Urinary examination may reveal sediment findings of pyelonephritis, with pyuria and white cells casts, as well as positive urine culture results. Bacteremia may or may not be present. Response to highly ionized water-soluble antibiotics is often favorable, as long as the isolated organism is sensitive to the drug. On the other hand, patients with cyst infection, also called pyocystis, usually have a discrete new area of tenderness over the involved kidney. These are usually more difficult to diagnose and manage. Cysts can originate from any part of the nephron, they often wall off from the tubule of origin, and ultimately no communication is left between the cyst and the collecting system. As urinalysis and urine culture do not reliably represent the composition of the cyst fluid, the absence of bacteriuria or negative urine culture results does not exclude cyst infection. Similarly, usual radiologic techniques are of limited value in diagnosing these conditions. In a retrospective study of 389 patients by Sallée et al., 33 patients had 41 episodes of cyst infection [8]. Microbiologic documentation was available for 3/4 of these episodes, and *Escherichia coli* accounted for 75% of the infections. Ultrasonography, CT, and MRI failed to detect infected cysts in 94%, 82%, and 60% of the cases. PET scan proved highly efficient in identification of infected cysts and is the best tool currently available to isolate infected cysts. Although characterized by superior sensitivity, PET has its own set of limitations. Often, it is not a readily available resource and may be associated with high diagnostic cost. The specificity of PET remains to be determined, in particular the ability to detect cyst hemorrhage, the major differential diagnosis of cyst infection.

While renoparenchymal and cyst infections are predominantly acquired through an ascending mechanism, a number of studies have also documented a high incidence of liver and kidney cyst infections in ADPKD patients undergoing hemodialysis, suggesting infectious spread through a hematogenous route in this specific subgroup [8, 9]. It is therefore emphasized that even in anuric ADPKD patients on hemodialysis presenting with abdominal pain and fever, the differential diagnosis of cyst infection has to be considered.

Management

Successful therapy depends on antibiotic penetration into the cyst fluid in order to achieve sufficient local concentrations to eradicate the infecting organisms. Delivery of antimicrobial agents has to occur through the cyst wall into the cyst lumen. Given the fact that cysts are often disconnected from the tubular system, antimicrobials that typically achieve high tubular concentrations by filtration and tubular secretion may not necessarily achieve high concentrations in cyst fluid [10]. In keeping with this hypothesis, commonly used polar water-soluble antibiotics (such as penicillins, cephalosporins, and aminoglycosides) have limited ability to penetrate into the cyst lumen. Lipid-soluble and nonpolar antibiotics are preferable as they can more easily equilibrate across cyst walls [11–14]. Due to these pharmacokinetic properties and their broad microbiologic coverage, fluoroquinolones are recommended as the first-line treatment for cyst infections [14]. Clindamycin, metronidazole, and trimethoprim-sulfamethoxazole are alternatives, if there is no response to initial quinolone therapy or if there is a prior history of infection with resistant organisms. It is important to note that the duration of treatment should be a minimum of 2 weeks and extended to 4 weeks if there is continued localized discomfort at the site of the original pain. Resistance to therapy cannot be presumed unless there are ongoing symptoms on prolonged therapy for 1 month or greater. As suggested above, beta-lactam antibiotics and aminoglycosides are unlikely to achieve therapeutic intra-cystic concentrations and are not recommended for localized cyst infections. However, additional broad-spectrum antibiotic coverage involving beta-lactams and aminoglycosides is highly appropriate, should a previously localized cyst infection evolve into bacteremia and a generalized sepsis syndrome.

While enteric organisms account for the vast majority of cyst infections, other organisms have been reported as well, including *Streptococcus* [15], *Staphylococcus* [16], *Clostridium perfringens* [17, 18], and *Candida albicans* [19]. Repeated antibiotic exposures can lead to development of multidrug-resistant organisms. In these cases, where the cyst infection may not respond to initial antibiotic therapy, exact bacteriologic documentation by cyst aspiration may be required to guide appropriate therapy. Aspiration of kidney cysts is the very last thing to be done and rarely needed (and should never be done routinely). However, larger infected cysts (>5 cm in diameter), in particular hepatic cysts, may benefit from early drainage as antibiotics alone cannot reliably cure these infections [8, 20]. Lastly, it is imperative that lower urinary tract infections be treated promptly to reduce complications related to infection spread to the upper urinary tract.

Cyst Rupture and Hemorrhage

Hemorrhage into a cyst and rupture of a cyst are common causes of acute flank pain. While gross hematuria is helpful in making the diagnosis of cyst rupture, its absence should not sway away from this diagnosis. Cysts are the result of aberrant tubulogenesis, becoming separate from the tubule of origin at an early stage (and invariably separated by the time they become detectable by imaging studies) [21]. Hemorrhage into a noncommunicating cyst often presents with pain without hematuria. Hematuria, following back pain, was the second most common reason (16.4%) that led to the diagnosis of ADPKD in a study cohort of 171 ADPKD patients [22]. Interestingly, only one third of these patients reported an association with back or abdominal pain, while hematuria was a painless event for the remaining two thirds. It is often recurrent; a precipitating event such as a urinary tract infection or strenuous activity is often reported [23, 24]. In a study of 191 adult ADPKD subjects, both kidney size and blood pressure were found to directly correlate with the frequency of hematuria [25]. These episodes also have prognostic significance, since increasing episodes of hematuria, as well as episodes early in life (before age 30), have been associated with worse renal outcomes [25, 26]. Similar to cyst infections, cyst rupture can occur after renal replacement therapy has been initiated [27].

Management

Bleeding episodes are usually self-limited, lasting 2–7 days. Similar to infected cysts, pain is often localized. Referred pain to another location can occur; for instance, hemorrhage into a large cyst at the upper pole of the right kidney can lead to diaphragmatic irritation and shoulder pain. Conservative management with bed rest and hydration is often effective for managing these episodes; occasionally bleeding can persist for weeks. Patients should be advised to avoid aspirin, nonsteroidal anti-inflammatory drugs, and physical activities. Judicious use of other pain medications, acetaminophen, and opioid analgesics (discussed in detail below) may be needed. Bleeding into a cyst on the surface of the kidneys can lead to formation of a subcapsular hematoma; these patients can have ongoing steady flank pain for weeks to months until the hematoma is resolved. If bleeding into the renal pelvis is significant, clots can form, which in turn can lead to obstruction and renal colic. Hospitalization may be necessary for pain control and close observation in these cases. Occasionally, blood transfusions are needed and rarely, renal arterial embolization and/or nephrectomy may be required for hemostasis. Although selective arterial embolization is less invasive than nephrectomy, subsequent renal parenchymal ischemia can lead to worsening pain. Nephrectomy should be the last resort after all other measures have been exhausted but may be considered earlier in an advanced chronic kidney disease or ESRD patient with recurrent episodes. Lastly, it is emphasized that the differential diagnosis of painless hematuria, particularly in the elderly patient, includes renal cell carcinoma and urothelial malignancies.

Nephrolithiasis

Symptomatic nephrolithiasis is reported in 20–30% of ADPKD patients [28, 29]. It is difficult to differentiate between cyst calcifications and renal calculi on unenhanced CT scans. Enhanced CT scan with and without contrast, when possible, is preferable but has its limitations in the patient with higher-stage chronic kidney disease. In a cross-sectional study of patients who had had both enhanced and unenhanced scans, 36% had evidence of nephrolithiasis; this is approximately ten times more common when compared to the general population [30].

Both anatomic and metabolic factors are implicated in the pathogenesis of stone formation. Patients who form stones are likely to have a higher cyst count and/or larger dominant cysts, suggesting that distortion of the collecting system and consequent fluid stasis within the intrarenal calyceal system contributes to the process. Multiple metabolic risk factors have been identified on 24 h urine collection specimens. Both magnesium and citrate are powerful inhibitors of crystal formation and aggregation. When compared to a normal daily citrate excretion of 520 mg/day, ADPKD patients have lower urinary citrate excretion. Hypocitraturia is more pronounced in ADPKD stone formers as compared to non-stone formers (247 mg/day vs. 337 mg/day) [28, 31]. Lower urinary magnesium excretion and lower urine volumes have also been documented in the stone-forming group [31]. Uric acid stones account for more than half of the calculi seen in this group [28, 32]. Since serum uric acid and renal urate handling are normal in the ADPKD population, the propensity for uric acid crystallization appears to be related to low urine pH. The average urine pH in 91 stone-forming ADPKD patients was 5.66 ± 0.05, significantly lower than 5.92 ± 0.03 in the control group [28]. There is evidence documenting overactivity of the renin angiotensin aldosterone system (RAAS) in PKD [33–35] that is related to the degree of local parenchymal ischemia as a consequence of cyst expansion. H^+ ATPase activity in the type A acid secreting intercalated cells is stimulated by aldosterone and angiotensin [36]. This upregulation may be one of the mechanisms responsible for urinary acidification and consecutive propensity for uric acid precipitation.

Beyond obtaining a thorough history, including details about prior episodes of stone disease, and careful physical examination, imaging is often needed to confirm the diagnosis. As in the general population, CT imaging has been shown to be superior to ultrasonography in the ADPKD population as well [37]. As noted earlier, renal calcifications can represent both calculi as well as cyst calcifications, and differentiation between the two based on unenhanced CT imaging can be challenging.

Management of Acute Renal Colic

The increase in intraluminal pressure from ureteric obstruction stretches the nerve endings in the mucosa, and the smooth muscle in the wall of the ureter contracts as it tries to move the stone, producing colicky pain [38]. If the stone is unable to move, muscle spasm leads to increased production of lactic acid, which irritates the sensory nerve fibers causing further pain. Prostaglandin-mediated preglomerular vasodilatation increases renal blood flow, leading to increased urine output, which causes further stretching of the calyceal system and pain exacerbation [39]. While time-honored management of renal colic includes opioid analgesia and antispasmodic therapy, randomized prospective studies comparing NSAIDs with morphine suggest that both agents provided comparable pain relief [40, 41]. The analgesic effect of NSAIDs is probably not only explained by local anti-inflammatory action but also mediated by their antidiuretic activity (through prevention of afferent arteriolar vasodilation and loss of inhibitory effects of prostaglandins on ADH effects). In PKD patients with advanced renal insufficiency, NSAIDs can induce renal failure through impairment of autoregulatory responses in the kidney and should be used with caution.

Early involvement of an experienced urologist may be essential during an acute episode of renal colic, particularly if there is evidence of hydronephrosis or acute kidney injury. Most patients with ADPKD who require urologic intervention for nephrolithiasis can be safely treated with careful use of extracorporeal shock wave lithotripsy, ureteroscopic procedures, or open nephrolithotomy, depending on the size and location of the stone. However, large cyst volume and kidney mass can cause traction and compression on the collecting system, making these procedures difficult. Also, the incidence of residual stones is higher than in patients without ADPKD [32, 37, 42–44].

Strategies for Prevention of Stone Formation

In patients with a high propensity for stone formation, the first step in the management of these patients is identifying their major risk factors through evaluation of a 24-h urine metabolic profile. Increased free water intake remains the basic tenet of treatment, no matter the cause for the recurrent stone formation. Prospective observational data shows that intake of 2.5 l/day is associated with a 29% risk reduction in first stone occurrence [45, 46]. In addition to a reduction in stone formation, increased free water intake may have a beneficial role with regard to reduction of cyst growth and preservation of renal function: Vasopressin enhances cyst expansion by increasing cyclic 3′-5′-adenosine monophosphate (cAMP) levels in the cystic epithelia. In the randomized double-blinded, placebo-controlled TEMPO 3:4 clinical trial of 1445 ADPKD patients with preserved eGFR followed for 3 years, the vasopressin receptor 2 (V2) antagonist, tolvaptan, was shown to alter the natural course of the disorder, with a statistically significant reduction in the annual kidney volume increment (2.8% growth in tolvaptan group vs. 5.5% in placebo group) over 3 years. Also, there was a significant slower rate of kidney function decline (reciprocal of the serum creatinine level, −2.61 ml/mg per year vs. −3.81 ml/mg per year) [47]. If a reduction in vasopressin levels can be achieved by increased water intake, without pharmacologic blockade, will there be the same effect on cyst growth and disease progression? While a large water intake has been shown to have some effect in rats [48], this hypothesis is yet to be tested in humans. In conclusion, while water therapy is sine qua non in treatment of stone disease, there may be additional distinct advantages in the ADPKD population [49].

Potassium citrate supplementation can be particularly helpful with management of uric acid nephrolithiasis, through both urinary alkalization and increasing urinary citrate concentration. While potassium citrate pills are available, as many as 8–12 tablets a day may be needed to achieve adequate urine citrate levels. This treatment regimen can be relatively expensive and cumbersome, and patients may find it difficult to comply. In our experience, use of lemon concentrate (which is potassium citrate) diluted in water has been effective; we recommend addition of three to four tablespoons of lemon concentrate to a liter of water and drinking it over the course of the day. Compliance with and response to prescribed measures should be assessed with a follow-up 24-h urine metabolic evaluation.

Prospective trials are needed to establish whether pharmacologic blockade of the RAAS (angiotensin-converting enzyme inhibitors, angiotensin receptor blockers, and aldosterone antagonists), with a consequent increase in urine pH, is sufficient to lower the incidence of uric acid nephrolithiasis.

Clinical Spectrum of Chronic Pain

Pain is a common symptom even before the diagnosis of PKD is established. In a pioneer study of 171 ADPKD patients by one of the authors (TIS), 40.9% reported pain before they received the diagnosis [22]. In fact, patient symptoms were the most common factor leading to diagnosis (37.4% cases); and back pain was the most common symptom (17.5%) during evaluation that established the diagnosis of ADPKD. Pain was often reported as occurring with increasing frequency after the definitive diagnosis was made; nearly three quarters (71.3%) experienced chronic back pain, and almost two thirds (61.4%) reported abdominal pain during the course of the disease. When patients were asked if they thought their pains were related to ADPKD, only a small minority (9.4%) answered in the affirmative. The vast majority was either not sure (53.8%) or did not believe their symptoms were related to their diagnosis (36.8%). The finding of pain commonly leading to the diagnosis of ADPKD was documented in another study that included over 400 patients [50]. In conclusion, pain occurs more frequently in this patient population than generally appreciated. Furthermore, there is no apparent relation between severity of kidney function and frequency and severity of pain. Pain often begins relatively early in the course of the disease, when renal function is preserved and does not directly correlate with total kidney volume (TKV) [51]. As will be highlighted in the following sections, a thorough history and physical examination, accompanied by judicious use of radiologic imaging, is needed to identify the etiology of pain that leads to targeted treatments.

Mechanical Back Pain

Low back pain is the most common complaint reported by ADPKD patients, 71.3% in the above mentioned study [22]. Pain intensity, as assessed by the visual analog scale (VAS), showed a bell-shaped distribution, with 37.7% having pain levels of 4 and 5 on a scale of 1–10. Almost two thirds of the patients with pain characterized it as constant or daily pain.

Although back pain related to degenerative spinal disease frequently affects the common population, the ADPKD population is particularly susceptible. Enlarging cysts cause an increase in abdominal girth. This leads to slowly progressive maladaptive postural changes, including increase of the pelvic tilt and lumbar lordosis. This places increasing mechanical strain on the lumbodorsal muscle groups. Over time, hypertrophy of these muscle groups ensues, along with progression of degenerative spine disease. These processes worsen as cysts grow and TKV increases, causing further worsening of lower back pain. In a personal observation by one of the authors (TIS), average lumbodorsal muscle thickness at L4–S1 level on abdominal MRI done to assess cyst volume was 38.7 mm, in contrast to 31.3 mm in ten matched individuals without ADPKD undergoing MRI for other reasons [52].

Since cyst enlargement can be asymmetric, the above mentioned changes can be more pronounced on one side compared to the other. When the liver is involved with enlarging cysts, the postural changes can be pronounced, leading to debilitating back pain. In contrast to those with degenerative spine disease not related to PKD, compression of lower lumbar or sacral nerves presented as lumbosacral radiculopathy or sciatica in 27% of the patients in the above-noted PKD cohort [22]. The burden of suffering is highlighted by the fact that 22.7%, 20.5%, and 27.3% of the ADPKD patients reported constant, daily, or once-a-week pain, respectively. 71.7% rated their pain between 3 and 6 on a VAS, with 4.3% needing some form of surgery for pain relief.

Pain Related to Enlarged Renal and Hepatic Cysts

As cysts grow in size, they can directly cause pain. Pain patterns can be due to stretching of the renal capsule, traction of the pedicle of the kidney, or compression of surrounding structures. Although pain severity usually correlates with cyst size, some patients with relatively small cysts can have marked pain, and others with very large cysts may have no discomfort. Clinically, pain directly related to cysts is distinct from mechanical back pain (a constant discomfort that is made worse by standing or walking). Pain from cysts is most often localized to the anterior abdomen, less frequently to the back. Patients are able to pinpoint the epicenter of pain with one finger. Localizing the culprit cyst is a critical part of management (as discussed below). We suggest using a skin marker over the point of maximum discomfort during an ultrasound procedure. If a cyst of 5 cm or greater in diameter is identified directly beneath the skin marker area, that is the likely source of pain. Laparoscopic decortication or unroofing of the culprit cyst(s) is a potential therapeutic option for these patients, and dramatic reduction or even total relief of pain has occurred in over 95% of our patient population who undergo this specific approach to diagnosis and treatment (personal observation, TIS). At our institution, we limit the unroofing procedure to no more than three cysts.

Pain related to enlarging cysts does not correlate with the degree of renal dysfunction. Severe discomfort is seen at all levels of chronic kidney disease, even after initiation of renal replacement therapy. When pain is the predominant complaint, it often begins early in the course of the disease. Cysts of any size can cause compression of surrounding structures, and pain symptoms do not necessarily correspond to the anatomic location of the largest cysts measured using various imaging techniques. Therefore, the cyst unroofing approach should be limited to the above mentioned criteria. External pressure on the greater curvature of the stomach or the duodenal loop by both kidney and liver cysts can lead to early satiety or nausea.

Cystic involvement of the liver is seen in about 30% of the ADKD patients at diagnosis. Liver cysts increase in frequency with advancing age and may eventually be noted in up to 80% of these patients. These cysts can grow freely into the abdominal cavity, producing severe (sometimes intractable) pain as well as symptoms of early satiety and nausea related to compression of the stomach and duodenum. The gastrointestinal symptoms tend to be more severe and occur more frequently with liver cysts as compared to kidney cysts. Females, more than males, are generally affected by large liver cysts, and a multiparous state (especially three or more pregnancies) is often associated with the greatest degree of total liver volume.

Other Patterns of Chronic Pain

Headaches

Given the association between PKD and cerebral aneurysms, headache in this population often generates anxiety and fear. Chronic headaches were reported by nearly half (48.5%) of the previously mentioned cohort [22]. In a study conducted by one of the authors (TIS), 40 consecutive PKD patients who reported chronic headaches on a questionnaire underwent evaluation by head CT scan or magnetic resonance imaging or magnetic resonance angiography (MRI/MRA). None of these patients had evidence of an intracranial aneurysm. There does not appear to be an association between chronic headache symptoms and presence of intracranial aneurysms. While 4–6% of ADPKD patients are estimated to have cerebral aneurysms, the pretest probability is much higher (16%) in the presence of a positive family history of aneurysms [53]. Multiple studies have shown an overall favorable prognosis of asymptomatic intracranial aneurysms [54–57]. Patients with a history of a previous rupture of an aneurysm are at increased risk for a recurrent hemorrhage, warranting lifelong screening. For asymptomatic individuals, the presence of a family history of a cerebral aneurysm remains the best predictor for increased individual risk. Hence, screening this particular subgroup is indicated [58]. Also, screening is warranted in the setting of a renal transplant evaluation or in patients working in a high-risk profession (i.e., airplane pilot, bus driver, heavy equipment operator).

Chest Pain

Varying quality and severity of chest pain was described by a significant proportion of the PKD patients (30.4%). While it is difficult to explain the association with PKD, thoracic aortic aneurysms are an infrequent occurrence in this population, and aortic dissection can present with these symptoms [59, 60].

Pancreas-Related Pain

Pancreatic cysts can be detected in 5–9% of the patients by ultrasound and in almost 19% by MRI [61]. These cysts can cause obstruction of pancreatic ducts leading to pancreatitis [62]. There are rare reports of intraductal papillary mucinous neoplasms in ADPKD patients [63, 64].

Sequential Approach to Chronic Pain Management

Chronic pain is a common health-care problem worldwide, and many general principles and approaches for pain control apply to pain management in ADPKD. For patients who suffer from chronic pain, it is critical to outline goals and expectations at initial visits. The goal is to decrease the severity of pain so that it least interferes with the patient's lifestyle. It is essential to realistically set expectations from treatment approaches and repeatedly emphasize that complete cure of pain is usually not possible. Patient disappointment and frustration can ensue if the point is not adequately delivered that complete relief from pain is unlikely. Self-medication is common in this population [22]. As noted earlier, patients may not associate their symptoms with ADPKD, and this may lead to underreporting of symptoms. These patients should be queried about symptoms and use of prescription and over-the-counter analgesics at their physician clinic visits. A stepwise approach for pain management is recommended, starting with non-pharmacologic measures, moving to progressively stronger systemic analgesics as needed, and reserving invasive and surgical measures for severe or refractory pain only.

Non-pharmacologic, Non- or Minimally Invasive Measures

There are no trials evaluating use of these techniques specifically in the ADPKD population. Extrapolating from other chronic pain syndromes, conservative measures are recommended for management for mild-to-moderate pain as the initial therapy before use of medications. Back strengthening exercises to counteract lumbar lordosis, along with proper posture when standing and walking, can provide long-term relief from the low back pain.

Alexander technique This is an educational process, rather than an exercise, that aims to change movement habits in everyday life. These lessons, when taught by an experienced instructor, help subjects identify, understand, and ultimately avoid their improper postural and movement habits. In particular, they focus on release of unnecessary tension from the axial muscles and have been shown to be very effective in the management of chronic back pain [65–67]. Patients should be warned that this is a slow and prolonged process, and months are often necessary before any benefit in symptoms is observed.

Heat and cold packs and massages This can facilitate exercises and assist with pain control.

Transcutaneous electric nerve stimulation (TENS) This is a noninvasive method of pain relief where low-voltage electrical impulses are transmitted through electrodes to the area that is in pain. Melzack and Wall described the gate control theory in 1965 [68]. Impulses from unmyelinated C fibers carrying pain signals and myelinated Aβ-fibers carrying light touch and pressure signals enter the dorsal horn of the spinal cord. When the electrical impulses from the C fibers outnumber those from the Aβ-fibers, the "gate opens" allowing transmission of nociceptive signals leading to sensation of pain. On the contrary, if Aβ-fibers are stimulated using TENS, the gate is closed, and pain sensation is suppressed. Benefit from TENS may not be seen in all individuals [69, 70]. We recommend a trial of at least 2 weeks. There are essentially no side effects associated with its use; if a patient reports symptom relief with its use, it can be used for long-term management.

Acupuncture This technique may be beneficial in some patients with mechanical back pain related to large kidney size and can be a useful adjunctive therapy.

Systemic Analgesics

Medications are often needed for pain control; and a slow and stepwise approach is recommended. Drug half-life and metabolism are affected by renal function; and drug-dosing guidelines should be carefully followed if renal function is impaired.

Acetaminophen is recommended as the first analgesic of choice in patients with preexisting kidney disease [71] but limits the use of this medication to no more than a few days of continued dosing. The initial dose is 500 mg or 650 mg every 4–6 h and may be escalated to 1000 mg every 6 h. In absence of concomitant liver disease or alcohol consumption (more than two to three drinks per day), a dose of 4000 mg per day is usually considered safe. It does not have any gastrointestinal side effects and can be used safely in patients on angiotensin-converting enzyme inhibitors and angiotensin receptor blockers, as well as in patients with advanced renal insufficiency.

Tramadol, although not a chemically clean opiate, exerts its analgesic activity as a μ-receptor agonist in the central nervous system, as well as a serotonin- and norepinephrine-reuptake inhibitor. These neurotransmitters are involved in the descending inhibitory pain pathway responsible for pain relief. It is slightly more potent than codeine but less effective than other commonly used opioids such as hydrocodone and morphine. Side effects include central nervous system depression and constipation, but the abuse potential is low, making this an overall safe drug. Starting dose is 50 mg once to twice daily; and it can be escalated to a maximum of 400 mg/day. Metabolites are excreted predominantly through the renal route making dose reduction necessary if the creatinine clearance is less than 30 ml/min. Moreover, extended release formulation should be avoided in those with advanced renal insufficiency. Acetaminophen and tramadol combination is well tolerated and can be an effective regimen for acute and chronic pain in these patients.

NSAIDs act through inhibition of constitutively expressed cyclooxygenase (COX-1) and inducible COX-2. In patients with chronic renal insufficiency, while occasional use of NSAIDs is reasonable, daily use for long-term management is not recommended. Given their antiplatelet properties, NSAIDs should be avoided when cyst rupture or intra-cystic hemorrhage is suspected. NSAIDs should not be used in patients with acute kidney injury, hemodynamic instability, those undergoing radiocontrast studies, or in combination with other potentially nephrotoxic medications. As mentioned earlier, paracrine effects of prostaglandins are in part responsible for the pain observed in renal colic. Hence, this class of drugs can be particularly effective in this scenario. We recommend that NSAID use should be limited to no more than 3 days in the PKD population, monitoring renal function closely at the same time.

Clonidine acts as an agonist at the α_2-adrenergic receptors in the central nervous system, resulting in reduced sympathetic outflow. While most analgesic data reflect effectiveness of intrathecal and epidural clonidine, oral and transdermal formulations have also been shown to have a modest effect. It is usually started at 0.1 mg once to twice daily; the dose can be uptitrated slowly over several weeks. Orthostatic dysregulation, hypotension, bradycardia, and sedation are the major dose-limiting side effects. The use of *gabapentin*, *pregabalin*, and *amitriptyline* has not been evaluated for pain control in the ADPKD population; they can be used as adjuvant therapies on a trial basis and continued if found to be effective [72]. Their clearance is predominantly renal, and dose reduction is necessary with renal insufficiency.

Opioids remain the last resort for patients with severe pain. Transdermal fentanyl and sustained release morphine can be used for chronic pain management, and short-acting or intravenous preparations should be reserved for breakthrough pain control [73]. Given the potential for abuse, severe side effects, and need for close monitoring, a narcotic agreement/contract should be established with the patient.

Invasive Measures

Spinal cord stimulation, autonomic plexus blockade, and neuraxial opioid administration are invasive procedures that should be reserved for patients with intractable pain not responding to conventional measures.

Spinal cord stimulation works on the same principle as TENS and is increasingly employed for chronic pain management. While long-term implantation of electrodes in the epidural space is needed, a stronger pain relief can be achieved. If satisfactory relief is obtained after an initial trial period of 5–7 days, the electrodes can be anchored to the interspinal ligaments to assist with long-term management. Likewise, an epidural or intrathecal catheter can be placed for continuous delivery of local anesthetic and/or opioids.

Celiac plexus block is another technique that is used for chronic nonmalignant pain. Local anesthetic agents, with or without steroids or adjuvant medications like clonidine, are injected into the celiac plexus. If initial treatment with these agents is effective, neurolytic blocks with alcohol, phenol, or glycerol can be used for longer-term relief.

Surgical Management of Pain

Surgery has a role in the management of severe pain related to cyst enlargement. As stated, the largest cysts are not always the source of pain, making identification of culprit cysts difficult. Pinpointing the source of pain from cysts and the diagnostic approach that eventually leads to laparoscopic unroofing of cysts was described earlier.

Percutaneous aspiration of cysts should not be done in an attempt to relieve cyst-derived pain, since cysts typically reaccumulate fluid with recurrence of symptoms and the patient is unnecessarily exposed to the procedural risks of injury, bleeding, and infection [74]. De-roofing and drainage of cysts were first described in non-ADPKD patients almost a century ago. However this procedure fell out of favor following reports of acceleration of renal damage after this procedure [75]. Subsequent more systematic case series demonstrated effective pain relief, with no adverse effect on renal function [76, 77]. Multiple recent studies have shown the effectiveness of laparoscopic surgery for cyst decortication and marsupialization [78–83]. As a very last resort, nephrectomy may be the only option left for a patient approaching ESRD. The presence of chronically infected cysts or massive kidney volumes that may represent a contraindication to renal transplantation are additional factors that may lead to the decision for nephrectomy in patients approaching ESRD. Since sensory nerves travel with autonomic nerve fibers, renal denervation through various techniques such as video-assisted thoracoscopic splanchnicectomy has been shown to provide immediate pain relief in case reports and small case series [84, 85]. Long-term results of this technique need validation [83].

To conclude, acute and chronic pain are common, yet underappreciated, problems in the patient with PKD. Careful history taking, physical examination, and goal-directed use of imaging techniques can help with identification of the etiology. A multidisciplinary approach involving nephrologists, urologists, primary care physicians, and pain specialists may be needed for effective pain control.

References

1. Gabow PA. Autosomal dominant polycystic kidney disease – more than a renal disease. Am J Kidney Dis. 1990;16(5):403–13.
2. Gabow PA. Autosomal dominant polycystic kidney disease. N Engl J Med. 1993;329(5):332–42. https://doi.org/10.1056/NEJM199307293290508.
3. Czarnecki PG, Steinman TI. Pain and pain management in polycystic kidney disease. In: Polycystic kidney disease: from bench to bedside: Future Medicine Ltd. London: Future Science Group, Unitec House; 2013. p. 114–28.
4. Gardner KD Jr, Evan AP. Cystic kidneys: an enigma evolves. Am J Kidney Dis. 1984;3(6):403–13. doi:S0272638684000147 [pii].
5. Simon HB, Thompson GJ. Congenital renal polycystic disease; a clinical and therapeutic study of three hundred sixty-six cases. J Am Med Assoc. 1955;159(7):657–62.
6. Idrizi A, Barbullushi M, Koroshi A, Dibra M, Bolleku E, Bajrami V, et al. Urinary tract infections in polycystic kidney disease. Med Arh. 2011;65(4):213–5.
7. Schwab SJ, Bander SJ, Klahr S. Renal infection in autosomal dominant polycystic kidney disease. Am J Med. 1987;82(4):714–8. doi:0002-9343(87)90005-2 [pii].
8. Sallee M, Rafat C, Zahar JR, Paulmier B, Grunfeld JP, Knebelmann B, et al. Cyst infections in patients with autosomal dominant polycystic kidney disease. Clin J Am Soc Nephrol. 2009;4(7):1183–9. https://doi.org/10.2215/CJN.01870309. CJN.01870309 [pii].
9. Christophe JL, van Ypersele de Strihou C, Pirson Y, The U.C.L. Collaborative Group. Complications of autosomal dominant polycystic kidney disease in 50 haemodialysed patients. A case-control study. Nephrol Dial Transplant. 1996;11(7):1271–6.
10. Grantham JJ. Polycystic kidney disease: a predominance of giant nephrons. Am J Phys. 1983;244(1):F3–10.
11. Bennett WM, Elzinga L, Pulliam JP, Rashad AL, Barry JM. Cyst fluid antibiotic concentrations in autosomal-dominant polycystic kidney disease. Am J Kidney Dis. 1985;6(6):400–4. doi:S0272638685001111 [pii].
12. Schwab S, Hinthorn D, Diederich D, Cuppage F, Grantham J. pH-dependent accumulation of clindamycin in a polycystic kidney. Am J Kidney Dis. 1983;3(1):63–6. doi:S0272638683000323 [pii].
13. Elzinga LW, Golper TA, Rashad AL, Carr ME, Bennett WM. Trimethoprim-sulfamethoxazole in cyst fluid from autosomal dominant polycystic kidneys. Kidney Int. 1987;32(6):884–8.
14. Basting RF, Bromberger G, Adam D. Ceftazidime concentrations in renal cysts. J Hosp Infect. 1990;15(Suppl A):77–9.
15. Hiyama L, Tang A, Miller LG. Levofloxacin penetration into a renal cyst in a patient with autosomal dominant polycystic kidney disease. Am J Kidney Dis. 2006;47(1):e9–13. doi:S0272-6386(05)01492-7 [pii]. https://doi.org/10.1053/j.ajkd.2005.09.021.
16. Chapman AB, Thickman D, Gabow PA. Percutaneous cyst puncture in the treatment of cyst infection in autosomal dominant polycystic kidney disease. Am J Kidney Dis. 1990;16(3):252–5. doi:S0272638690001123 [pii].
17. Erkoc R, Sayarlioglu H, Ceylan K, Dogan E, Kara PS. Gas-forming infection in a renal cyst of a patient with autosomal dominant polycystic kidney disease. Nephrol Dial Transplant. 2006;21(2):555–6. doi:gfi174 [pii]. https://doi.org/10.1093/ndt/gfi174.
18. Van Zijl PS, Chai TC. Gas-forming infection from Clostridium perfringens in a renal cyst of a patient with autosomal dominant polycystic kidney disease. Urology. 2004;63(6):1178–9. https://doi.org/10.1016/j.urology.2004.01.027. S0090429504001268 [pii].
19. Hepburn MJ, Pennick GJ, Sutton DA, Crawford GE, Jorgensen JH. Candida krusei renal cyst infection and measurement of amphotericin B levels in cystic fluid in a patient receiving AmBisome. Med Mycol. 2003;41(2):163–5.
20. Telenti A, Torres VE, Gross JB Jr, Van Scoy RE, Brown ML, Hattery RR. Hepatic cyst infection in autosomal dominant polycystic kidney disease. Mayo Clin Proc. 1990;65(7):933–42.
21. Grantham JJ. The etiology, pathogenesis, and treatment of autosomal dominant polycystic kidney disease: recent advances. Am J Kidney Dis. 1996;28(6):788–803. doi:S0272-6386(96)90378-9 [pii].
22. Bajwa ZH, Sial KA, Malik AB, Steinman TI. Pain patterns in patients with polycystic kidney disease. Kidney Int. 2004;66(4):1561–9. https://doi.org/10.1111/j.1523-1755.2004.00921.x. KID921 [pii].
23. Mufarrij AJ, Hitti E. Acute cystic rupture and hemorrhagic shock after a vigorous massage chair session in a patient with polycystic kidney disease. Am J Med Sci. 2011;342(1):76–8. https://doi.org/10.1097/MAJ.0b013e31821a50c5.
24. Kim HG, Bae SR, Lho YS, Park HK, Paick SH. Acute cyst rupture, hemorrhage and septic shock after a shockwave lithotripsy in a patient with autosomal dominant polycystic kidney disease. Urolithiasis. 2013;41(3):267–9. https://doi.org/10.1007/s00240-013-0550-2.
25. Gabow PA, Duley I, Johnson AM. Clinical profiles of gross hematuria in autosomal dominant polycystic kidney disease. Am J Kidney Dis. 1992;20(2):140–3. doi:S0272638692000969 [pii].

26. Johnson AM, Gabow PA. Identification of patients with autosomal dominant polycystic kidney disease at highest risk for end-stage renal disease. J Am Soc Nephrol. 1997;8(10):1560–7.
27. Tarrass F, Benjelloun M. Acute abdomen caused by spontaneous renal cyst rupture in an ADPKD haemodialysed patient. Nephrology (Carlton). 2008;13(2):177–8. https://doi.org/10.1111/j.1440-1797.2007.00902.x. NEP902 [pii].
28. Torres VE, Erickson SB, Smith LH, Wilson DM, Hattery RR, Segura JW. The association of nephrolithiasis and autosomal dominant polycystic kidney disease. Am J Kidney Dis. 1988;11(4):318–25. doi:S0272638688000563 [pii].
29. Dimitrakov D, Simeonov S. Studies on nephrolithiasis in patients with autosomal dominant polycystic kidney disease. Folia Med (Plovdiv). 1994;36(3):27–30.
30. Levine E, Grantham JJ. Calcified renal stones and cyst calcifications in autosomal dominant polycystic kidney disease: clinical and CT study in 84 patients. AJR Am J Roentgenol. 1992;159(1):77–81. https://doi.org/10.2214/ajr.159.1.1609726.
31. Grampsas SA, Chandhoke PS, Fan J, Glass MA, Townsend R, Johnson AM, et al. Anatomic and metabolic risk factors for nephrolithiasis in patients with autosomal dominant polycystic kidney disease. Am J Kidney Dis. 2000;36(1):53–7. doi:S0272-6386(00)27988-2 [pii]. https://doi.org/10.1053/ajkd.2000.8266.
32. Ng CS, Yost A, Streem SB. Nephrolithiasis associated with autosomal dominant polycystic kidney disease: contemporary urological management. J Urol. 2000;163(3):726–9. doi:S0022-5347(05)67792-0 [pii].
33. Kocyigit I, Yilmaz MI, Unal A, Ozturk F, Eroglu E, Yazici C, et al. A link between the intrarenal renin angiotensin system and hypertension in autosomal dominant polycystic kidney disease. Am J Nephrol. 2013;38(3):218–25. https://doi.org/10.1159/000354317. 000354317 [pii].
34. Chapman AB, Stepniakowski K, Rahbari-Oskoui F. Hypertension in autosomal dominant polycystic kidney disease. Adv Chronic Kidney Dis. 2010;17(2):153–63. https://doi.org/10.1053/j.ackd.2010.01.001. S1548-5595(10)00002-9 [pii].
35. Loghman-Adham M, Soto CE, Inagami T, Cassis L. The intrarenal renin-angiotensin system in autosomal dominant polycystic kidney disease. Am J Physiol Ren Physiol. 2004;287(4):F775–88. https://doi.org/10.1152/ajprenal.00370.2003. 00370.2003 [pii].
36. Pech V, Zheng W, Pham TD, Verlander JW, Wall SM. Angiotensin II activates H+-ATPase in type A intercalated cells. J Am Soc Nephrol. 2008;19(1):84–91. https://doi.org/10.1681/ASN.2007030277. 19/1/84 [pii].
37. Nishiura JL, Neves RF, Eloi SR, Cintra SM, Ajzen SA, Heilberg IP. Evaluation of nephrolithiasis in autosomal dominant polycystic kidney disease patients. Clin J Am Soc Nephrol. 2009;4(4):838–44. https://doi.org/10.2215/CJN.03100608. CJN.03100608 [pii].
38. Shokeir AA. Renal colic: new concepts related to pathophysiology, diagnosis and treatment. Curr Opin Urol. 2002;12(4):263–9.
39. Zwergel U, Zwergel T, Ziegler M. Effects of prostaglandins and prostaglandin synthetase inhibitors on acutely obstructed kidneys in the dog. Urol Int. 1991;47(2):64–9.
40. Cordell WH, Larson TA, Lingeman JE, Nelson DR, Woods JR, Burns LB, et al. Indomethacin suppositories versus intravenously titrated morphine for the treatment of ureteral colic. Ann Emerg Med. 1994;23(2):262–9. doi:S0196064494002957 [pii].
41. Hetherington JW, Philp NH. Diclofenac sodium versus pethidine in acute renal colic. Br Med J (Clin Res Ed). 1986;292(6515):237–8.
42. Torres VE, Wilson DM, Hattery RR, Segura JW. Renal stone disease in autosomal dominant polycystic kidney disease. Am J Kidney Dis. 1993;22(4):513–9. doi:S0272638693001969 [pii].
43. Delakas D, Daskalopoulos G, Cranidis A. Extracorporeal shockwave lithotripsy for urinary calculi in autosomal dominant polycystic kidney disease. J Endourol. 1997;11(3):167–70.
44. Chen WC, Lee YH, Huang JK, Chen MT, Chang LS. Experience using extracorporeal shock-wave lithotripsy to treat urinary calculi in problem kidneys. Urol Int. 1993;51(1):32–8.
45. Taylor EN, Stampfer MJ, Curhan GC. Dietary factors and the risk of incident kidney stones in men: new insights after 14 years of follow-up. J Am Soc Nephrol. 2004;15(12):3225–32. doi:15/12/3225 [pii]. https://doi.org/10.1097/01.ASN.0000146012.44570.20.
46. Curhan GC, Willett WC, Knight EL, Stampfer MJ. Dietary factors and the risk of incident kidney stones in younger women: Nurses' Health Study II. Arch Intern Med. 2004;164(8):885–91. https://doi.org/10.1001/archinte.164.8.885. 164/8/885 [pii].
47. Torres VE, Chapman AB, Devuyst O, Gansevoort RT, Grantham JJ, Higashihara E, et al. Tolvaptan in patients with autosomal dominant polycystic kidney disease. N Engl J Med. 2012;367(25):2407–18. https://doi.org/10.1056/NEJMoa1205511.
48. Nagao S, Nishii K, Katsuyama M, Kurahashi H, Marunouchi T, Takahashi H, et al. Increased water intake decreases progression of polycystic kidney disease in the PCK rat. J Am Soc Nephrol. 2006;17(8):2220–7. doi:ASN.2006030251 [pii]. https://doi.org/10.1681/ASN.2006030251.
49. Wang CJ, Grantham JJ, Wetmore JB. The medicinal use of water in renal disease. Kidney Int. 2013;84(1):45–53. https://doi.org/10.1038/ki.2013.23.
50. Bourquia A. Autosomal dominant polycystic kidney disease (ADPKD) in Morocco. Multicenter study about 308 families. Nephrologie. 2002;23(2):93–6.
51. Nishiura JL, Eloi SR, Heilberg IP. Pain determinants of pain in autosomal dominant polycystic kidney disease. J Bras Nefrol. 2013;35(3):242–3. https://

doi.org/10.5935/0101-2800.20130038. S0101-28002013000300012 [pii].
52. Bajwa ZH, Gupta S, Warfield CA, Steinman TI. Pain management in polycystic kidney disease. Kidney Int. 2001;60(5):1631–44. doi:985 [pii]. https://doi.org/10.1046/j.1523-1755.2001.00985.x.
53. Pirson Y, Chauveau D, Torres V. Management of cerebral aneurysms in autosomal dominant polycystic kidney disease. J Am Soc Nephrol. 2002;13(1):269–76.
54. Gibbs GF, Huston J 3rd, Qian Q, Kubly V, Harris PC, Brown RD Jr, et al. Follow-up of intracranial aneurysms in autosomal-dominant polycystic kidney disease. Kidney Int. 2004;65(5):1621–7. https://doi.org/10.1111/j.1523-1755.2004.00572.x. KID572 [pii].
55. Belz MM, Fick-Brosnahan GM, Hughes RL, Rubinstein D, Chapman AB, Johnson AM, et al. Recurrence of intracranial aneurysms in autosomal-dominant polycystic kidney disease. Kidney Int. 2003;63(5):1824–30. doi:kid918 [pii]. https://doi.org/10.1046/j.1523-1755.2003.00918.x.
56. Schrier RW, Belz MM, Johnson AM, Kaehny WD, Hughes RL, Rubinstein D, et al. Repeat imaging for intracranial aneurysms in patients with autosomal dominant polycystic kidney disease with initially negative studies: a prospective ten-year follow-up. J Am Soc Nephrol. 2004;15(4):1023–8.
57. Irazabal MV, Huston J 3rd, Kubly V, Rossetti S, Sundsbak JL, Hogan MC, et al. Extended follow-up of unruptured intracranial aneurysms detected by presymptomatic screening in patients with autosomal dominant polycystic kidney disease. Clin J Am Soc Nephrol. 2011;6(6):1274–85. https://doi.org/10.2215/CJN.09731110. CJN.09731110 [pii].
58. Rinkel GJ. Intracranial aneurysm screening: indications and advice for practice. Lancet Neurol. 2005;4(2):122–8. doi:S1474442205009932 [pii]. https://doi.org/10.1016/S1474-4422(05)00993-2.
59. Osawa Y, Omori S, Nagai M, Obayashi H, Maruyama H, Gejyo F. Thoracic aortic dissection in a patient with autosomal dominant polycystic kidney disease treated with maintenance hemodialysis. J Nephrol. 2000;13(3):193–5.
60. Paynter HE, Parnham A, Feest TG, Dudley CR. Thoracic aortic dissection complicating autosomal dominant polycystic kidney disease. Nephrol Dial Transplant. 1997;12(8):1711–3.
61. Torra R, Nicolau C, Badenas C, Navarro S, Perez L, Estivill X, et al. Ultrasonographic study of pancreatic cysts in autosomal dominant polycystic kidney disease. Clin Nephrol. 1997;47(1):19–22.
62. Malka D, Hammel P, Vilgrain V, Flejou JF, Belghiti J, Bernades P. Chronic obstructive pancreatitis due to a pancreatic cyst in a patient with autosomal dominant polycystic kidney disease. Gut. 1998;42(1):131–4.
63. Naitoh H, Shoji H, Ishikawa I, Watanabe R, Furuta Y, Tomozawa S, et al. Intraductal papillary mucinous tumor of the pancreas associated with autosomal dominant polycystic kidney disease. J Gastrointest Surg. 2005;9(6):843–5. doi:S1091-255X(05)00325-2 [pii]. https://doi.org/10.1016/j.gassur.2005.01.290.
64. Sato Y, Mukai M, Sasaki M, Kitao A, Yoneda N, Kobayashi D, et al. Intraductal papillary-mucinous neoplasm of the pancreas associated with polycystic liver and kidney disease. Pathol Int. 2009;59(3):201–4. https://doi.org/10.1111/j.1440-1827.2009.02352.x. PIN2352 [pii].
65. Beattie A, Shaw A, Yardley L, Little P, Sharp D. Participating in and delivering the ATEAM trial (Alexander technique lessons, exercise, and massage) interventions for chronic back pain: a qualitative study of professional perspectives. Complement Ther Med. 2010;18(3–4):119–27. https://doi.org/10.1016/j.ctim.2010.05.037. S0965-2299(10)00074-9 [pii].
66. Woodman JP, Moore NR. Evidence for the effectiveness of Alexander Technique lessons in medical and health-related conditions: a systematic review. Int J Clin Pract. 2012;66(1):98–112. https://doi.org/10.1111/j.1742-1241.2011.02817.x.
67. Yardley L, Dennison L, Coker R, Webley F, Middleton K, Barnett J, et al. Patients' views of receiving lessons in the Alexander technique and an exercise prescription for managing back pain in the ATEAM trial. Fam Pract. 2010;27(2):198–204. https://doi.org/10.1093/fampra/cmp093. cmp093 [pii].
68. Melzack R, Wall PD. Pain mechanisms: a new theory. Science. 1965;150(3699):971–9.
69. Johnson M, Martinson M. Efficacy of electrical nerve stimulation for chronic musculoskeletal pain: a meta-analysis of randomized controlled trials. Pain. 2007;130(1–2):157–65. doi:S0304-3959(07)00073-5 [pii]. https://doi.org/10.1016/j.pain.2007.02.007.
70. Nnoaham KE, Kumbang J. Transcutaneous electrical nerve stimulation (TENS) for chronic pain. Cochrane Database Syst Rev. 2008(3):CD003222. https://doi.org/10.1002/14651858.CD003222.pub2.
71. Henrich WL, Agodoa LE, Barrett B, Bennett WM, Blantz RC, Buckalew VM Jr, et al. Analgesics and the kidney: summary and recommendations to the Scientific Advisory Board of the National Kidney Foundation from an Ad Hoc Committee of the National Kidney Foundation. Am J Kidney Dis. 1996;27(1):162–5.
72. Hogan MC, Norby SM. Evaluation and management of pain in autosomal dominant polycystic kidney disease. Adv Chronic Kidney Dis. 2010;17(3):e1–e16. https://doi.org/10.1053/j.ackd.2010.01.005. S1548-5595(10)00006-6 [pii].
73. Chou R, Fanciullo GJ, Fine PG, Adler JA, Ballantyne JC, Davies P, et al. Clinical guidelines for the use of chronic opioid therapy in chronic noncancer pain. J Pain. 2009;10(2):113–30. https://doi.org/10.1016/j.jpain.2008.10.008. S1526-5900(08)00831-6 [pii].
74. Bennett WM, Elzinga L, Golper TA, Barry JM. Reduction of cyst volume for symptomatic management of autosomal dominant polycystic kidney disease. J Urol. 1987;137(4):620–2.
75. Bricker NS, Patton JF. Renal-function studies in polycystic disease of the kidneys with observations on the effects of surgical decompression. N Engl

J Med. 1957;256(5):212–4. https://doi.org/10.1056/NEJM195701312560504.
76. He SZ, An SY, Jiang HM, Yang R, Cao YF. Cyst decapitating decompression operation in polycystic kidney: preliminary report of 52 cases. Chin Med J. 1980;93(11):773–8.
77. Elzinga LW, Barry JM, Torres VE, Zincke H, Wahner HW, Swan S, et al. Cyst decompression surgery for autosomal dominant polycystic kidney disease. J Am Soc Nephrol. 1992;2(7):1219–26.
78. Brown JA, Torres VE, King BF, Segura JW. Laparoscopic marsupialization of symptomatic polycystic kidney disease. J Urol. 1996;156(1):22–7. doi:S0022-5347(01)65927-5 [pii].
79. Teichman JM, Hulbert JC. Laparoscopic marsupialization of the painful polycystic kidney. J Urol. 1995;153(4):1105–7. doi:S0022-5347(01)67520-7 [pii].
80. Rubenstein SC, Hulbert JC, Pharand D, Schuessler WW, Vancaillie TG, Kavoussi LR. Laparoscopic ablation of symptomatic renal cysts. J Urol. 1993;150(4):1103–6.
81. Nieh PT, Bihrle W 3rd. Laparoscopic marsupialization of massive renal cyst. J Urol. 1993;150(1):171–3.
82. Lifson BJ, Teichman JM, Hulbert JC. Role and long-term results of laparoscopic decortication in solitary cystic and autosomal dominant polycystic kidney disease. J Urol. 1998;159(3):702–5; discussion 5–6. doi:S0022-5347(01)63704-2 [pii].
83. Elashry OM, Nakada SY, Wolf JS Jr, McDougall EM, Clayman RV. Laparoscopy for adult polycystic kidney disease: a promising alternative. Am J Kidney Dis. 1996;27(2):224–33. doi:S0272-6386(96)90545-4 [pii].
84. Resnick M, Chang AY, Casale P. Laparoscopic renal denervation and nephropexy for autosomal dominant polycystic kidney disease related pain in adolescents. J Urol. 2006;175(6):2274–6.; ; discussion 6. doi:S0022-5347(06)00336-3 [pii]. https://doi.org/10.1016/S0022-5347(06)00336-3.
85. Chapuis O, Sockeel P, Pallas G, Pons F, Jancovici R. Thoracoscopic renal denervation for intractable autosomal dominant polycystic kidney disease-related pain. Am J Kidney Dis. 2004;43(1):161–3. doi:S0272638603013659 [pii].
86. Ansell J, Gee W, Bonica J. Management of pain. In: Bonica J, editor. Diseases of the kidney and ureter, vol. 2. 2nd ed. Philadelphia: Lea and Febiger; 1990.

10 Extrarenal Manifestations of Autosomal Dominant Polycystic Kidney Disease: Polycystic Liver Disease

Fouad T. Chebib and Marie C. Hogan

Introduction

The liver is the commonest extrarenal site of disease involvement in autosomal dominant polycystic kidney disease (ADPKD). Both liver cysts and parenchymal enlargement are responsible for most complications associated with polycystic liver disease (PLD), but other manifestations may occasionally be encountered, including congenital hepatic fibrosis and segmental dilation of the biliary tract [1–3]. Most individuals remain asymptomatic, but some experience chronic manifestations related to progressive liver enlargement leading to disability and severely impacting their quality of life.

Epidemiology

Hepatic cysts are seen in a heterogeneous group of disorders that differ in etiology, prevalence, and clinical manifestations. The prevalence of simple cysts increases with age and ranges between 2.5% and 24% [4]. Simple cysts tend to be more prevalent in women and occur mostly in the right lobe; they also tend to be solitary, but two to three simple cysts may be present in up to 25% of these patients. In contrast to common simple hepatic cysts, polycystic liver disease (PLD) is arbitrarily defined where >20 cysts are present, is a rare condition, and is seen as part or all of the phenotype of two inherited disorders, ADPKD (Fig. 10.1a, b, e) and ADPLD (Fig. 10.1c, d, f) (autosomal dominant polycystic liver disease) (Table 10.1). ADPKD, the most prevalent inherited genetic renal disorder in adults leading to end-stage renal disease, has a prevalence of 0.1% [1]. In addition to ADPKD, and ADPLD, conditions associated with hepatic cysts include other genetic disorders, tuberous-sclerosis complex, von Hippel-Lindau disease, and oral-facial-digital syndrome type I, and acquired disorders associated with the development of cysts of the hepatic hilus, such as portal hypertension and biliary obstruction as well as parasitic and neoplastic cysts.

In ADPKD, hepatic cysts tend to develop later than renal cysts. They are rare in children, and their frequency increases with age and might have been underestimated by ultrasound and CT studies [1]. Using MRI (3 mm slice thickness), prevalence in a large cohort study (*C*onsortium for *R*adiologic *I*maging *S*tudies of *P*olycystic Kidney Disease; CRISP) was 58% in 15–24-year-old, 85% in 25–34-year-old, and 94% in 35–46-year-old participants [5]. There are several known risk

F. T. Chebib, MD · M. C. Hogan, MD, PhD (✉)
Mayo Medical School, Division of Nephrology & Hypertension, Department of Internal Medicine, Mayo Clinic, Rochester, MN, USA
e-mail: Chebib.fouad@mayo.edu; hogan.marie@mayo.edu

B. D. Cowley, Jr., J. J. Bissler (eds.), *Polycystic Kidney Disease*,
https://doi.org/10.1007/978-1-4939-7784-0_10

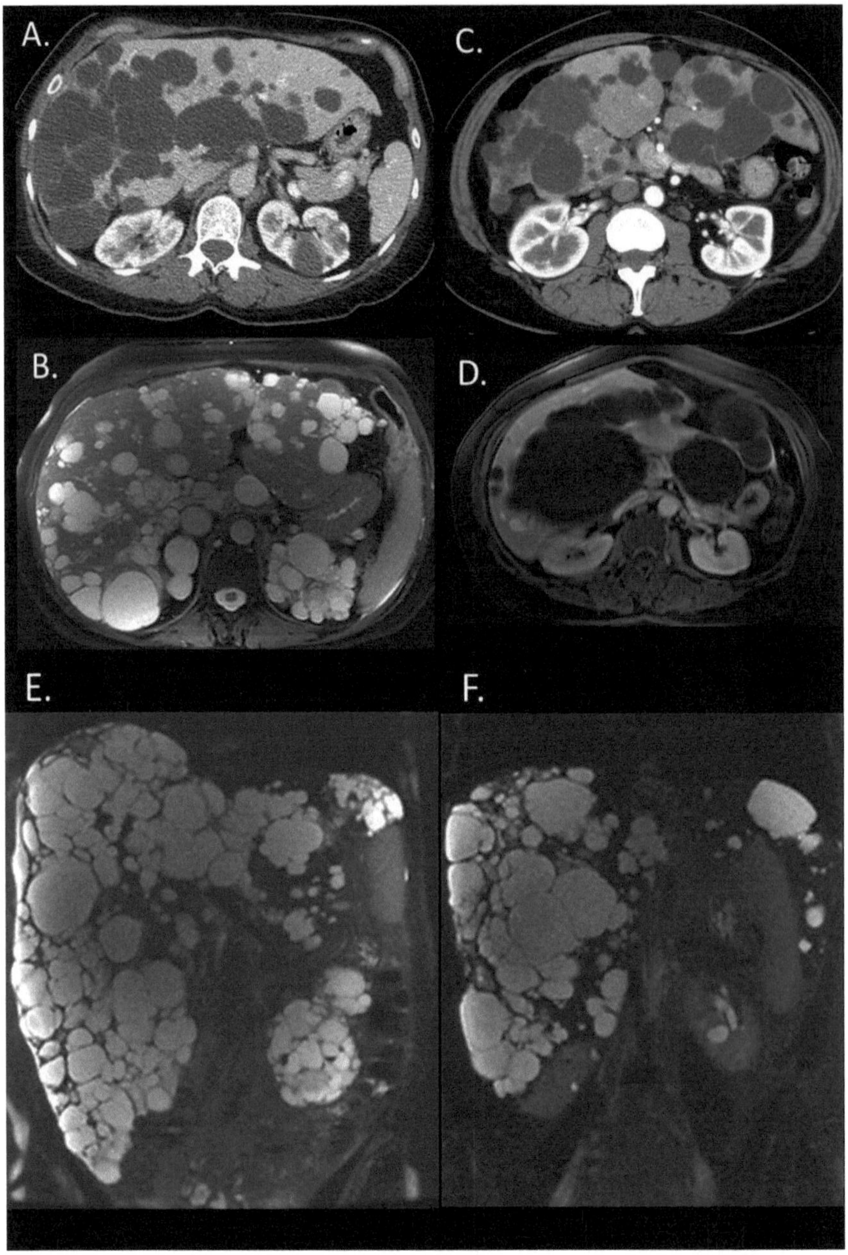

Fig. 10.1 Representative cases of APDKD with PLD and ADPLD. (**a**) Sagittal CT and (**b**) sagittal MRI polycystic liver disease cases with ADPKD; (**c**) sagittal CT and (**d**) sagittal MRI showing autosomal dominant polycystic liver disease. (**e**) Coronal magnetic resonance imaging sections of polycystic liver disease in an individual with ADPKD and (**f**) autosomal dominant polycystic liver disease

factors that influence PLD severity (Table 10.2) including female gender, parity, and exogenous estrogen exposure. Cysts are more prevalent, and cyst volume is generally higher in women than in men [5–7]. Women who have multiple pregnancies or who have used oral contraceptive drugs or estrogen replacement therapy have worse disease, suggesting an estrogen effect on hepatic cyst growth [6, 8]. In fact, 1 year of estrogen use in postmenopausal females with ADPKD selectively increased total liver volume by 7%, whereas total kidney volume remained unaffected in a case-control study [8, 9]. Data from two major cohort studies (in the HALT and CRISP studies) in ADPKD show that there was only a weak correlation of liver cyst and kidney cyst volumes, indicating there are separate genetic and environmental factors that influence the PLD severity compared with kidney disease severity reflected by total kidney volume [5, 7]. Massive PLD develops in a minority of ADPKD/ ADPLD cases (mostly females). Familial aggregation of massive PLD is thought to be uncommon.

ADPLD a genetically distinct disease with few or absent renal cysts (Fig. 10.1c, d, f). The prevalence of ADPLD is not known but appears to be underreported with median age at diagnosis of 47 years and the majority being female [10]. The presence of renal cysts can often confuse the diagnosis of ADPLD with ADPKD, but the absence of a family history of end-stage renal disease in these families and the relatively few numbers of renal cysts can reassure the patient and the physician of the ADPLD diagnosis as can genetic testing (although this is not routinely performed). Similar to ADPKD, ADPLD is a genetically heterogeneous disease, with one-third to one-half of isolated ADPLD cases being accounted by four genes identified to date (*PRKCSH*, *SEC63*, *LRP5*, and *GANAB*) [11–15]. Thus, other genetic loci not yet identified are likely also implicated. The protein products of these genes (hepatocystin, sec63p, low-density lipoprotein receptor-related protein 5, and glucosidase II, alpha subunit, respectively) act in concert to achieve proper topology, folding and quality control of integral membrane or secreted glycoproteins in the endoplasmic reticulum (ER) [16]. Selective loss of *PRKCSH* and *SEC63* leads

Table 10.1 Risk factors for liver cyst growth

Risk factors for liver cyst growth
Older age
Female gender
Higher number of pregnancies
Previous use of exogenous estrogens as oral contraceptives or estrogen replacement therapy
Larger renal cysts

Table 10.2 Mutated genes and proteins of polycystic liver diseases

Mutated genes	Protein	Localization	Function
ADPLD (−1:100,000)			
PRKCSH 19p13.2	Glucosidase 2 subunit ß, protein kinase C substrate 80K-H, or hepatocystin	Endoplasmic reticulum	N-linked glycan-processing enzyme in the endoplasmic reticulum
SEC63 6q21	Translocation protein SEC 63 homolog	Endoplasmic reticulum	Translocation of proteins in the endoplasmic reticulum
LRP5 11q13.2	Low-density lipoprotein receptor-related protein 5	Plasma membrane	Canonical Wnt signaling
GANAB 11q12.3	Catalytic α subunit of glucosidase II	Endoplasmic reticulum	Quality control and maturation of N-linked glycoproteins including PC1 and PC2
ADPKD (−1: 400–1000)			
PKD1 16 p13.3	Polycystin-1	Primary cilium, plasma membrane, and cell junctions	Mechanoreceptor involved in calcium signaling
PKD2 4q21	Polycystin-2	Primary cilium and endoplasmic reticulum	Nonselective calcium channel
GANAB 11q12.3	Catalytic α subunit of glucosidase II	Endoplasmic reticulum	Quality control and maturation of N-linked glycoproteins including PC1 and PC2
ARPKD (−1/20,000)			
PKHD1	Fibrocystin	Primary cilium	Tubulogenesis and/or maintenance of bile duct architecture

to both hepatic and renal cyst formation [17]. The products of both of these genes are required for adequate expression of polycystin-1 and polycystin-2. LRP5 is involved in canonical Wnt signal transduction. The rate-limiting component appears to be polycystin-1 with an inverse dose-response relationship with cystic dilation [17].

Pathogenesis

Malformation of the ductal plate of medium-size ducts during embryonic development appears to give rise to liver cysts. Ductal plate malformations are a group of pathological abnormalities ranging from biliary hamartoma to PLD, Caroli's disease, and congenital hepatic fibrosis [18]. These diseases can exist as individual conditions or in combinations. Phenotypes depend on the level affected in the biliary tree (intrahepatic and/or extrahepatic biliary ducts; large, medium, or smaller intrahepatic biliary ducts) during embryogenesis. Remodeling of the ductal plate begins in utero extending from the hilum to the periphery of the liver, and the normal remodeling process leads to the formation of bile ducts and ductules via epithelial proliferation and apoptosis, with subsequent resorption of the remaining ductal plate elements. Premature arrest or interruption in this process leads to the persistence of excessive embryonic bile duct structures in the ductal plate complex leading to ductal plate malformations. Normal bile ducts arise from the ductal plate through growth and apoptosis. The bile ducts normally comprise 2–4% of the liver cell mass and serve to dilute and alkalinize bile in the liver. Biliary microhamartomas are small clusters of bile ductules surrounded by fibrous tissue. Intrahepatic cysts containing bile duct epithelial cells (peribiliary glands) are thought to be derived by progressive dilatation of biliary microhamartomas leading to cysts in PLD. Abnormalities in biliary cell proliferation, apoptosis, enhanced fluid secretion, cholangiocyte cilia length, centrosomal dysfunction, disturbed signaling pathways, and aberrant protein and miRNA expression are thought to be major factors in the pathogenesis of PLD (Figs. 10.2 and 10.3) [13, 19, 20]. Cyst fluid resembles the bile salt-independent fraction of bile. Cyst walls are usually thin and are composed of a single layer of cuboidal or flat epithelial cells and variable amounts of connective tissue. Multiple intracellular signaling routes are involved in hepatic cystogenesis. Secretin stimulates cAMP-dependent Cl^- and $HCO3^-$ secretion by biliary epithelia. Liver cysts continue to have a secretory function (Fig. 10.2).

Altered cell-matrix interaction and remodeling also contribute to cyst formation. Alterations in intracellular homeostasis and 3′–5′ cAMP stimulate mitogen-activated protein kinase-mediated cell proliferation and cystic fibrosis transmembrane conductance regulator-driven chloride and fluid secretion [21]. Cyst growth is enhanced by growth factors and cytokines secreted into the cyst fluid [22]. Downstream

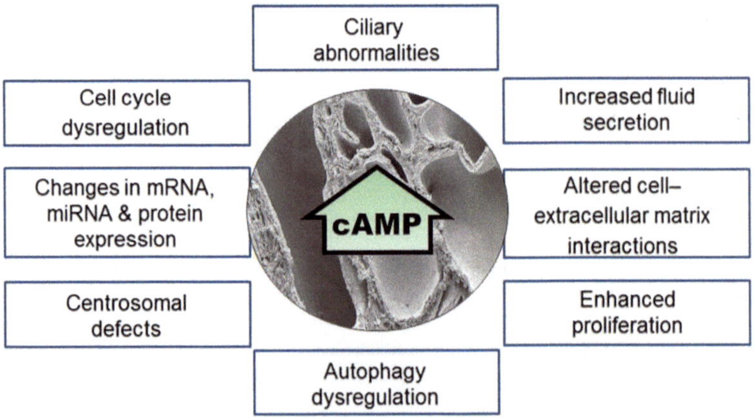

Fig. 10.2 Mechanisms of hepatic cystogenesis: many different mechanisms are involved in liver cyst development (Used with permission of Mayo Foundation for Medical Education and Research, all rights reserved)

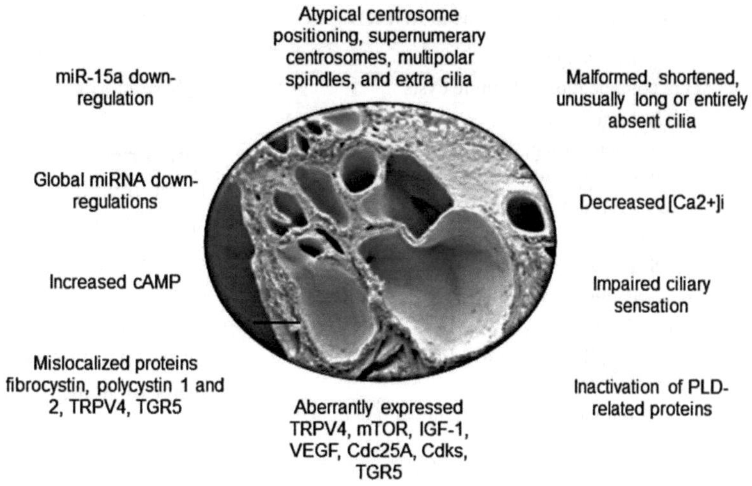

Fig. 10.3 Hepatic cystogenesis is associated with ciliary abnormalities, centrosomal dysfunction, disturbed signaling pathways, and aberrant protein and miRNA expression. Image shows hepatic cysts in liver parenchyma of PCK rats. Scale bar, 100 mm (Reprinted from Ref. [109] with permission from Elsevier)

activation of mTOR likely contributes to cystogenesis [23]. Cholangiocytes bordering the cyst can secrete vascular endothelial growth factor (VEGF), which stimulates the growth of liver cysts through autocrine and paracrine mechanisms [24]. Another important factor that affects cholangiocyte proliferation is the intracellular calcium concentration. Cystic cholangiocytes have decreased intracellular calcium concentrations, which is associated with hyperproliferation of cholangiocytes [19]. The expression of mammalian target of rapamycin (mTOR) is reported to be increased in the epithelium lining of cysts in PLD patients, suggesting that the mTOR pathway might have a role in liver cysts growth modulation. mTOR has significant roles in protein translation, cell growth, and cell proliferation [23].

In ADPLD patients, the primary cilia are structurally intact, suggesting that the pathology of cilia function and cilia structure is not solely responsible for PLD, but rather other mechanisms are disrupted, such as protein trafficking and the protein quality control processes within the cell [25]. Polycystin-1, the product of the PKD1 gene, seems to be involved in both renal and hepatobiliary embryogenesis. This is strongly supported by the finding that polycystin-1 is more highly expressed in fetal than in adult kidney and is also overexpressed in the liver and the biliary fetal system, but it is speculative to postulate that an abnormal polycystin-1 may fully account for abnormal biliary organogenesis and early-onset renal disease [6, 26–29].

Symptoms

Although ADPLD and ADPKD are genetically distinct, the clinical course of liver disease in these diseases is similar. The course of PLD is progressive, with continuous growth in the number and size of liver cysts [13]. On the basis of data from the placebo arms of three randomized clinical trials, the polycystic liver growth rate is estimated at 0.9–1.6% in 6–12 months [30–32]. One study found that patients with ADPLD have greater numbers of liver cysts and cysts with larger volumes than individuals with ADPKD with polycystic livers, and ADPLD cases with confirmed mutations in either *PRKCSH* or *SEC63* showed a more severe disease course than those without a known mutation [10, 13, 33, 34]. Initially, PLD is asymptomatic, but symptoms have become more common as the lifespan of patients with polycystic kidney and liver disease has lengthened with interventions such as improved blood pressure control (that positively influences cardiovascular complications), dialysis, and transplantation. Complications might be either acute or chronic and might be related or unrelated to liver cysts (Table 10.3). The minority with symptomatic

Table 10.3 Liver complications in ADPKD

Related to hepatic cysts
Acute complications of single cysts
1. Cyst infection
2. Cyst hemorrhage (intracystic or hemoperitoneum)
3. Cyst rupture
4. Cyst torsion
5. Obstructive jaundice
6. Ascending cholangitis
Massive PLD
1. Uncomplicated massive PLD (abdominal mass/distention)
Abdominal (usually right upper quadrant) pain/fullness
Anorexia/nausea (due to stomach compression)
GERD/regurgitation
Dyspnea
Early satiety
Back pain
Abdominal hernia
Mild abnormalities in liver function
Complications superimposed upon massive PLD
(a). Ascites
(b). Hepatic venous outflow obstruction
(c). Portal hypertension with variceal bleeding
(d). IVC compression
(e). Bile duct compression: jaundice
(f). Pleural effusion
(g). Organ displacement:
Kidneys
Uterine prolapse
Constipation
(h). Loss of mobility
(i). Loss of muscle mass
(j). Failure to thrive and malnutrition
2. Budd-Chiari syndrome
3. Progressive hepatic failure (rare)
Unrelated to hepatic cysts
Isolated common bile duct dilatation
Congenital hepatic fibrosis or biliary fibroadenomatosis, focal or diffuse
Others
Idiopathic dilation of the intra- or extrahepatic biliary tract (Caroli syndrome)
Cholangiocarcinoma

PLD complains of heartburn due to gastroesophageal reflux, early satiety, abdominal pain, abdominal distention, etc. (Table 10.3). These symptoms may not be queried or recognized as being related to PLD in individuals with ADPKD who are concerned about renal function and kidney-related symptoms.

Imaging

Liver imaging to determine the extent of PLD should be included in the initial assessment of all ADPKD patients (Figs. 10.4, 10.5, and 10.6) [35]. There is currently no consensus as to the frequency or necessity of repeat imaging for PLD unless patients develop symptoms and in situations of acute pain and/or fever where there is suspicion of hemorrhage into a cyst or torsion or cyst infection [35]. Two qualitative and one quantitative imaging classification systems are described in Table 10.4; Gigot's classification categorizes PLD according to the number and size of liver cysts and the amount of remaining liver parenchyma [36] and is useful in describing the severity of PLD. Individuals with Gigot type I (<10 large cysts) have the mildest disease. Gigot II includes cases with diffuse involvement of liver parenchyma by multiple medium-sized cysts with large areas of noncystic liver parenchyma remaining, and Gigot type III includes individuals with large numbers of small- and medium-sized liver cysts spread diffusely through the liver parenchyma with few remaining areas of normal parenchyma. Highly symptomatic patients are usually Gigot stage II or III. The Mayo Clinic PLD classification is useful in that it stratifies patients for operative procedure selection [37]. (Table 10.4) CT or MRI volumetry currently only available as a research tool is the most accurate method to quantitate PLD using organ volume and/or cyst volumes. Both MR- and CT-based volumetric imaging have been used as a research tool to quantitate disease severity using total liver volume. The third classification uses data from liver volumes (assessed by MRI in a cohort with early-stage ADPKD in the HALT study in >500 individuals with ADPKD) noting that the average liver weight (or volume in a normal adult) is 1500 g (or 1500 ml) and is useful in providing cross-sectional analysis of liver volumes in a population with mostly mild PLD and provides a reference point for liver volume as a quantitative measure of disease severity [38]

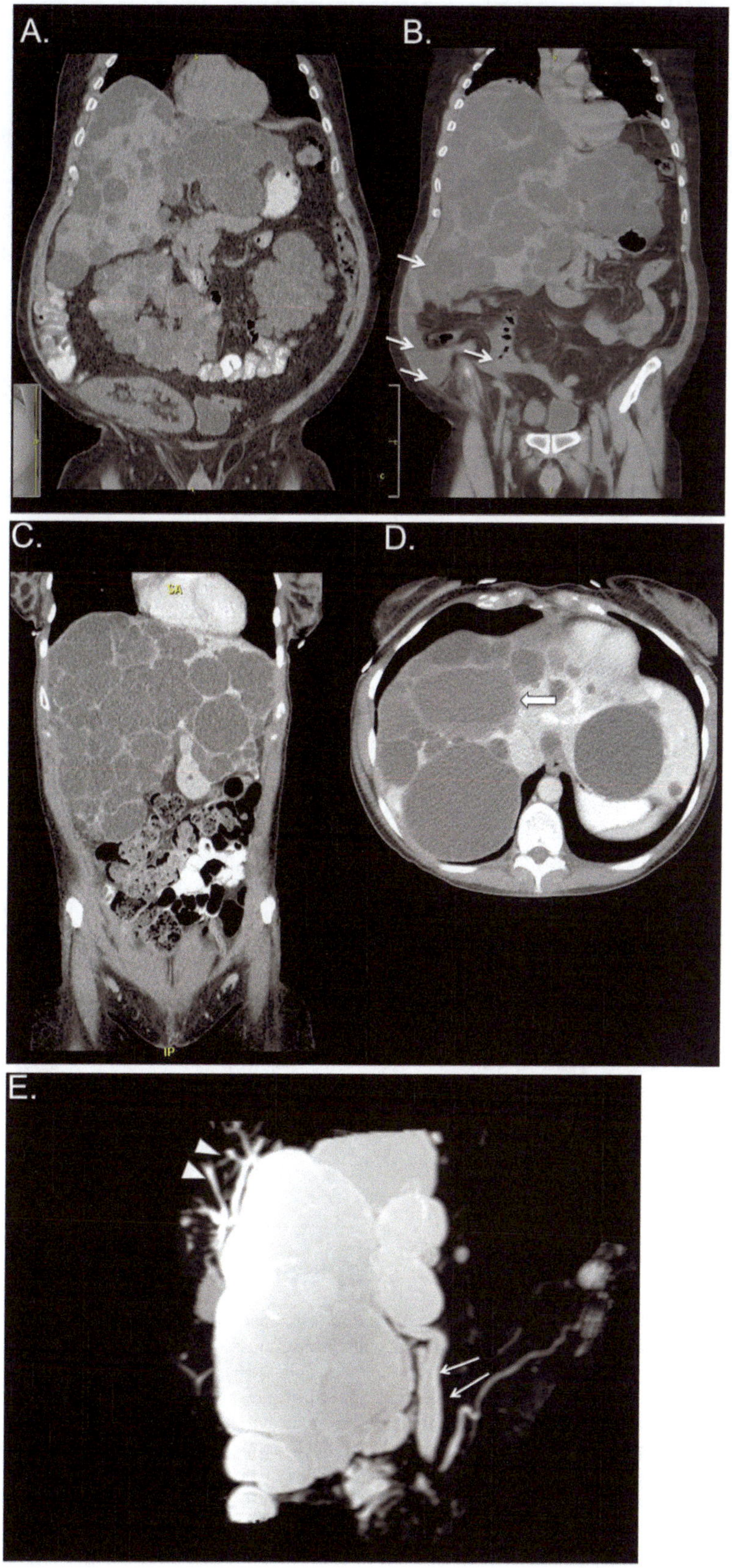

Fig. 10.4 Complications associated with PLD: (**a**) This man with ADPKD also has symptomatic PLD. (**b**) Abdominal CT in the same individual at the time of hospitalization showed evidence of new-onset abdominal ascites (arrows). He had probably ruptured a liver cyst presenting with abdominal pain. Note he also has a kidney transplant in the right lower quadrant. (**c**) A woman with known polycystic liver disease who developed acute right upper quadrant pain. A CT abdomen was performed in the emergency room. (**d**) An acute hemorrhage into a liver cyst is seen (arrowed) on contrast CT. (**e**) MRCP showing asymptomatic 7-mm common bile duct dilatation (arrowed) in another PLD patient who previously had a left hepatectomy and cholecystectomy). Mild dilatation of the right intrahepatic biliary ducts secondary to compression by a large cyst is also seen (arrowheads)

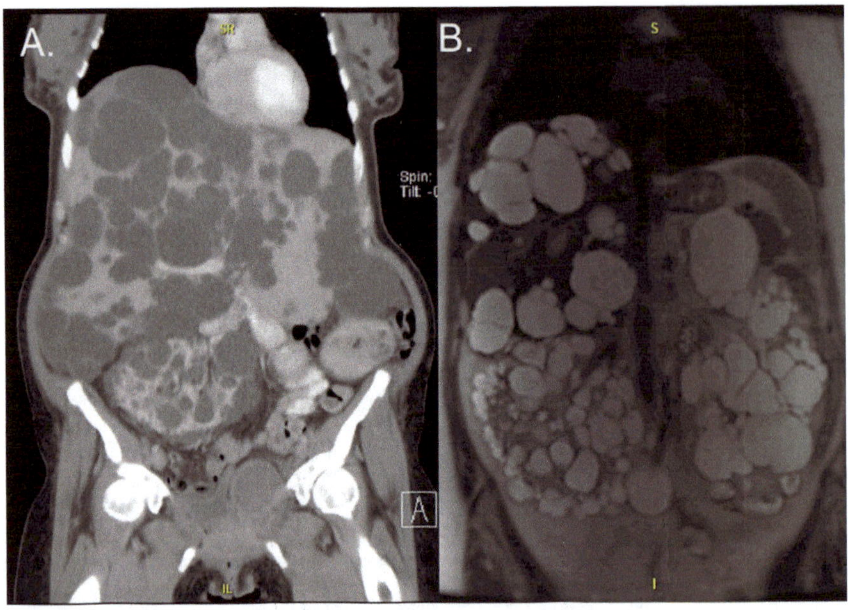

Fig. 10.5 (**a**) Massive symptomatic polycystic liver disease in a woman with ADPKD (contrast CT coronal view) (note the right kidney is malrotated). This individual required total parenteral nutrition for several months before liver reductive surgery. She underwent left hepatectomy, shown in (**b**).

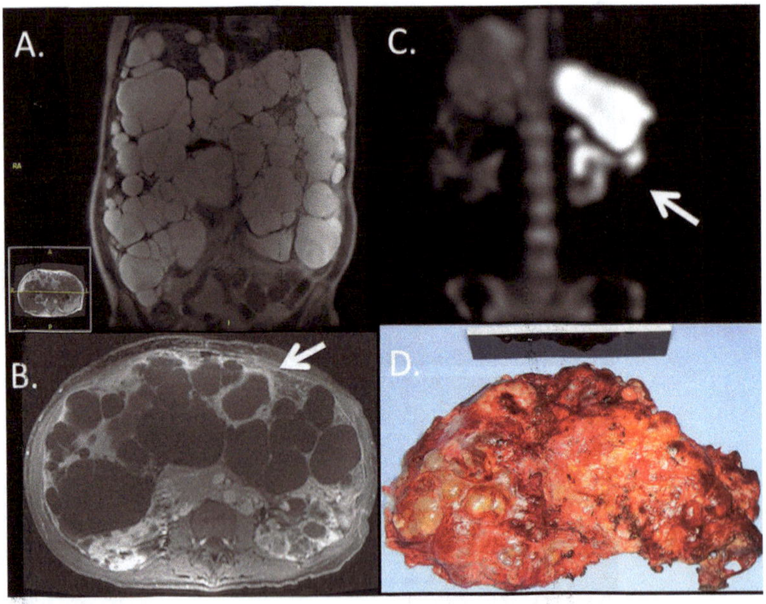

Fig. 10.6 Liver cyst infections. (**a**) Magnetic resonance imaging of the abdomen without and with intravenous gadolinium in a woman with polycystic liver and kidney disease who was experiencing right upper quadrant abdominal pain and fevers. (**b**) There is an abnormal-appearing cyst in the left lobe of the liver which demonstrates increased internal T1 signal and enhancement of the cyst wall on post-gadolinium images. To the left, adjacent to this enhancing cyst are few smaller cysts with similar characteristics. (**c**) Post-scan 4-h planar and SPECT/CT In-111 WBC images of the abdomen were obtained centered on the liver. There is intense-labeled WBC activity correlating with the multiple abnormal cysts within the left hepatic lobe demonstrated on the MRI. This would include the largest abnormal cyst within the anterior left hepatic lobe (arrowed in **b**).

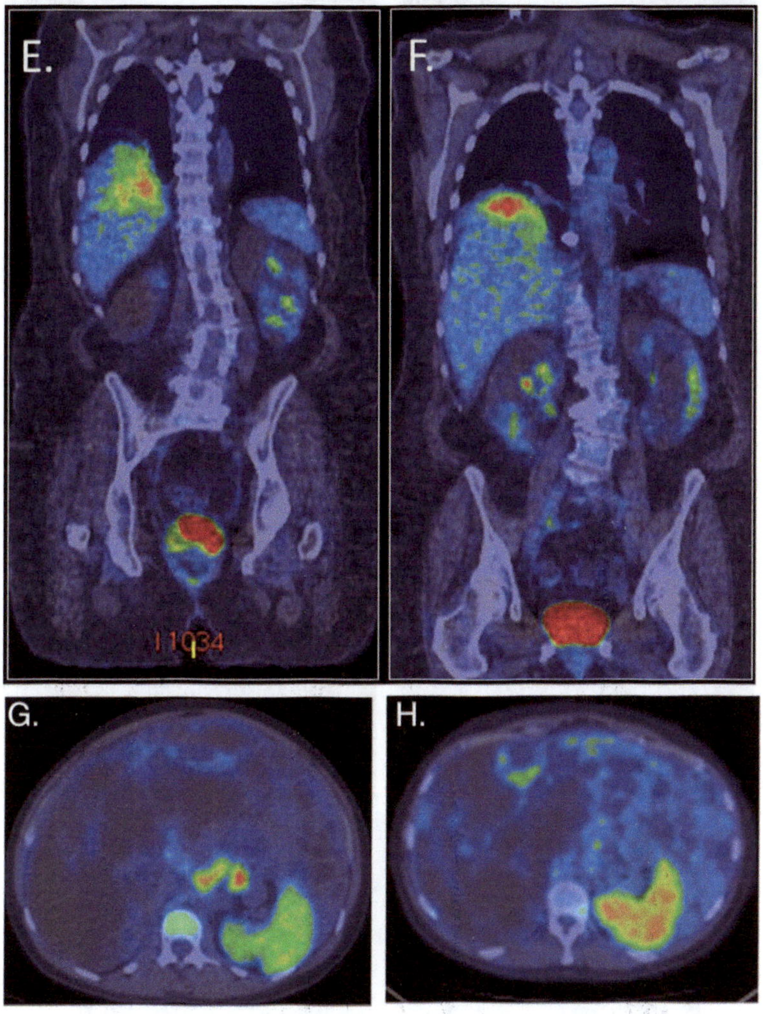

Fig. 10.6 (continued) Continuous with this infected cyst or directly adjacent is another more superior cyst demonstrating intense WBC localization (not shown). There is intense abnormal white blood cell localization in the abnormal-appearing cysts on MRI to the left of the dominant infected cyst along the anterior margin of the left hepatic lobe. Findings correlate with at least four if not five infected left hepatic lobe cysts. The remaining WBC localization to the liver appears physiologic and correlated with residual normal liver parenchyma predominantly in the right hepatic lobe. The degree of WBC localization in these areas is far less than within the infected cysts. Normal physiologic WBC localization was seen in the spleen also shown. (**d**) Left hepatectomy tissue containing the resected infected cysts. (**e**) PET-CT of a woman who had right upper quadrant pain and recurrent gram negative bacteremia with mild polycystic liver (and kidney) disease. Her presentation was preceded by a surgical procedure for evaluation of a possible episode of cholangitis where she underwent ERCP and sphincterotomy. She later presented with infected cysts in hepatic segment IV and an infected fluid collection in the dome of the liver (**f**) demonstrated on PET-CT scan. She required liver resection of the affected liver tissue and recurrent intravenous antibiotics followed by suppressive oral antibiotics. (**g–m**) A 39-year-old female with known PLD and ADPKD presented with fever and severe right upper quadrant pain radiating to her shoulder and was found to have *K. pneumonia* bacteremia. C-reactive protein was 325 mg/L (normal <8 mg/L). Focal areas of severe infection within the inferior celiac lymph node and adjacent superior portion of the caudate lobe of the liver were identified on PET-CT. She completed a 2-week intravenous antibiotic course and was reassessed with PET-CT several weeks later. Because of persistent malaise abdominal pain and elevated C-reactive protein infection (**j**, **k**), she underwent CT-guided aspiration (**l**, **m**) of the cysts corresponding to the areas of persistent infection on repeat PET-CT followed by a second course of intravenous antibiotics and subsequent suppressive long-term oral antibiotic therapy without further recurrence of cyst infections

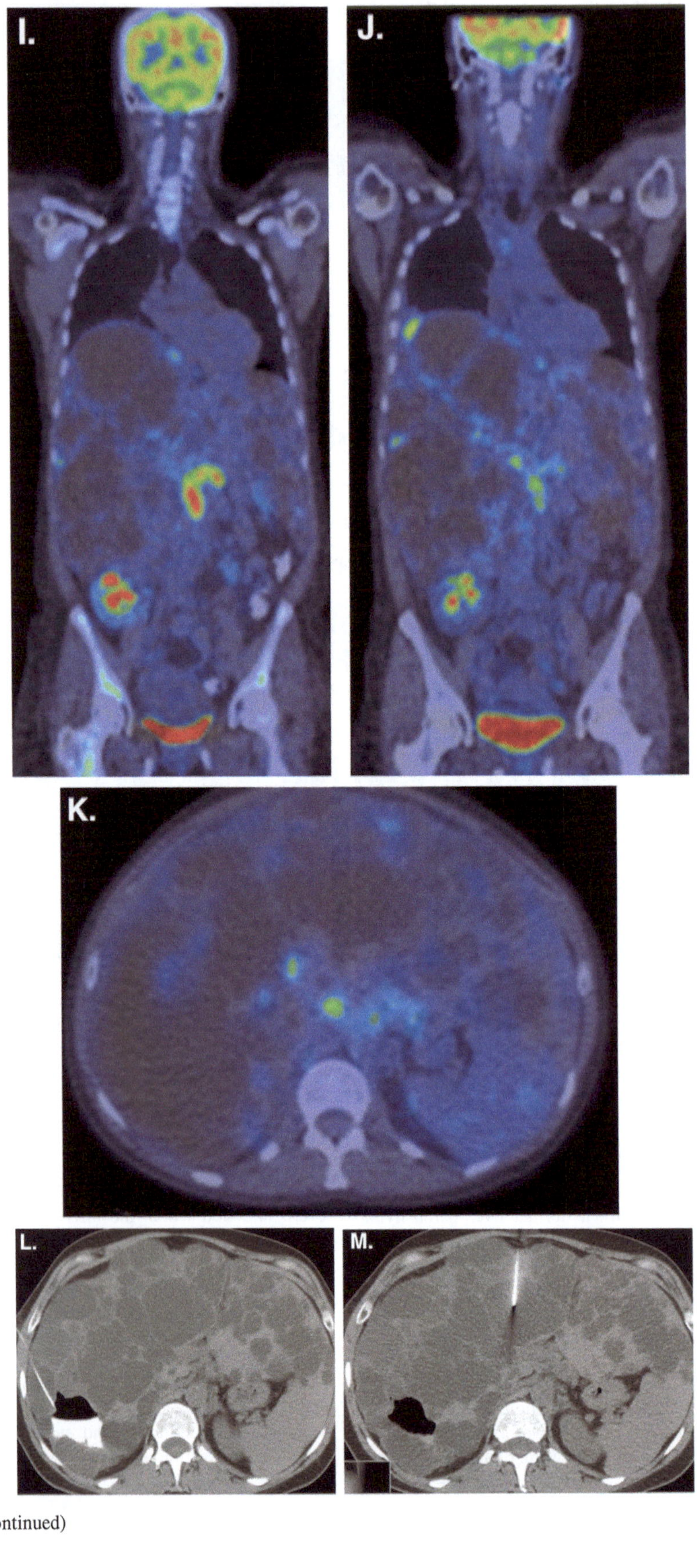

Fig. 10.6 (continued)

(Table 10.4). It is hoped that routine liver and kidney volume measurements using automated segmentation will soon become more routinely available for clinical monitoring [39].

Special Complications of PLD

Acute Complications

New-onset right upper quadrant pain usually denotes an acute complication such as cyst hemorrhage, rupture, or torsion (Fig. 10.4a–d). A detailed history and clinical examination can usually narrow the etiology of the complication and help determine the most optimal form of imaging that will help confirm the etiology of the symptoms.

Hepatic Cyst Infection

Hepatic cyst infections are relatively less common than infected kidney cysts, and diagnosis and management can be challenging (Fig. 10.6a–m). Three retrospective case series (and many case reports) describe their evaluation and management with the largest (a retrospective analysis) reporting 14 cases [40–42]. Right upper quadrant abdominal pain associated with fever with or without focal hepatic tenderness should raise suspicion of cyst infection (a potentially life-threatening complication), especially if concurrent liver function abnormalities coexist [40, 41]. Patients may have only vague symptoms of malaise without localizing symptoms, and therefore, there should be a high index of suspicion of infected cyst(s). It has been proposed that liver cyst infections result from either hematogenous seeding or by retrograde traffic of enteric pathogens via the biliary tract [40, 43, 44]. While cyst infection can complicate percutaneous liver cyst fluid aspiration, this should rarely occur if performed by experienced personnel [2]. Other risk factors include recent abdominal surgery, kidney transplantation (on immunosuppression), and chronic dialysis patients. Leukocytosis and elevated alkaline phosphatase can be seen [40, 42]. Elevated AST or bilirubin is uncommon.

When all four of the following criteria are concomitantly met (temperature >38 °C for >3 days, liver/loin tenderness, C-reactive protein (CRP) >5 mg/dL, and no evidence of intracystic bleeding on CT (suggested by spontaneous intracystic density >25 Hounsfield units)), then either liver or kidney infection is probable (Figs. 10.7c–f and 10.8) [42]. Episodes with two or three elements of these criteria might be labeled as "fever of unknown origin" [45]. Localization of the infected liver cysts(s) can be difficult as conventional imaging modalities such as MRI may be inconclusive [45, 46]. Debris within a cyst with a thick wall (Fig. 10.6b) and/or distal acoustic enhancement detected in at least one cyst are specific to infected cysts [42]. Positron emission tomography-CT appears to be superior to conventional imaging techniques for the detection and localization of infected cysts (Fig. 10.6e–j) [42, 43, 46–48]. In a recent series, ultrasound, computed tomography scan, and MRI failed to detect the infected cyst in 94%, 82%, and 60% of cases, respectively [41]. Indium white blood-labeled scans (Fig. 10.6c) are also helpful in localizing the site of an infection or abscess, especially if PET-CT is not available and is not limited in sensitivity by the presence of renal failure [49–52].

Liver cyst infections are usually monomicrobial with *Enterobacteriaceae. Escherichia coli* or *Klebsiella pneumoninga* accounting for the majority of reports [35, 40] (Figs. 10.6, 10.7, and 10.8). Urine and blood cultures should also be promptly obtained. Early drainage and cyst fluid analysis (which will reveal bacteria and neutrophils), in combination with intravenous antibiotics that concentrate in the biliary tree and penetrate the cysts, such as sulfamethoxazole-trimethoprim or ciprofloxacin [40], are recommended, especially if the suspected cyst is large (>5 cm) [42]. Cyst fluid cultures often remain positive despite several days of antibiotics and should permit directed antibiotic therapy. Gas can also be seen on imaging if the cyst has been previously punctured or if there is a communication with the bile ducts [40]. In some cases, surgical resection of the affected lobe(s) is required (Fig. 10.6a–d). Episodes with two or three elements

Table 10.4 Clinical and volumetric classifications for PLD severity [36–38]

Mayo classification [37]	**Type A**	**Type B**	**Type C**	**Type D**
Symptoms	Absent/mild	Moderate/severe	Moderate/severe	Moderate/severe
Cyst characteristics	Any	Limited no. large cysts	Any	Any
Areas of relative normal liver parenchyma	Any	≥2 sectors	≥1 sectors	<1 sector
Isosectoral portal vein or hepatic vein occlusion of preserved sector	Any	Absent	Absent	Present
Treatment	Observation/medical treatment	Cyst fenestration	Partial hepatectomy with remnant cyst fenestration	Liver transplantation
Gigot classification [36]	**Type I**	**Type II**	**Type III**	
	<10 large cysts (>10 cm) Does not classify as PLD	Diffuse involvement of liver parenchyma by multiple medium-sized cysts with large areas of noncystic liver parenchyma remaining	Large numbers of small- and medium-sized liver cysts are present and spread diffusely through the liver parenchyma. Few areas of normal liver parenchyma are present	
Volumetric classification (height adjusted LV) of PLD severity [38]	Mild	Moderate	Severe	
	Liver volume <1000 ml/m	Liver volume 1000–1800/m	Liver volume >1800/m	

of these criteria might be labeled as "fever of unknown origin" [43, 45]. Carbohydrate antigen 19-9 (CA19-9) has been proposed as a biomarker for hepatic cyst infection, but in our experience, this biomarker has very limited or no role in diagnosis or management [45, 53, 54]. Currently there are limited evidence-based guidelines for choice and duration of antibiotic therapy in treatment of hepatic cyst infection in PLD. Ciprofloxacin concentration in the hepatic cysts is severalfold relative to the concentration in the serum. Sallee et al. concluded from their experience in treating renal and hepatic cyst infections, that fluoroquinolones may be superior to beta-lactams, and initial use of dual antibiotics superior to monotherapy, until the organism is identified [42]. By extrapolation from treating pyogenic liver abscess, empiric antibiotic therapy may consist of monotherapy with a beta-lactam/beta-lactamase inhibitor or a combination of third-generation cephalosporin and metronidazole. Alternatively, a combination of fluoroquinolone and metronidazole or monotherapy with a carbapenem may be used.

Fig. 10.7 (continued) 200 cc of feculent-appearing and feculent-smelling fluid was aspirated, some of which was sent for cultures. The limited postprocedural scan demonstrated no immediate complications. The catheter was positioned centrally within the larger posterior infected hepatic segment VIII cyst passing through the infected cyst just anterior to it. *K. pneumonia*, sensitive to third-generation cephalosporins, was identified and symptoms resolved with treatment. In this case, her blood cultures were indeterminate. (**g**) Pre- and (**h**) postoperative coronal CT scan of a patient who underwent a combined liver/kidney transplant (the renal allograft is in the right pelvis)

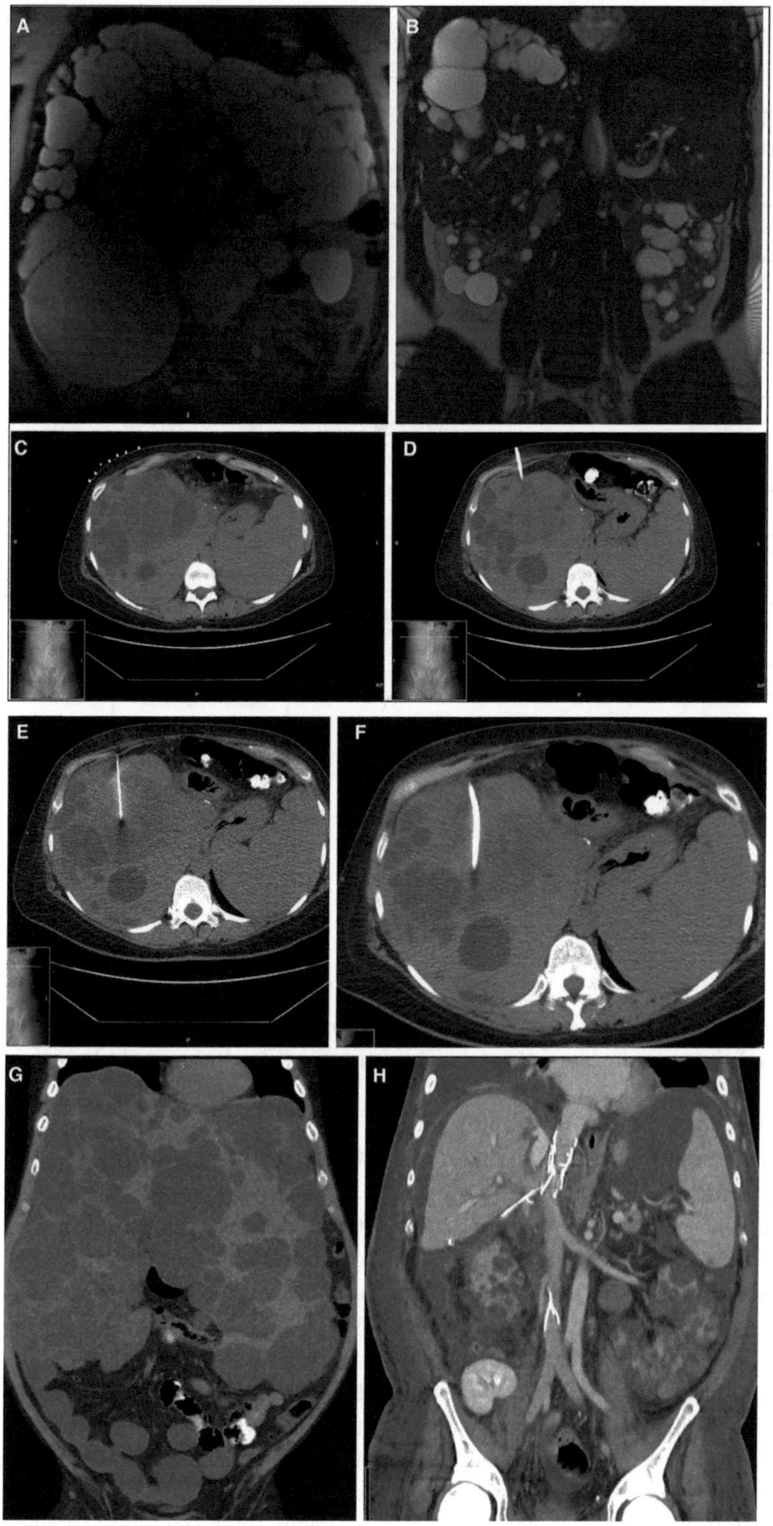

Fig. 10.7 MRI images in a PLD case who presented with increasing abdominal girth and shortness of breath. Pre-(**a**) and (**b**) post-left hepatectomy, cholecystectomy, and fenestration of multiple right lobe liver cysts; note there is also splenomegaly. Note also her right kidney was displaced caudally in the preoperative MRI. (**c**–**f**) Infected liver cyst in a 47-year-old woman who had a hepatic resection 4 months prior; a 10 French percutaneous pigtail drainage catheter was placed into the adjacent cysts within hepatic segment VIII that appeared complicated/infected on a prior MRI.

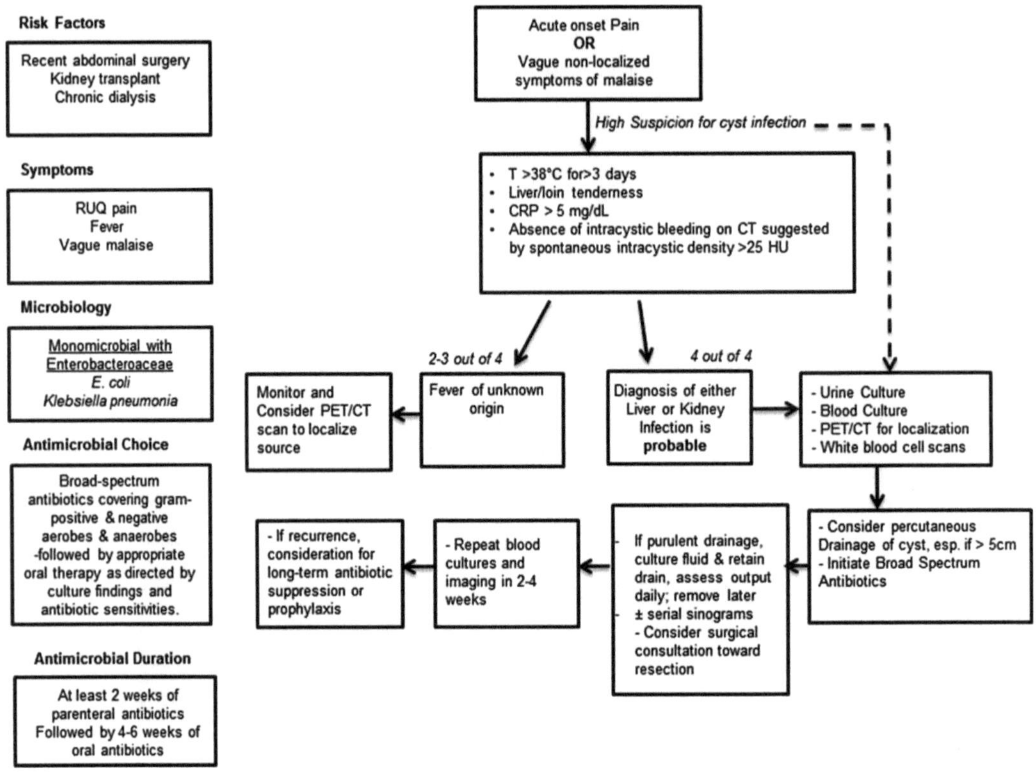

Fig. 10.8 Algorithm for evaluation and management of hepatic cyst infection in PLD

Optimal treatment duration of parenteral and subsequent oral therapy remains unknown. This may be directed by the extent of the infection, response to initial therapy, trend of clinical indicators such as fever, white cell count and CRP, and imaging. Antibiotics should be directed at gram-positive and gram-negative aerobes and anaerobes initially. Parenteral antibiotics should be administered for up to 2 weeks, followed by appropriate oral therapy for another 4–6 weeks as directed by culture findings and antibiotic sensitivities. A repeat blood culture in 2–4 weeks is strongly recommended. When treatment with antibiotics fails, percutaneous drainage or hepatic resection should be considered (Figs. 10.6, 10.7, and 10.8) [3, 40]. Repeated antibiotic courses, drainage, and surgical procedures may lead to emergence of nosocomial bacterial strains; therefore, long-term oral antibiotic suppression or prophylaxis should be reserved for those patients with confirmed relapse or recurrences (Fig. 10.6g–m) [42].

Obstructive Jaundice

Obstructive jaundice caused by cysts is a rare complication of PLD and should be diagnosed only after other causes have been excluded [55]. When cysts are implicated in the etiology, they are usually located at the porta hepatis and may be of biliary or peribiliary gland origin, and there may be intrahepatic biliary dilatation on imaging which can be confused with a group of small cysts [56, 57]. Endoscopic retrograde pancreatography (with stenting) and magnetic resonance pancreatography or Tc-99m hepatobiliary imaging may be useful in confirming there is obstruction and the level at which it is present [58]. If the obstruction is confirmed to be caused by a cyst or cysts, these can be aspirated, sclerosed with alcohol, or surgically (preferentially laparoscopically) removed [59, 60]. Budd-Chiari syndrome (hepatic venous outflow tract obstruction) and acute hepatic vein thrombosis are reported in ADPKD patients post uni- or bilateral nephrectomy [61]. Progressive hepatic failure is rare but has been reported [62].

Cyst Hemorrhage or Torsion

Severe hemorrhage of liver cysts may present with symptoms that mimic those of infected liver, but this complication occurs less frequently [63]. Cyst torsion is also reported [3]. Symptoms at onset (usually right upper quadrant pain) may be debilitating, and affected individuals will seek urgent medical evaluation as the pain can require management with opiate pain medications and support with intravenous fluids and hospitalization. These evaluations will often take place in an emergency room where providers may have limited experience with the condition or its management, and thus, guidance should be offered to the emergency room physician evaluating individuals presenting in these circumstances by the polycystic kidney disease physician. MRI is the most sensitive diagnostic modality to differentiate the hemorrhagic liver cyst from other liver complications. Hemorrhage is associated with hyperintense signal in T-1 and T-2 images. On rare occasions, acute pain is associated with torsion or rupture of a massive liver cyst with hemoperitoneum [64]. Pain following cyst hemorrhage or rupture can take several weeks to resolve, and there may sometimes be a case for short-term nonsteroidal anti-inflammatory analgesia, tramadol, or opiates (for a few weeks) for pain control. If possible, opiate medications are to be avoided due to side effects and risk of dependence.

Chronic Complications

Massive liver enlargement may be associated with a variety of symptoms including a sensation of abdominal heaviness or distention, bloating, and dull, sharp, intermittent, or continuous pain (Table 10.3). Mechanical compression by the liver can restrict mobility of the hemidiaphragm leading to dyspnea, orthopnea, early satiety, gastroesophageal reflux, umbilical and ventral hernias, and uterine prolapse. The mass effect can lead also to mechanical low back pain [3].

Complications Superimposed on Massive PLD

Ascites

In polycystic patients, ascites and variceal bleeding are relatively uncommon. Evaluation of ascitic fluid should be initiated to exclude infective processes and should be followed by endoscopy of the upper gastrointestinal tract. In cases where there is intrahepatic or inferior vena caval compression leading to ascites and or lower extremity edema, stenting of the vessel may be indicated [65].

Hepatic Venous Outflow Obstruction

In patients with severe cystic disease, hepatic venous outflow obstruction (HVOO or Budd-Chiari syndrome) should be suspected and is probably underrecognized as a cause of portal hypertension, ascites, and liver dysfunction in PLD. Portal hypertension is likely caused by compression of the hepatic vein or inferior vena cava [66, 67]. Exudative ascites with high protein content due to high protein permeability of the dilated sinusoidal walls occurs. Hepatic venous or IVC thrombosis may be occasionally superimposed and is associated with rapid onset of acute ascites and tender hepatomegaly. The mechanism involves mechanical compression of hepatic veins by the cysts and possibly thrombi formation in small hepatic vein tributaries [66–68]. These patients will improve with stenting of the occluded vessels.

Malnutrition

In a minority of severe cases, further worsening of the disease may lead to debility and malnutrition. Low albumin and total cholesterol correlate with poor nutritional status (Fig. 10.5).

In general, hepatic parenchyma and function remain preserved irrespective of the liver size. Liver failure symptoms should trigger an evaluation of a diagnosis other than PLD. However, massive PLD might be associated with a moderate increase in gamma-glutamyl transferase or alkaline phosphatase with a range of two to five times the upper normal limit. These derangements might be noticed in two-thirds and half of patients, respectively. Elevation of serum aminotransferase and bilirubin is noted in <20% of cases [2].

Portal Hypertension

If portal hypertension is suspected, the differential diagnosis would depend on the size of hepatic cysts and the patient's age. In young patients (<30 years of age) with few or no liver cysts, congenital hepatic fibrosis or liver cirrhosis should be excluded. In patients with large liver cysts, portal hypertension can be secondary to mechanical compression of portal venous flow which affects the main portal vein or intrahepatic portal vessel radicles.

Congenital Hepatic Fibrosis

While congenital hepatic fibrosis (CHF) is a classic feature of ARPKD, several families have been described in which siblings had ADPKD with CHF; however, there are no reports of families in which both a parent and child have been seen with both ADPKD and CHF [69–74]. Currently, it is believed that ADPKD-CHF is caused by *PKD1* mutations, with a probable contribution from modifier gene(s) which as of yet have to be identified. CHF can also be associated with Caroli's syndrome (best visualized on MR cholangiography). Portal hypertension should be considered and monitored for in these cases, and beta-blockers should be strongly considered. Splenomegaly and variceal bleeding, both sequelae of portal hypertension and cholangitis, a life-threatening complication, may occur more often in advanced CHF cases.

Cholangiocarcinoma

Cases of cholangiocarcinoma in PLD have been rarely reported and may be resectable [75–77]. It is believed these tumors develop following the occurrence of dysplasia and carcinomatous transformation in peribiliary cysts.

Treatment of Massive PLD

Most patients with PLD are asymptomatic and do not require treatment [1, 6]. The principal aim of treatment of PLD is to reduce symptoms by decreasing liver volume. Options for management include conservative management and medical, radiological, or invasive surgical measures.

Aspiration of Cysts and Sclerotherapy

Cyst aspiration is indicated for large symptomatic liver cysts (Figs. 10.6 and 10.7) [13]. Percutaneous aspiration should always be followed by injection of a sclerosing agent that causes destruction of the epithelial lining inhibiting fluid production [78, 79]. The most commonly used sclerosing agent is ethanol, but minocycline and tetracycline are also used [13]. It is recommended to select a dominant cyst that is likely to be responsible for the symptoms. Typically, cysts larger than 5 cm and that are superficial are good candidates [13]. The technique involves puncture of the cyst with an aspiration needle, aspiration of the total content of the cyst, and then injection of the sclerosing agent (volume varies from 10% to 25% of aspirated cyst fluid) for a predetermined time [13, 80]. Drenth et al. reviewed a total of 34 articles with a total of 292 patients and showed that aspiration sclerotherapy caused total regression of cysts in 22% and partial regression in 19% [13]. The effect of this therapy seems to extend beyond the first few weeks, and a continuous decrease in the volume of the liver cyst might be noted over the course of 4–6 months but may not fully resolve following this procedure. Without sclerosant, the cyst fluid immediately reaccumulates, but aspiration alone can help determine if the cause of pain is the cyst [81]. In patients with cyst recurrence, multiple sessions might be needed, but it is suggested to avoid repeating procedures within 6 months as the effect is enduring and due to the increased risk of infection [82].

Fenestration

Fenestration is a technique that combines surgical deroofing of multiple cysts in a single procedure. Its aim is to reduce the liver volume [83]. The major advantage is that multiple cysts can be treated simultaneously [25]. A laparoscopic approach is preferred over laparotomy because of the lower complication rates (29% versus 40%). Patients with cranially located cysts are not ideal candidates for this approach [84]. Reported complications are ascites, pleural effusion, arterial or venous bleeding, and biliary leakage. Morbidity and mortality was 23% and 2%, respectively. Causes of death might be irreversible shock, hepatic abscesses, and acute kidney injury [13].

Segmental Hepatic Resection

Segmental hepatic resection (with or without cyst fenestration) should be considered in individuals with symptomatic disease and/or massive hepatomegaly, who harbor cyst-rich segments and have at least one segment with unaffected liver parenchyma (Fig. 10.5) [13, 82, 85]. Careful preoperative selection and imaging is needed to select appropriate patients. Preoperative imaging (usually with MRI with gadolinium enhancement or contrast CT) is usually required to evaluate the presence or absence of intrahepatic vein, inferior vena cava, and portal vein compression and to evaluate the amount of residual noncystic parenchyma in the liver. The choice of right or left hepatectomy and/or cyst fenestration depends on the distribution of the disease, venous and arterial anatomy, and residual hepatic function. The reduction in liver volume following this procedure can be both significant and durable for selected patients and relief of symptoms is usually achieved. This procedure can be associated with significant morbidity and mortality, and complications relate to the experience of the surgical team with surgery in PLD cases, which is limited to only a few medical centers [37, 85]. Morbidity is higher in patients who underwent prior surgery or those on immunosuppressive drugs and included ascites, pleural effusion, biliary leakage, and hemorrhage. Hepatic resection is associated with significant perioperative risk, but with successful procedures, quality of life improves or normalizes.

Liver Transplantation

Liver transplantation is the only curative therapeutic option and is warranted in patients with extremely debilitating symptoms, seriously compromised functional status and reduced quality of life, untreatable complications such as portal hypertension, and severe malnutrition with bilobar extensive cystic liver disease lacking adequate areas of parenchymal sparing (Fig. 10.7g, h). Concomitant renal evaluation is mandatory in PKD [86]. The surgery is technically difficult because of the distortion and compression of vascular and biliary structures. In addition, high morbidity rates have been reported with massive postoperative ascites or hemorrhage. In light of the shortage of liver donors, offering liver transplantation has to be considered carefully, especially since PLD is not associated with excess liver-related mortality and since hepatocellular function remains preserved even in advanced disease. Since PLD patients have essentially normal liver function, calculated MELD scores are low or normal which makes organ allocation more difficult [87]. Appeals through regional review boards are possible. Due to their disadvantage in graft allocation, caval sparing hepatectomy and subsequent living donor liver transplantation might provide a potential alternative for highly selected patients [87]. Survival has improved (5-year survival is ~90%) (Table 10.5) after

Table 10.5 Summary of reported outcomes in liver transplantation for PLD

Author (year)	Patients	Mortality (%)	Morbidity (%)	Follow-up (Mo.)	Symptom-free (%)
Kwok and Lewin (1988) [110]	1	100%	–	–	–
Starzl (1990) [111]	4	25%	N.S.	29	75%
Washbun (1996) [112]	5	20%	20%	38	80%
Lang (1997) [113]	17	30%	N.S.	12	91%
Swenson (1998) [114]	9	11%	33%	29	89%
Pirenne (2001) [62]	16	13%	–	18–120	
Gustafson (2003) [115]	7	0	?	4	N.S.
Demirci (2003) [116]	17	18%	?	49	
Ueno (2006) [117]	14	7%	86%	?	92%
Kirchner (2006) [88]	36	16%		626	91%
Krohn (2008) [118]	14	7%	23%	55	86%
Schnelldorfer (2009) [37]	7	29%	57%	60	N.S.
Taner (2009) [119]	13	23%	82%	25	82%
Aussilhou (2010) [120]	27	15%	85%	36	100%
Coquillard, (liver-kidney) [89]	107	1.9% (liver-kidney transplant) 9.2% liver alone	N.S.	60	N.S.

Legend: *N.S* Not shown

deceased donor liver or combined liver-kidney transplantation to a level comparable with that of an age-matched group of people from the general population [10, 37, 88, 89]. In individuals with eGFR <30 ml/min or end-stage renal disease, simultaneous deceased donor liver or combined liver-kidney transplant is the most optimal approach (Fig. 10.8) [62, 90].

Transcatheter Arterial Embolization

Hepatic Arterial Embolization

Because liver cysts are mostly supplied from hepatic arteries but not from portal veins, transcatheter arterial embolization (TAE) of the hepatic artery branches that supply major hepatic cysts can lead to shrinkage of the cyst and liver size. This technique aims to selectively embolize the hepatic artery branches that supply the major liver cysts and is an option for individuals who are not good surgical candidates for partial hepatectomy [91–95].

Medical Therapies

Sirolimus

The immunosuppressive agent sirolimus may decrease PLD volume, possibly via an antiproliferative effect [96]. In a retrospective analysis of kidney transplant recipients, liver volume was assessed in seven individuals with PLD given sirolimus-mycophenolate-prednisone and nine recipients given tacrolimus-mycophenolate-prednisone [96]. At 19 months, the sirolimus-based regimen resulted in a decrease in mean TLV of ~12%, while it increased by 14% in those taking the tacrolimus regimen. Further studies are required to understand the role of sirolimus in this setting.

Somatostatin Analogs

Based on positive results of octreotide LAR in experimental animal studies of PLD, several clinical trials have examined the effects of somatostatin analogs in symptomatic PLD (Table 10.6) [97]. Van Kiempema et al. reported that 27 patients treated with lanreotide for 6 months

Table 10.6 Clinical trials of medical therapies in polycystic liver diseases

Study	Patient randomization	Dose	Treatment duration	Route of administration	Liver volume reduction
Octreotide (targets cAMP)					
Caroli et al. (2010) [31]	ADPKD, $n = 12$ (5 treated, 7 placebo)	40 mg every 28 days	6 months	Intramuscular	4.5% (vs 0.9% increase in placebo)
Hogan et al. (2010) [32]	ADPKD and ADPLD, $n = 42$	40 mg every 28 (±5) days	12 months	Intramuscular	4.95% (vs 0.92% increase in placebo)
Hogan et al. (2012) [99]	Extension study: ADPKD and ADPLD, $n = 41/42$ (all received treatment)	40 mg every 28 (±5) days	Additional 12 months (24 months total)	Intramuscular	No significant changes (−0.77%) after an additional year of therapy
Hogan et al. (2015) [100]	Extension study ADPKD and ADPLD (on and off somatostatin LAR (25/42))	40 mg every 28 (±5) days	48 months of treatment (average 8 months off therapy)	Intramuscular	Off OctLAR, TLVs increased 3.4%+/− 8.2% per year; after resuming OctLAR, TLVs decreased 4.7%+/− 6.1% per year
Pisani et al. (ALADIN) [101]	RCT followed by 2 years observation off somatostatin ($n = 27$; 14 treated; 13 placebo)	40 mg every 28 (±5) days	36 months followed by 24-month observation off therapy	Intramuscular	OctLAR reduced LV while on drug (−7.8 ± 7.4%) and increased by (6.1 ± 14.1%) continued residual treatment effect in OctLAR group seen in the 2 years off treatment
Lanreotide (targets cAMP)					
Van Keimpema et al. (2009) [30]	ADPKD and ADPLD, $n = 54$ (28 treated, 27 placebo)	120 mg every 28 days	24 weeks	Subcutaneous	2.9% (vs 1.6% increase in placebo)
Temmerman et al. (2013) [121](LOCKCSYT I and II and open label extension pooled analysis	ADPKD and ADPLD, $n = 132$ (106 treated, 26 placebo)	90 ($n = 55$) or 120 mg ($n = 51$) every 28 days	6 months	Subcutaneous	1.4% (LAN 90 mg)
					2.8% (LAN 120 mg) (vs 1.1% increase in placebo)
					LAN 90 mg had fewer adverse effects
Chrispijn et al. (2012) [98]	Extension study: ADPKD and ADPLD, $n = 41/54$ (All received treatment)	120 mg every 28 days	12 months	Subcutaneous	4% decrease first 6 months and the beneficial effect was maintained in the following 6 months. Stopping resulted in PLD growth
Sirolimus vs tacrolimus (targets mTOR)					
Qian et al. (2008) [98]	ADPKD (sirolimus $n = 8$, tacrolimus $n = 9$)	5–10 mg daily (sirolimus)	Retrospective analysis 19.4 months	Oral	11.9% decrease with sirolimus vs 14.1% increase with tacrolimus
		3 mg twice a day (tacrolimus)			
Everolimus alone or in combination with octreotide (targets cAMP and mTOR)					
Chrispijn et al. (2013) [103]	ADPKD and ADPLD, $n = 44$ (23 received octreotide and 21 received octreotide + everolimus)	40 mg octreotide every 4 weeks, 2.5 mg everolimus daily	48 weeks	Intramuscular (octreotide) and oral (everolimus)	3.5 ± 5.2% octreotide monotherapy vs 3.8 ± 4.7% in the octreotide/everolimus group (in response to octreotide, everolimus does not further reduce liver volume)

Legend: *LAN* Lanreotide therapy

experienced a reduction of 2.9% in total liver volume (TLV), while those on placebo (n = 27) experienced a 1.6% increase [30]. In the subsequent 12-month open-label extension, an overall 4% decrease in TLVs was further observed in 41 participants [98]. Caroli et al. described a 4.5% reduction in TLV in response to octreotide LAR in 12 ADPKD patients after 6 months of treatment [31]. We randomized 42 patients to octreotide LAR (n = 28) or placebo (n = 14) treatment for 12 months [32]. As a result, liver growth decreased 4.95% in the octreotide LAR group compared to a 0.9% increase in the placebo group. A total of 41 patients participated in an open-label extension study for an additional 12 months [99]. In subjects initially randomized to placebo, TLV decreased by 7.66% but was sustained in patients initially treated with octreotide. In pooled analysis, after 12 months of octreotide treatment, TLV declined by ~6%. This study was extended again for an additional 24 months after an average of 8.3-month period off therapy (where again there was increase in liver growth) [100]. Twenty-four individuals who underwent 2 further years of treatment experienced a mean ± SD reduction of 4.7% ± 6.1% per year in TLV. Therefore, after 4 years of octreotide LAR therapy, liver growth declined by 11.8% [100]. Similarly in a population with mild PLD, there was halting in LV growth in the octreotide LAR arm over 5 years (3 years on treatment and 2 years off therapy) [101]. In addition, two other non-placebo-controlled studies showed beneficial effects of somatostatin analogs in PLD [98, 102]. Therefore, the conclusions from these studies are (i) treatment with somatostatin analogs for 6–12 months decreases TLV; (ii) reduction in liver volume is sustained beyond 12 months of therapy; (iii) response to treatment varies among patients with some (~15%) nonresponders; (iv) once therapy is stopped, liver volume starts to increase toward baseline suggesting that long-term treatment may be required; (vi) somatostatin analogs are well tolerated and improve quality of life; and (vii) similar changes in liver volume in response to treatment occur in patients with ADPKD-associated PLD or isolated ADPLD. Thus, somatostatin analogues have become the standard of care for symptomatic patients with PLD or those who want to avoid surgical interventions. The addition of everolimus to octreotide LAR provided no additional benefit [103].

Other promising therapeutic targets include histone deacetylase inhibitors, vitamin K, and the bile salt ursodeoxycholic acid [104–107]. The future holds the promise of drug screening in animal models that appropriately represent the disease such as mouse, rat, and zebrafish models [108].

References

1. Torres VE, Harris PC, Pirson Y. Autosomal dominant polycystic kidney disease. Lancet. 2007;369(9569):1287–301.
2. Chauveau D, Pirson Y, Le Moine A, Franco D, Belghiti J, Grunfeld JP. Extrarenal manifestations in autosomal dominant polycystic kidney disease. Adv Nephrol Necker Hosp. 1997;26:265–89.
3. Chauveau D, Fakhouri F, Grunfeld JP. Liver involvement in autosomal-dominant polycystic kidney disease: therapeutic dilemma. J Am Soc Nephrol. 2000;11(9):1767–75.
4. Gaines PA, Sampson MA. The prevalence and characterization of simple hepatic cysts by ultrasound examination. Br J Radiol. 1989;62(736):335–7.
5. Bae KT, Zhu F, Chapman AB, Torres VE, Grantham JJ, Guay-Woodford LM, et al. Magnetic resonance imaging evaluation of hepatic cysts in early autosomal-dominant polycystic kidney disease: the Consortium for Radiologic Imaging Studies of Polycystic Kidney Disease cohort. Clin J Am Soc Nephrol. 2006;1(1):64–9.
6. Kanaan N, Devuyst O, Pirson Y. Renal transplantation in autosomal dominant polycystic kidney disease. Nat Rev Nephrol. 2014;10(8):455–65.
7. Torres VE, Chapman AB, Perrone RD, Bae KT, Abebe KZ, Bost JE, et al. Analysis of baseline parameters in the HALT polycystic kidney disease trials. Kidney Int. 2012;81(6):577–85.
8. Sherstha R, McKinley C, Russ P, Scherzinger A, Bronner T, Showalter R, et al. Postmenopausal estrogen therapy selectively stimulates hepatic enlargement in women with autosomal dominant polycystic kidney disease. Hepatology. 1997;26(5):1282–6.
9. van Keimpema L, Nevens F, Adam R, Porte RJ, Fikatas P, Becker T, et al. Excellent survival after liver transplantation for isolated polycystic liver disease: an European Liver Transplant Registry study. Transplant Int: Off J Eur Soc Organ Transplant. 2011;24(12):1239–45.

10. Van Keimpema L, De Koning DB, Van Hoek B, Van Den Berg AP, Van Oijen MG, De Man RA, et al. Patients with isolated polycystic liver disease referred to liver centres: clinical characterization of 137 cases. Liver Int. 2011;31(1):92–8.
11. Reynolds DM, Falk CT, Li A, King BF, Kamath PS, Huston J 3rd, et al. Identification of a locus for autosomal dominant polycystic liver disease, on chromosome 19p13.2-13.1. Am J Hum Genet. 2000;67(6):1598–604.
12. Davila S, Furu L, Gharavi AG, Tian X, Onoe T, Qian Q, et al. Mutations in SEC63 cause autosomal dominant polycystic liver disease. Nat Genet. 2004;36(6):575–7.
13. Drenth JP, Chrispijn M, Nagorney DM, Kamath PS, Torres VE. Medical and surgical treatment options for polycystic liver disease. Hepatology. 2010;52(6):2223–30.
14. Cnossen WR, te Morsche RHM, Hoischen A, Gilissen C, Chrispijn M, Venselaar H, et al. Whole-exome sequencing reveals LRP5 mutations and canonical Wnt signaling associated with hepatic cystogenesis. Proc Natl Acad Sci. 2014;111(14):5343–8.
15. Porath B, Gainullin VG, Cornec-Le Gall E, Dillinger EK, Heyer CM, Hopp K, et al. Mutations in GANAB, encoding the glucosidase II alpha subunit, cause autosomal-dominant polycystic kidney and liver disease. Am J Hum Genet. 2016;98(6):1193–207.
16. Xu C, Ng DT. Glycosylation-directed quality control of protein folding. Nat Rev Mol Cell Biol. 2015;16(12):742–52.
17. Fedeles SV, Tian X, Gallagher AR, Mitobe M, Nishio S, Lee SH, et al. A genetic interaction network of five genes for human polycystic kidney and liver diseases defines polycystin-1 as the central determinant of cyst formation. Nat Genet. 2011;43(7):639–47.
18. Desmet VJ. Congenital diseases of intrahepatic bile ducts: variations on the theme "ductal plate malformation". Hepatology. 1992;16(4):1069–83.
19. Gradilone SA, Masyuk TV, Huang BQ, Banales JM, Lehmann GL, Radtke BN, et al. Activation of Trpv4 reduces the hyperproliferative phenotype of cystic cholangiocytes from an animal model of ARPKD. Gastroenterology. 2010;139(1):304–14 e2.
20. Perugorria MJ, Masyuk TV, Marin JJ, Marzioni M, Bujanda L, LaRusso NF, et al. Polycystic liver diseases: advanced insights into the molecular mechanisms. Nat Rev Gastroenterol Hepatol. 2014;11(12):750–61.
21. Torres VE, Harris PC. Autosomal dominant polycystic kidney disease: the last 3 years. Kidney Int. 2009;76(2):149–68.
22. Fabris L, Cadamuro M, Fiorotto R, Roskams T, Spirli C, Melero S, et al. Effects of angiogenic factor overexpression by human and rodent cholangiocytes in polycystic liver diseases. Hepatology. 2006;43(5):1001–12.
23. Chen J, Futami K, Petillo D, Peng J, Wang P, Knol J, et al. Deficiency of FLCN in mouse kidney led to development of polycystic kidneys and renal neoplasia. PLoS One. 2008;3(10):e3581.
24. Spirli C, Okolicsanyi S, Fiorotto R, Fabris L, Cadamuro M, Lecchi S, et al. Mammalian target of rapamycin regulates vascular endothelial growth factor-dependent liver cyst growth in polycystin-2-defective mice. Hepatology. 2010;51(5):1778–88.
25. van Keimpema L, Ruurda JP, Ernst MF, van Geffen HJ, Drenth JP. Laparoscopic fenestration of liver cysts in polycystic liver disease results in a median volume reduction of 12.5%. J Gastrointest Surg : Off J Soc Surg Aliment Tract. 2008;12(3):477–82.
26. Geng L, Segal Y, Pavlova A, Barros EJ, Lohning C, Lu W, et al. Distribution and developmentally regulated expression of murine polycystin. Am J Phys. 1997;272(4 Pt 2):F451–9.
27. Ibraghimov-Beskrovnaya O, Dackowski WR, Foggensteiner L, Coleman N, Thiru S, Petry LR, et al. Polycystin: in vitro synthesis, in vivo tissue expression, and subcellular localization identifies a large membrane-associated protein. Proc Natl Acad Sci. 1997;94(12):6397–402.
28. Griffin MD, Torres VE, Grande JP, Kumar R. Immunolocalization of polycystin in human tissues and cultured cells. Proc Assoc Am Phys. 1996;108(3):185–97.
29. Griffin MD, O'Sullivan DA, Torres VE, Grande JP, Kanwar YS, Kumar R. Expression of polycystin in mouse metanephros and extra-metanephric tissues. Kidney Int. 1997;52(5):1196–205.
30. van Keimpema L, Nevens F, Vanslembrouck R, van Oijen MG, Hoffmann AL, Dekker HM, et al. Lanreotide reduces the volume of polycystic liver: a randomized, double-blind, placebo-controlled trial. Gastroenterology. 2009;137(5):1661–8 e1–2.
31. Caroli A, Antiga L, Cafaro M, Fasolini G, Remuzzi A, Remuzzi G, et al. Reducing polycystic liver volume in ADPKD: effects of somatostatin analogue octreotide. Clin J Am Soc Nephrol. 2010;5(5):783–9.
32. Hogan MC, Masyuk TV, Page LJ, Kubly VJ, Bergstralh EJ, Li X, et al. Randomized clinical trial of long-acting somatostatin for autosomal dominant polycystic kidney and liver disease. J Am Soc Nephrol. 2010;21(6):1052–61.
33. Waanders E, te Morsche RH, de Man RA, Jansen JB, Drenth JP. Extensive mutational analysis of PRKCSH and SEC63 broadens the spectrum of polycystic liver disease. Hum Mutat. 2006;27(8):830.
34. Hoevenaren IA, Wester R, Schrier RW, McFann K, Doctor RB, Drenth JP, et al. Polycystic liver: clinical characteristics of patients with isolated polycystic liver disease compared with patients with polycystic liver and autosomal dominant polycystic kidney disease. Liver Int: Off J Int Assoc Study Liver. 2008;28(2):264–70.
35. Chapman AB, Devuyst O, Eckardt K-U, Gansevoort RT, Harris T, Horie S, et al. Autosomal-dominant polycystic kidney disease (ADPKD): executive summary from a Kidney Disease: Improving Global

Outcomes (KDIGO) controversies conference. Kidney Int. 2015;88(1):17–27.
36. Gigot JF, Jadoul P, Que F, Van Beers BE, Etienne J, Horsmans Y, et al. Adult polycystic liver disease: is fenestration the most adequate operation for long-term management? Ann Surg. 1997;225(3):286–94.
37. Schnelldorfer T, Torres VE, Zakaria S, Rosen CB, Nagorney DM. Polycystic liver disease: a critical appraisal of hepatic resection, cyst fenestration, and liver transplantation. Ann Surg. 2009;250(1):112–8.
38. Hogan MC, Abebe K, Torres VE, Chapman AB, Bae KT, Tao C, et al. Liver involvement in early autosomal dominant polycystic kidney disease. Clin Gastroenterol Hepatol: Off Clin Pract J Am Gastroenterol Assoc. 2015;13(1):155–64.e6.
39. Bae KT, Giger ML, Chen CT, Kahn CE. Automatic segmentation of liver structure in CT images. Med Phys. 1993;20(1):71–8.
40. Telenti A, Torres VE, Gross JB Jr, Van Scoy RE, Brown ML, Hattery RR. Hepatic cyst infection in autosomal dominant polycystic kidney disease. Mayo Clin Proc. 1990;65(7):933–42.
41. Bistritz L, Tamboli C, Bigam D, Bain VG. Polycystic liver disease: experience at a teaching hospital. Am J Gastroenterol. 2005;100(10):2212–7.
42. Sallee M, Rafat C, Zahar JR, Paulmier B, Grunfeld JP, Knebelmann B, et al. Cyst infections in patients with autosomal dominant polycystic kidney disease. Clin J Am Soc Nephrol: CJASN. 2009;4(7):1183–9.
43. Jouret F, Lhommel R, Devuyst O, Annet L, Pirson Y, Hassoun Z, et al. Diagnosis of cyst infection in patients with autosomal dominant polycystic kidney disease: attributes and limitations of the current modalities. Nephrol Dial Transplant. 2012;27(10):3746–51.
44. Carrim ZI, Murchison JT. The prevalence of simple renal and hepatic cysts detected by spiral computed tomography. Clin Radiol. 2003;58(8):626–9.
45. Jouret F, Lhommel R, Beguin C, Devuyst O, Pirson Y, Hassoun Z, et al. Positron-emission computed tomography in cyst infection diagnosis in patients with autosomal dominant polycystic kidney disease. Clin J Am Soc Nephrol. 2011;6(7):1644–50.
46. Bleeker-Rovers CP, de Sevaux RG, van Hamersvelt HW, Corstens FH, Oyen WJ. Diagnosis of renal and hepatic cyst infections by 18-F-fluorodeoxyglucose positron emission tomography in autosomal dominant polycystic kidney disease. Am J Kidney Dis. 2003;41(6):E18–21.
47. Hsu CT, Chang HR, Lee JK, Weng JH, Kao PF. FDG PET/CT repeatedly demonstrated hepatic cyst infection in a patient with autosomal dominant polycystic kidney disease. Clin Nucl Med. 2013;38(4):e188–90.
48. Banzo J, Ubieto MA, Gil D, Prats E, Razola P, Tardin L, et al. 18F-FDG PET/CT diagnosis of liver cyst infection in a patient with autosomal dominant polycystic kidney disease and fever of unknown origin. Rev Esp Med Nucl Imagen Mol. 2013;32(3):187–9.
49. Lahiri SA, Halff GA, Speeg KV, Esterl RM Jr. In-111 WBC scan localizes infected hepatic cysts and confirms their complete resection in adult polycystic kidney disease. Clin Nucl Med. 1998;23(1):33–4.
50. Kwok CG, McDougall IR. Persistent fever in a patient with polycystic kidney and liver diseases and bilateral hip prostheses. J Nucl Med: Off Publ Soc Nucl Med. 1996;37(12):2062–5.
51. Even-Sapir E, Barnes DC, Iles SE. Remnants of normal tissue in polycystic disease of the liver. A cause for difficulty in the interpretation of indium-111 white blood cell study. Clin Nucl Med. 1993;18(11):967–9.
52. Bretan PN Jr, Price DC, McClure RD. Localization of abscess in adult polycystic kidney by indium-111 leukocyte scan. Urology. 1988;32(2):169–71.
53. Pirson Y, Kanaan N. Infectious complications in autosomal dominant polycystic kidney disease. Nephrol Therapeutique. 2015;11(2):73–7.
54. Kanaan N, Goffin E, Pirson Y, Devuyst O, Hassoun Z. Carbohydrate antigen 19-9 as a diagnostic marker for hepatic cyst infection in autosomal dominant polycystic kidney disease. Am J Kidney Dis. 2010;55(5):916–22.
55. Macutkiewicz C, Plastow R, Chrispijn M, Filobbos R, Ammori BA, Sherlock DJ, et al. Complications arising in simple and polycystic liver cysts. World J Hepatol. 2012;4(12):406–11.
56. Johnson DK, Panchili S, Kolasseri S, Mavali RT. Polycystic liver disease presenting as pruritus. Ann Gastroenterol: Q Publ Hell Soc Gastroenterol. 2014;27(1):76–8.
57. Terada T, Nakanuma Y. Pathological observations of intrahepatic peribiliary glands in 1,000 consecutive autopsy livers. III. Survey of necroinflammation and cystic dilatation. Hepatology. 1990;12(5):1229–33.
58. Salam M, Keeffe EB. Liver cysts associated with polycystic kidney disease: role of Tc-99m hepatobiliary imaging. Clin Nucl Med. 1989;14(11):803–7.
59. Ergun H, Wolf BH, Hissong SL. Obstructive jaundice caused by polycystic liver disease. Radiology. 1980;136(2):435–6.
60. Dumot JA, Fields MS, Meyer RA, Shay SS, Conwell DL, Brzezinski A. Alcohol sclerosis for polycystic liver disease and obstructive jaundice: use of a nasobiliary catheter. Am J Gastroenterol. 1994;89(9):1555–7.
61. Clive DM, Davidoff A, Schweizer RT. Budd-Chiari syndrome in autosomal dominant polycystic kidney disease: a complication of nephrectomy in patients with liver cysts. Am J Kidney Dis. 1993;21(2):202–5.
62. Pirenne J, Aerts R, Yoong K, Gunson B, Koshiba T, Fourneau I, et al. Liver transplantation for polycystic liver disease. Liver Transpl. 2001;7(3):238–45.
63. Dofferhoff AS, Sluiter HE, Geerlings W, de Jong PE. Complications of liver cysts in patients with adult polycystic kidney disease. Nephrol Dial Transplant: Off Publ Eur Dial Transplant Assoc – Eur Ren Assoc. 1990;5(10):882–5.
64. Chung T, Chen K, Yen C, Chen H, Cherng W, Fang K. Acute abdomen in a haemodialysed patient with

polycystic kidney disease – rupture of a massive liver cyst. Nephrol Dial Transplant. 1998;13(7):1840–2.
65. Grams J, Teh SH, Torres VE, Andrews JC, Nagorney DM. Inferior vena cava stenting: a safe and effective treatment for intractable ascites in patients with polycystic liver disease. J Gastrointest Surg: Off J Soc Surg Aliment Tract. 2007;11(8):985–90.
66. Torres VE, Rastogi S, King BF, Stanson AW, Gross JB Jr, Nogorney DM. Hepatic venous outflow obstruction in autosomal dominant polycystic kidney disease. J Am Soc Nephrol. 1994;5(5):1186–92.
67. Uddin W, Ramage JK, Portmann B, Wilson P, Benjamin I, Tan KC, et al. Hepatic venous outflow obstruction in patients with polycystic liver disease: pathogenesis and treatment. Gut. 1995;36(1):142–5.
68. Schwaller KH, Pirovino M. Budd-Chiari syndrome in polycystic kidney disease. Praxis. 2001;90(17):738–40.
69. Cobben JM, Breuning MH, Schoots C, ten Kate LP, Zerres K. Congenital hepatic fibrosis in autosomal-dominant polycystic kidney disease. Kidney Int. 1990;38(5):880–5.
70. O'Brien K, Font-Montgomery E, Lukose L, Bryant J, Piwnica-Worms K, Edwards H, et al. Congenital hepatic fibrosis and portal hypertension in autosomal dominant polycystic kidney disease. J Pediatr Gastroenterol Nutr. 2012;54(1):83–9.
71. Torra R, Badenas C, Darnell A, Bru C, Escorsell A, Estivill X. Autosomal dominant polycystic kidney disease with anticipation and Caroli's disease associated with a PKD1 mutation. Rapid Commun Kidney Int. 1997;52(1):33–8.
72. Kanaheswari Y, Hamzaini AH, Wong SW. Congenital hepatic fibrosis in a child with autosomal dominant polycystic kidney disease. Med J Malaysia. 2008;63(3):251–3.
73. Klinkert J, Koopman MG, Wolf H. Pregnancy in a patient with autosomal-dominant polycystic kidney disease and congenital hepatic fibrosis. Eur J Obstet Gynecol Reprod Biol. 1998;76(1):45–7.
74. Matsuda O, Ideura T, Shinoda T, Shiigai T, Takeuchi H, Chen WC, et al. Polycystic kidney of autosomal dominant inheritance, polycystic liver and congenital hepatic fibrosis in a single kindred. Am J Nephrol. 1990;10(3):237–41.
75. Imamura M, Miyashita T, Tani T, Naito A, Tobe T, Takahashi K. Cholangiocellular carcinoma associated with multiple liver cysts. Am J Gastroenterol. 1984;79(10):790–5.
76. Sasaki M, Katayanagi K, Watanabe K, Takasawa K, Nakanuma Y. Intrahepatic cholangiocarcinoma arising in autosomal dominant polycystic kidney disease. Virchows Archiv: Int J Pathol. 2002;441(1):98–100.
77. Burns CD, Kuhns JG, Wieman TJ. Cholangiocarcinoma in association with multiple biliary microhamartomas. Arch Pathol Lab Med. 1990;114(12):1287–9.
78. Bean WJ, Rodan BA. Hepatic cysts: treatment with alcohol. AJR Am J Roentgenol. 1985;144(2):237–41.
79. Saini S, Mueller PR, Ferrucci JT Jr, Simeone JF, Wittenberg J, Butch RJ. Percutaneous aspiration of hepatic cysts does not provide definitive therapy. AJR Am J Roentgenol. 1983;141(3):559–60.
80. vanSonnenberg E, Wroblicka JT, D'Agostino HB, Mathieson JR, Casola G, O'Laoide R, et al. Symptomatic hepatic cysts: percutaneous drainage and sclerosis. Radiology. 1994;190(2):387–92.
81. Larssen TB, Rosendahl K, Horn A, Jensen DK, Rorvik J. Single-session alcohol sclerotherapy in symptomatic benign hepatic cysts performed with a time of exposure to alcohol of 10 min: initial results. Eur Radiol. 2003;13(12):2627–32.
82. Gevers TJ, Drenth JP. Diagnosis and management of polycystic liver disease. Nat Rev Gastroenterol Hepatol. 2013;10:101–8.
83. Russell RT, Pinson CW. Surgical management of polycystic liver disease. World J Gastroenterol. 2007;13(38):5052–9.
84. Martin AP, Bartels M, Kiehle A, Hauss J, Fangmann J. Polycystic liver and kidney disease: post-transplant kidney function in patients receiving pre-emptive kidney transplantation. Transplant Int : Off J Eur Soc Organ Transplant. 2008;21(3):263–7.
85. Chebib FT, Harmon A, Irazabal Mira MV, Jung YS, Edwards ME, Hogan MC, et al. Outcomes and durability of hepatic reduction after combined rartial hepatectomy and cyst fenestration for massive polycystic liver disease. J Am Coll Surg. 2016;223:118–26.
86. Everson GT, Taylor MR, Doctor RB. Polycystic disease of the liver. Hepatology. 2004;40(4):774–82.
87. Mekeel KL, Moss AA, Reddy KS, Douglas DD, Vargas HE, Carey EJ, et al. Living donor liver transplantation in polycystic liver disease. Liver Transplant : Off Publ Am Assoc Study Liver Dis Int Liver Transplant Soc. 2008;14(5):680–3.
88. Kirchner GI, Rifai K, Cantz T, Nashan B, Terkamp C, Becker T, et al. Outcome and quality of life in patients with polycystic liver disease after liver or combined liver-kidney transplantation. Liver Transpl. 2006;12(8):1268–77.
89. Coquillard C, Berger J, Daily M, Shah M, Mei X, Marti F, et al. Combined liver-kidney transplantation for polycystic liver and kidney disease: analysis from the UNOS dataset. Liver Int: Off J Int Assoc Study Liver. 2016;36(7):1018–25.
90. Eason JD, Gonwa TA, Davis CL, Sung RS, Gerber D, Bloom RD. Proceedings of consensus conference on Simultaneous Liver Kidney Transplantation (SLK). Am J Transplant: Off J Am Soc Transplant Am Soc Transplant Surg. 2008;8(11):2243–51.
91. Fujita T, Tanabe M, Uchiyama K, Matsuyama H, Matsunaga N. Symptomatic polycystic liver disease treated with transcatheter hepatic arterial embolization and inferior vena cava stenting: a case report. Exp Clin Transplant: Off J Middle East Soc Org Transplant. 2014;12(4):377–80.
92. Wang MQ, Duan F, Liu FY, Wang ZJ, Song P. Treatment of symptomatic polycystic liver dis-

ease: transcatheter super-selective hepatic arterial embolization using a mixture of NBCA and iodized oil. Abdom Imaging. 2013;38(3):465–73.
93. Park HC, Kim CW, Ro H, Moon JY, Oh KH, Kim Y, et al. Transcatheter arterial embolization therapy for a massive polycystic liver in autosomal dominant polycystic kidney disease patients. J Korean Med Sci. 2009;24(1):57–61.
94. Takei R, Ubara Y, Hoshino J, Higa Y, Suwabe T, Sogawa Y, et al. Percutaneous transcatheter hepatic artery embolization for liver cysts in autosomal dominant polycystic kidney disease. Am J Kidney Dis. 2007;49(6):744–52.
95. Ubara Y, Takei R, Hoshino J, Tagami T, Sawa N, Yokota M, et al. Intravascular embolization therapy in a patient with an enlarged polycystic liver. Am J Kidney Dis. 2004;43(4):733–8.
96. Qian Q, Du H, King BF, Kumar S, Dean PG, Cosio FG, et al. Sirolimus reduces polycystic liver volume in ADPKD patients. J Am Soc Nephrol. 2008;19(3):631–8.
97. Masyuk TV, Masyuk AI, Torres VE, Harris PC, Larusso NF. Octreotide inhibits hepatic cystogenesis in a rodent model of polycystic liver disease by reducing cholangiocyte adenosine 3′,5′-cyclic monophosphate. Gastroenterology. 2007;132(3):1104–16.
98. Chrispijn M, Nevens F, Gevers TJ, Vanslembrouck R, van Oijen MG, Coudyzer W, et al. The long-term outcome of patients with polycystic liver disease treated with lanreotide. Aliment Pharmacol Ther. 2012;35(2):266–74.
99. Hogan MC, Masyuk TV, Page L, Holmes DR 3rd, Li X, Bergstralh EJ, et al. Somatostatin analog therapy for severe polycystic liver disease: results after 2 years. Nephrol Dial Transplant : Off Publ Eur Dial Transplant Assoc – Eur Ren Assoc. 2012;27(9):3532–9.
100. Hogan MC, Masyuk T, Bergstralh E, Li B, Kremers WK, Vaughan LE, et al. Efficacy of 4 years of octreotide long-acting release therapy in patients with severe polycystic liver disease. Mayo Clin Proc. 2015;90(8):1030–7.
101. Pisani A, Sabbatini M, Imbriaco M, Riccio E, Rubis N, Prinster A, et al. Long-term effects of octreotide on liver volume in patients with polycystic kidney and liver disease. Clin Gastroenterol Hepatol: Off Clin Pract J Am Gastroenterol Assoc. 2016;14:1022–30.
102. Temmerman F, Ho TA, Vanslembrouck R, Coudyzer W, Billen J, Dobbels F, et al. Lanreotide reduces liver volume, but might not improve muscle wasting or weight loss, in patients with symptomatic polycystic liver disease. Clin Gastroenterol Hepatol: Off Clin Pract J Am Gastroenterol Assoc. 2015;13(13):2353–9 e1.
103. Chrispijn M, Gevers TJ, Hol JC, Monshouwer R, Dekker HM, Drenth JP. Everolimus does not further reduce polycystic liver volume when added to long acting octreotide: results from a randomized controlled trial. J Hepatol. 2013;59(1):153–9.
104. Iijima T, Hoshino J, Suwabe T, Sumida K, Mise K, Kawada M, et al. Ursodeoxycholic acid for treatment of enlarged polycystic liver. Ther Apher Dial: Off Peer-Rev J Int Soc Apher Jpn Soc Apher Jpn Soc Dial Ther. 2016;20(1):73–8.
105. Munoz-Garrido P, Marin JJ, Perugorria MJ, Urribarri AD, Erice O, Saez E, et al. Ursodeoxycholic acid inhibits hepatic cystogenesis in experimental models of polycystic liver disease. J Hepatol. 2015;63(4):952–61.
106. Gradilone SA, Habringer S, Masyuk TV, Howard BN, Masyuk AI, Larusso NF. HDAC6 is overexpressed in cystic cholangiocytes and its inhibition reduces cystogenesis. Am J Pathol. 2014;184(3):600–8.
107. Masyuk TV, Radtke BN, Stroope AJ, Banales JM, Masyuk AI, Gradilone SA, et al. Inhibition of Cdc25A suppresses hepato-renal cystogenesis in rodent models of polycystic kidney and liver disease. Gastroenterology. 2012;142(3):622–33 e4.
108. Tietz Bogert PS, Huang BQ, Gradilone SA, Masyuk TV, Moulder GL, Ekker SC, et al. The zebrafish as a model to study polycystic liver disease. Zebrafish. 2013;10(2):211–7.
109. Masyuk TV, Huang BQ, Masyuk AI, Ritman EL, Torres VE, Wang X, et al. Biliary dysgenesis in the PCK rat, an orthologous model of autosomal recessive polycystic kidney disease. Am J Pathol. 2004;165(5):1719–30.
110. Kwok MK, Lewin KJ. Massive hepatomegaly in adult polycystic liver disease. Am J Surg Pathol. 1988;12(4):321–4.
111. Starzl TE, Reyes J, Tzakis A, Mieles L, Todo S, Gordon R. Liver transplantation for polycystic liver disease. Arch Surg. 1990;125(5):575–7.
112. Washburn WK, Johnson LB, Lewis WD, Jenkins RL. Liver transplantation for adult polycystic liver disease. Liver Transpl Surg. 1996;2(1):17–22.
113. Lang H, Jv W, Oldhafer KJ, Behrend M, Schlitt HJ, Nashan B, et al. Liver transplantation in patients with polycystic liver disease. Transplant Proc. 1997;29(7):2832–3.
114. Swenson K, Seu P, Kinkhabwala M, Maggard M, Martin P, Goss J, et al. Liver transplantation for adult polycystic liver disease. Hepatology. 1998;28(2):412–5.
115. Gustafsson BI, Friman S, Mjornstedt L, Olausson M, Backman L. Liver transplantation for polycystic liver disease – indications and outcome. Transplant Proc. 2003;35(2):813–4.
116. Demirci G, Becker T, Nyibata M, Lueck R, Bektas H, Lehner F, et al. Results of combined and sequential liver-kidney transplantation. Liver Transplant: Off Publ Am Assoc Study Liver Dis Int Liver Transplant Soc. 2003;9(10):1067–78.
117. Ueno T, Barri YM, Netto GJ, Martin A, Onaca N, Sanchez EQ, et al. Liver and kidney transplantation for polycystic liver and kidney-renal function and outcome. Transplantation. 2006;82(4):501–7.
118. Krohn PS, Hillingsø JG, Kirkegaard P. Liver transplantation in polycystic liver disease: a relevant

treatment modality for adults? Scand J Gastroenterol. 2008;43(1):89–94.
119. Taner B, Willingham DL, Hewitt WR, Grewal HP, Nguyen JH, Hughes CB. Polycystic liver disease and liver transplantation: single-institution experience. Transplant Proc. 2009;41(9):3769–71.
120. Aussilhou B, Doufle G, Hubert C, Francoz C, Paugam C, Paradis V, et al. Extended liver resection for polycystic liver disease can challenge liver transplantation. Ann Surg. 2010;252(5):735–43.
121. Temmerman F, Gevers T, Ho TA, Vanslembrouck R, Coudyzer W, van Pelt J, et al. Safety and efficacy of different lanreotide doses in the treatment of polycystic liver disease: pooled analysis of individual patient data. Aliment Pharmacol Ther. 2013;38(4):397–406.

11 Other Extrarenal Manifestations of Autosomal Dominant Polycystic Kidney Disease

Charles L. Edelstein

ADPKD is a systemic disease with extrarenal as well as renal manifestations. Extrarenal manifestations (Table 11.1) that will be discussehd in this chapter are (1) intracranial aneurysms, (2) cardiac valve abnormalities, (3) vascular abnormalities, (4) diverticular disease and diverticulitis, (5) abdominal hernias, and (6) bronchiectasis.

Intracranial Aneurysms (ICA) in ADPKD

Demographics

The prevalence of asymptomatic ICA in ADPKD is about 8%, which is 3–4× higher than the general population [1, 2]. The prevalence is higher (16%) in patients with a family history of an ICA [1, 2]. Ninety percent of the ICA are in the anterior circulation, just like the general population. The majority of ICA are small, <6 mm in diameter. Besides the family history of an ICA, the clinical features of ADPKD (e.g., HTN, CKD) are no different in patients with or without unruptured ICA or ICA rupture. The average age of rupture is 41 years old, which is similar to that observed in other familial forms of ICA but 10 years earlier than reported in sporadic ICA.

In the general population, cigarette smoking and hypertension are risk factors for the development and rupture of sporadic or familial ICA. It is unknown if these risk factors apply to ADPKD. Size, location in posterior circulation, and a previous history of SAH from another ICA are risk factors for rupture in the general population [3].

Genetics

The familial clustering of ICA suggests that genetic factors are important in the etiology. A genotype-phenotype study was performed in which mutations were characterized in 58 ADPKD families with vascular complications; 51 were PKD1 (88%) and 7 PKD2 (12%). The median position of the PKD1 mutation was significantly more in the five prime (aminoterminal) regions in patients with ICA, whether ruptured or not, compared to controls. This study demonstrated that the position, but not the type, of a germline mutation in Pkd1 is an important factor in who develops aneurysms [4].

Clinical Features of ICA [1, 2, 5]

A ruptured ICA results in subarachnoid hemorrhage (SAH). The symptoms of SAH are headache variably described as “the worst headache of my life,” diffuse, radiating over the whole

C. L. Edelstein, MD, PhD, FAHA (✉)
Division of Renal Diseases and Hypertension, University of Colorado at Denver, Aurora, CO, USA
e-mail: Charles.edelstein@ucdenver.edu

B. D. Cowley, Jr., J. J. Bissler (eds.), *Polycystic Kidney Disease*,
https://doi.org/10.1007/978-1-4939-7784-0_11

Table 11.1 Extrarenal manifestations of ADPKD

Abnormality	% of patients
Intracranial aneurysms	8%
Cardiac valve abnormalities:	
MVP/MVR	18–31%
AVR	8–19%
Vascular abnormalities:	Unknown
Endothelial dysfunction, increased carotid intimal, and medial thickness	
Biventricular diastolic dysfunction	
Activation of the RAAS	
Arterial dissections	
Diverticulosis – pre-ESRD	14%
Diverticulitis:	
ESRD on HD	20–85%
Posttransplant	3.5–12%
Abdominal hernias:	
Pre-ESRD	13%
ESRD not on PD	33–46%
ESRD on PD	45%
Bronchiectasis	37%

RAAS renin-angiotensin-aldosterone system, *MVP* mitral valve prolapse, *MVR* mitral valve regurgitation, *AVR* aortic valve regurgitation, *ESRD* end-stage renal disease, *PD* peritoneal dialysis

head. However, headache may be less severe, and there may be "warning headaches" for weeks due to a small leak of blood from the ICA. A change in the pattern of pre-existing chronic headaches may be a warning of SAH. Other symptoms of SAH may include nausea, vomiting, photophobia, and neck stiffness. Clinical signs of SAH include neck stiffness and focal neurological deficits, especially a third cranial nerve palsy presenting with a unilateral fixed eye position, a drooped eyelid, and a dilated pupil. CT of the head without contrast is the initial diagnostic test of choice for suspected SAH. Lumbar puncture is reserved for approximately 5% of patients with a strong suspicion of SAH in which CT scan shows no SAH. The presence of a yellowish discoloration of CSF (xanthochromia) is more definitive of SAH than red blood cells in the CSF. Cerebral angiography is the test of choice to identify or rule out an ICA, although CT angiography or MR angiography has also been used.

Medical Therapy of ICA

Cerebral artery vasospasm is a major cause of morbidity and mortality. Nimodipine, a calcium channel blocker, has been shown to improve outcome after SAH. In patients who develop vasospasm or new neurological defects, triple-H therapy is used (hypertension, hypervolemia, hemodilution) [5].

Invasive Therapy of ICA

There are three options for treating an ICA: observation, craniotomy with clipping of the aneurysm, and endovascular occlusion using coiling. The time of intervention and type of intervention depends on the severity grading scale of the ICA and is discussed in detail elsewhere [5].

In the International Subarachnoid Aneurysm Trial (ISAT), 2143 patients with ruptured anterior ICA, good clinical status, and aneurysm <10 mm were randomly assigned to endovascular coiling vs. neurosurgical clipping [6–8]. Endovascular coiling had significantly less death or dependent complications (reduction in lifestyle) at 1 year (23% vs. 30%), less seizures/cognitive impairment, but more rebleeding. The major criticism of the ISAT trial is that the trial included only 2143 patients out of a total of 9559 with aneurysmal SAH. Part 2 of the study will include all patients with SAH. The ISAT concluded that endovascular coiling should be considered if expertise is available on an emergency basis and that endovascular coiling is becoming more widely used in unruptured aneurysms.

Screening of ADPKD Patients for ICA (Table 11.2)

Indications for screening include (1) family history of aneurysm or SAH; (2) family history of stroke before age 50; (3) previous aneurysm rupture; (4) preparation for major elective surgery; (5) high-risk occupations, e.g., airline pilots; (6) patient

Table 11.2 Indications for screening ADPKD patients for ICA

Family history of aneurysm or SAH
Family history of stroke before age 50
Previous aneurysm rupture
Preparation for major elective surgery
High-risk occupations, e.g., airline pilots
Patient anxiety
New onset or change in headaches

anxiety; and (7) new onset or change in headaches. The strongest indications for screening are a family history of ICA or SAH, or a family history suspicious of ICA or SAH, especially in family members before the age of 50, or a new onset or change in the pattern of headaches [1, 2, 9].

MR angiography is the best screening technique [2, 10]. A skilled neuroradiologist can detect 100% of ICA >5 mm, 88% of ICA >4 mm, 68% of ICA >3 mm, and 56% of ICA >2 mm without false-positive results [10]. The MRA is low risk and can be done without gadolinium. Because of advances in MR technology, it is likely that most aneurysms >2 mm can be detected [2, 10].

Repeat Imaging for ICA

There has been one study of repeat imaging for ICA in ADPKD patients with an initially negative study [11]. Seventy-six patients with an initial negative study were studied. Fifty-seven percent of patients had a negative family history. More than 50% were smokers and had hypertension. Only 2/76 had an ICA after 10 year follow-up of which 1/76 who had a clinically significant ICA had a FH. It was concluded that those with a FH of ruptured ICA could be rescreened at 10 years, but if they were not rescreened, only 1/76 who had an ICA would be missed.

Management of ICA in ADPKD Patients

The risk of enlargement is very low in small (<7 mm) aneurysms. Conservative management is suggested in aneurysms <7 mm. However, repeat imaging after 1 year to document stability of the ICA is suggested [1, 2]. In addition, stopping smoking and aggressive treatment of hypertension and hyperlipidemia are suggested. The natural history of unruptured ICA in ADPKD is largely unknown. However, the risk of rupture of ICA in ADPKD patients is similar to that from the International Study of Unruptured Intracranial Aneurysm (ISUIA) [3]. In the ISUIA, 1692 patients were followed for 4 years. Optimum size cut point for defining low risk of rupture was 7 mm. With increasing ICA size over 7 mm, the risk of aneurismal SAH increases proportionally. For anterior circulation aneurysms, the 5-year rates of rupture were 2.6% for 7–12 mm, 14.5% for 13–24 mm, and 40% for >25 mm. In patients without a history of previous SAH, risk of rupture of ICA <10 mm was as low as 0.05% per year. In patients with a history of previous SAH, risk of rupture of ICA<10 mm was 0.5% per year (ten times higher). The likelihood of rupture of ICA >10 mm in diameter was <1% per year. The ISUIA also assessed the risk of clipping aneurysms. The 1-year outcomes of elective surgery were a 1–4% mortality, and the morbidity was approximately 15%. However, the optimal management of both ruptured and unruptured ICA has not been fully determined [5].

It is unknown whether the low risk of rupture of small ICA seen in the ISUIA applies to ADPKD patients. In a study of ICA in ADPKD patients diagnosed by MRA, 15 asymptomatic ICA measuring from 1.5 to 6.5 mm in diameter were followed for a mean of 30 months. No change in aneurysm size or development of new aneurysms was detected [12]. In an extended follow-up study of presymptomatic ICA in ADPKD patients, 45 aneurysms of which 38 aneurysms were from 31 families were followed for a cumulative follow-up period of 243 years. The mean size of the ICA was 3.5 mm, 84% were in the anterior circulation, and the median age was 49 years. None of the ICA ruptured, and two increased slightly in size. The conclusion of the study was that growth and rupture of ICA in ADPKD patients is not higher than general population [13].

ICA Dolichoectasia

ICA dolichoectasia refers to elongation and dilatation of an arterial segment. ICA dolichoectasia was found in 2% of ADPKD patients vs. 0.06% in general population [14]. ICA dolichoectasia may be the sequela of dissection and may cause stroke [14].

Other Vascular Abnormalities

Other rare arterial abnormalities that have been reported in PKD patients include dissections of cervico-encephalic arteries and the thoracic aorta, coronary artery aneurysms, and central retinal vein/artery occlusions [14].

Summary of ICA (Table 11.3)

Asymptomatic patients with a family history suggestive of an ICA or SAH or ADPKD patients with a previous ruptured ICA should be screened.

Table 11.3 ICA in ADPKD patients

Asymptomatic patients with a FH suggestive of an ICA or SAH or a previous ruptured ICA should be screened
Best screening technique is MR angiography
Conservative management is recommended with ICA less than 7 mm
After an initial negative study, rescreening after 10 years

The best screening technique is MR angiography. Conservative management is recommended with ICA less than 7 mm. After an initial negative study, rescreening is not recommended for at least 10 years.

Cardiac Valve Abnormalities (Table 11.4)

Echocardiography, including Doppler analysis, was performed to assess the prevalence of cardiac abnormalities in 163 patients with ADPKD, 130 unaffected family members, and 100 control subjects. In these three groups, the prevalence of mitral valve prolapse was 26%, 14%, and 2%, respectively. There was also a higher prevalence of mitral incompetence (31%, 14%, and 9%, respectively), aortic incompetence (8%, 3%, and 1%, respectively), tricuspid incompetence (15%, 7%, and 4%, respectively), and tricuspid valve prolapse (6%, 2%, and 0%, respectively) in patients with ADPKD [15].

In a combined retrospective and prospective study, 11 patients with autosomal dominant polycystic kidney disease were studied. Seven patients had aortic regurgitation and two patients required aortic valve replacement. Mitral regurgitation was present in three patients, of whom one had mitral valve prolapse. Histologic analysis of available aortic and mitral valve tissue demonstrated myxomatous degeneration with loss and disruption of collagen [16].

Table 11.4 Cardiac valvular abnormalities in ADPKD

No of patients	%	Abnormality	Reference
228	25	MVP	[19]
	30/19	MVR/AVR	
	35	LVH after 10 years	
109 Pkd 1 mutation	26	MVP	[18]
	13	MVR grade 2 or 3	
154 children	12	MVP	[17]
62	18	MV histological abnormality	[16]
	27	AV histological abnormality	
163	26	MVP	[15]
	31	MVR	
	8	AVR	

Echocardiography was performed in 154 children of 66 families in which one parent had ADPKD. Eighty-six children with ADPKD and 68 children without ADPKD were evaluated by echocardiography in a prospective, single-blinded manner. There was a 12% incidence of mitral valve prolapse in the affected children compared with only 3% of the unaffected children ($P < 0.05$) [17].

To determine cardiac abnormalities in patients with the Pkd1 mutation, M-mode and color Doppler echocardiography was performed on 109 patients from 16 families with Pkd 1 gene mutations. The echocardiographic findings were compared with 73 unaffected family members and 73 healthy controls. Mitral valve prolapse was found in 26% of patients with PKD1, 14% of unaffected relatives, and 10% of control subjects. The prevalence of hemodynamically significant mitral regurgitation (grade 2 or 3) was 13%, 4%, and 3%, respectively. Prevalences of grade 2 or 3 aortic regurgitation and tricuspid regurgitation were not significantly different among the three groups [18].

Clinical, electrocardiographic and echocardiographic data were compared in 228 patients with ADPKD versus 146 unaffected family members and 181 controls. Mitral valve prolapse was more frequent in ADPKD patients and unaffected family members (25% and 20%, respectively) compared to control subjects (2%). Aortic valve regurgitation was more frequent in ADPKD patients and unaffected family members (19% and 17%, respectively) compared to control subjects (5%) [19].

In summary, mitral valve prolapse and mitral valve regurgitation are the most common cardiac valve abnormalities in ADPKD occurring in 18–31% of adults and 12% of children (Table 11.4). In one study 19% of patients had aortic valve regurgitation, and in an autopsy study, 27% of ADPKD patients had abnormalities of the aortic root, annulus, or valve. The cardiac valve abnormalities, especially myxomatous degeneration with loss and disruption of collagen, seen in one autopsy study reflect the systemic nature of ADPKD and may support the hypothesis that the cardiac abnormalities in ADPKD involve a defect in the extracellular matrix and a defect in collagen.

Vascular Abnormalities (Table 11.5)

There is evidence that the vascular abnormalities in ADPKD are caused by blood vessel alterations linked to Pkd1 or 2 gene mutations. The gene products of the *Pkd* 1 and 2 genes, polycystin 1 and polycystin 2, are detected in vascular smooth muscle cells and endothelial cells of all major vessels including intracranial arteries. Animal models of ADPKD duplicate the vascular abnormalities in humans with a gene dosage effect [20]. Pkd 1 or 2 −/− mice die *in utero* from massive hemorrhage caused by vascular leaks and vessel rupture. Histological analysis of tissues from Pkd1 −/− mouse embryos showed red blood cells outside of blood vessels, gross hemorrhage around blood vessels, red blood cells traversing the endothelial cell lining of blood

Table 11.5 Vascular abnormalities in ADPKD patients

Endothelial dysfunction
Impaired acetylcholine (ACh)-induced endothelium-dependent relaxation
Improvement of endothelial dysfunction with simvastatin
Increased carotid intima-media thickness
Decreased coronary flow velocity reserve
Biventricular diastolic dysfunction
Activation of the renin-angiotensin-aldosterone system (RAAS) that precedes hypertension
Decrease in vascular endothelial nitric oxide synthase (eNOS) early in the course of ADPKD
Arterial dissections
Aortic abdominal aneurysms

vessels, and a leak of intravascularly injected fluorescent dextran into the extravascular interstitium [20]. Mice with reduced PC-1 expression have arterial dissections. Pkd 2 +/− mice develop ICA when induced to develop HTN. These studies suggest that the vascular abnormalities in PKD are linked to the *Pkd* gene mutations.

Vascular abnormalities have been demonstrated in ADPKD patients [21–26]. There is endothelial dysfunction and increased carotid intimal and medial thickness in normotensive ADPKD patients with preserved kidney function [23] and improvement of endothelial dysfunction with simvastatin [23]. Normotensive patients with ADPKD with well-preserved renal function have significantly increased carotid intimal and medial thickness and significantly decreased coronary flow velocity reserve compared with healthy subjects. These findings suggest that atherosclerosis starts at an early stage in the course of ADPKD [22].

There is impaired endothelium-dependent relaxation and eNOS activity in isolated blood vessels from PKD rats and patients [27]. Acetylcholine (ACh)-induced endothelium-dependent relaxation (EDR) and constitutive nitric oxide synthase (cNOS) activity was determined in subcutaneous resistance vessels in normal control patients, patients with ADPKD, or patients with essential hypertension. EDR was decreased significantly in normotensive ADPKD patients but was more decreased in hypertensive ADPKD patients or those with CKD. Vascular cNOS activity and renal NOS excretion were reduced in patients with all categories of ADPKD and especially in ADPKD patients with hypertension. The study concluded that EDR in resistance vessels from patients with ADPKD is impaired even in the absence of hypertension or CKD but becomes more marked as hypertension develops. The patients with ADPKD had defective nitric oxide generation from diminished cNOS activity.

Arterial dissections in the thoracic and abdominal aorta, coronary arteries, and cervical and vertebral arteries have been reported in ADPKD patients [28]. The association between abdominal aortic aneurysms (AAA) and ADPKD is controversial. Aortic diameters measured in 139 ADPKD patients and 149 healthy patients were the same [29]. Aortic diameter was increased (2.7 cm) in 14 ADPKD patients compared to 200 other non-PKD ESRD patients [30]. In 100 patients with AAA and 100 age and sex-matched controls without an AAA, 54% of the AAA patients had renal cysts compared to only 30% in the control group [31]. Thus the data is mixed as to whether there is an increased incidence of AAA in ADPKD patients.

It has been suggested that the vascular abnormalities, cardiac valve abnormalities, ICA, and diverticular disease seen in ADPKD represent a systemic defect in basement membrane collagen and other basement membrane proteins. Several studies support the idea of a basement membrane collagen defect in ADPKD. Abnormal basement membrane in kidney biopsies was seen in both early- and late-stage human PKD kidneys [32]. Hybrid dilated blood vessels with red blood cell extravasation surrounded by excessive matrix accumulation were seen in human PKD kidney [33]. Matrix abnormalities in ADPKD kidneys during development and regression of tubular cysts have also been seen [34]. Thickened, laminated basement membrane, increased expression of alpha 1 type IV collagen and laminins B1 and B2, and changes in heparin sulfate proteoglycan and fibronectin have been seen in mouse models of PKD [35]. To prove mechanistically that defects of laminin cause PKD, it was demonstrated that laminin −/− mice develop PKD [36].

Does the Presence of ICA or MVP Affect the Progression of Kidney Disease in ADPKD?

Gabow et al. showed that factors associated with worse renal function were the PKD1 gene, younger age at diagnosis, male gender, hypertension, left ventricular hypertrophy (LVH), increased number of pregnancies, hematuria, hepatic cysts, and renal size. Factors not associated with the course of renal function were MVP, ICA, and any pregnancy [37].

Does the Presence of ICA or MVP Affect Survival After ESRD in ADPKD Patients?

Perrone et al. studied 9435 ADPKD patients and 9435 patients with other causes of ESRD. ADPKD patients had a better survival than nondiabetic controls. The survival after transplant was similar to controls. ADPKD-specific causes of death, such as valvular disease, ICA, or bowel perforation, but not polycystic liver disease, were lower in ADPKD patients. The major causes of death in ADPKD were myocardial infarction and congestive heart failure (36%) or infection (24%). This study does not support the assumption that cardiac valvular disease, ICA, or bowel perforation in ADPKD contribute to excess mortality [38].

Diverticular Disease and Diverticulitis (Table 11.6)

Diverticular disease in ADPKD patients can occur pre-ESRD, in ESRD patients on dialysis, and after kidney transplant.

Pre-ESRD

There has been only one study of diverticular disease in pre-ESRD patients. Sharp et al. studied 55 patients with ADPKD who were not receiving renal replacement therapy compared with 12 unaffected family members and 59 random control patients who had undergone barium enemas [39]. All patients underwent a double-contrast barium enema after administration of glucagon. There was no significant difference among the groups in regard to sex or age. There was no significant difference in the percentage of patients with diverticula (47% in ADPKD patients, 58% in unaffected family members, and 59% in controls). There was no significant difference in the mean number of diverticula in patients with diverticulosis or the size of the largest diverticula. There was no significant difference in these variables between the patients with ADPKD with a creatinine clearance greater than or less than 70 mL/min/. Thus, this study did not show a greater prevalence of diverticular disease in CKD patients with ADPKD not yet on dialysis compared with the general population.

Table 11.6 Diverticulosis or diverticulitis in ADPKD patients

Stage	Number	Complication	Reference
Pre-ESRD	55 PKD	14% diverticulosis	[39]
	59 Random controls	10% diverticulosis	
ESRD on HD	12 PKD	85% diverticulosis	[40]
	31 No PKD	32% diverticulosis	
ESRD on HD	14 PKD	50% diverticulosis	[41]
	86 No PKD	15% diverticulosis	
ESRD on HD	59 PKD	20% diverticulosis	[42]
	125 No PKD	3% diverticulosis	
Transplant	114 PKD	3.5% diverticulitis	[45]
	760 No PKD	0% diverticulitis	
Transplant	91 PKD	6.6% diverticulitis	[44]
	1046 No PKD	0.6% diverticulitis	
Transplant	145 PKD	12% GI complication	[43]
	1322 No PKD	6% GI complication	
Transplant	46 PKD	53% diverticulosis	[46]
	1082 No PKD	53% diverticulosis	

ESRD Patients on Hemodialysis

There have been three studies of diverticular disease in ESRD patients on hemodialysis that demonstrate a higher incidence of diverticular disease or diverticulitis. Scheff studied 12 of 151 hemodialysis patients with ADPKD [40]. Ten (83%) of these patients had diverticulosis, and four of these patients developed gross colonic perforation secondary to diverticulitis. Barium enemas on 31 CKD patients without polycystic kidney disease from the same dialysis unit showed diverticulosis in 10 (32%), and none had diverticulitis. Barium enemas in 120 age-matched nonrenal failure control patients showed diverticulosis in 45 (38%). McCune screened 1019 ESRD patients older than age 50 for diverticular disease prior to transplant [41]. There were significantly more PKD patients with diverticular disease than non-PKD patients. Lederman retrospectively reviewed ESRD patients from a single nephrology group practice [42]. The incidence and severity of diverticulitis in these patients was compared to a similar cohort of patients with ESRD due to other etiologies. Twelve (20%) of 59 patients with PKD had a history of active diverticulitis, whereas only 4 of 125 (3%) of the non-PKD controls had diverticulitis ($P = 0.0003$). Six of the 12 PKD patients required surgical intervention. This study demonstrated that ESRD patients with ADPKD have a significantly higher rate of diverticulitis than do non-ADPKD ESRD patients.

Post-Kidney Transplant

There have been four studies of diverticulitis after kidney transplant, of which three have shown an increased risk of diverticulitis. In 1467 renal transplant recipients, 145 patients had ADPKD. There was no significant difference in mortality between PKD and non-PKD patients. PKD patients had had a better long-term graft survival [43]. However, the PKD group had a higher incidence of gastrointestinal complications requiring surgery (e.g., appendicitis, small bowel ischemia, cholecystitis, diverticulitis) within 90 days of transplant (12.4% vs. 6.2%). In a retrospective study of 91 PKD patients and 1046 non-PKD patients after kidney transplant, 6.6% of PKD patients and 0.6% of non-PKD patients had diverticulitis [44]. Hadimeri studied 114 ADPKD patients after kidney transplant and control patients matched for sex, age, and donor type. 3.5% of the PKD patients versus 0% of the non-PKD patients had diverticulitis [45]. In a study of 46 PKD patients and 1082 non-PKD patients after transplant, the number of patients with diverticulosis or sigmoid perforation was not different [46]. In summary, three studies demonstrate a higher incidence of diverticulitis in PKD patients versus non-PKD patients after kidney transplant. However, the higher incidence of diverticulitis did not result in increased mortality. Nonetheless, diverticulitis is an important part of the differential diagnosis of abdominal pain in ADPKD patients on dialysis of posttransplant.

Abdominal Hernias

Compared to non-PKD family members, ADPKD patients have an increased incidence of inguinal hernias (13% vs. 4%) or umbilical hernias (7% vs. 2%) [47]. In a retrospective study of 85 ADPKD patients, the prevalence of inguinal, incisional, or paraumbilical hernias was 45% in ADPKD patients compared to 8% for other causes of ESRD and 4% for general surgical controls [48]. In patients on peritoneal dialysis (PD), abdominal wall hernias were more common in ADPKD patients than controls (33% vs. 7%) [49]. In another study of 142 PD patients, advanced age, PKD, and high body mass index were independent risk factors for abdominal hernias [50]. In this study, 61% of ADPKD patients on continuous ambulatory peritoneal dialysis (CAPD) had an abdominal wall complication. In another study, 6/13 (46.2%) CAPD patients with ADPKD developed bilateral indirect inguinal hernia compared to 1/30 (3.3%) CAPD patients without ADPKD [51]. Possible reasons for increased abdominal wall hernias in ADPKD patients include the pressure of large polycystic kidneys on abdominal organs and the abdominal wall or the "collagen defect" as previously discussed. The correlation between kidney size and abdominal hernias has not been studied.

Bronchiectasis

CT scans from 95 ADPKD and 95 non-PKD CKD controls were retrospectively reviewed for the presence of bronchiectasis using defined criteria.

There was a threefold increased prevalence of bronchiectasis (37%) compared to the control group (13%) [52]. Immunostaining demonstrated polycystin-1 expression in the motile cilia of non-ADPKD airway epithelial cells. The association between ADPKD and bronchiectasis suggests that patients with primary cilia-associated diseases may be at risk for bronchiectasis.

References

1. Pirson Y. Extrarenal manifestations of autosomal dominant polycystic kidney disease. Adv Chronic Kidney Dis. 2010;17:173–80.
2. Pirson Y, Chauveau D, Torres V. Management of cerebral aneurysms in autosomal dominant polycystic kidney disease. J Am Soc Nephrol. 2002;13:269–76.
3. Wiebers DO, Whisnant JP, Huston J III, et al. Unruptured intracranial aneurysms: natural history, clinical outcome, and risks of surgical and endovascular treatment. Lancet. 2003;362:103–10.
4. Rossetti S, Chauveau D, Kubly V, et al. Association of mutation position in polycystic kidney disease 1 (PKD1) gene and development of a vascular phenotype. Lancet. 2003;361:2196–201.
5. Brisman JL, Song JK, Newell DW. Cerebral aneurysms. N Engl J Med. 2006;355:928–39.
6. Molyneux A, Kerr R, Stratton I, et al. International Subarachnoid Aneurysm Trial (ISAT) of neurosurgical clipping versus endovascular coiling in 2143 patients with ruptured intracranial aneurysms: a randomised trial. Lancet. 2002;360:1267–74.
7. Molyneux AJ, Kerr RS, Birks J, et al. Risk of recurrent subarachnoid haemorrhage, death, or dependence and standardised mortality ratios after clipping or coiling of an intracranial aneurysm in the International Subarachnoid Aneurysm Trial (ISAT): long-term follow-up. Lancet Neurol. 2009;8:427–33.
8. Molyneux AJ, Kerr RS, Yu LM, et al. International subarachnoid aneurysm trial (ISAT) of neurosurgical clipping versus endovascular coiling in 2143 patients with ruptured intracranial aneurysms: a randomised comparison of effects on survival, dependency, seizures, rebleeding, subgroups, and aneurysm occlusion. Lancet. 2005;366:809–17.
9. Grantham JJ. Clinical practice. Autosomal dominant polycystic kidney disease. N Engl J Med. 2008;359:1477–85.
10. Huston J III, Nichols DA, Luetmer PH, et al. Blinded prospective evaluation of sensitivity of MR angiography to known intracranial aneurysms: importance of aneurysm size. AJNR Am J Neuroradiol. 1994;15:1607–14.
11. Schrier RW, Belz MM, Johnson AM, et al. Repeat imaging for intracranial aneurysms in patients with autosomal dominant polycystic kidney disease with initially negative studies: a prospective ten-year follow-up. J Am Soc Nephrol. 2004;15:1023–8.
12. Huston J III, Torres VE, Wiebers DO, Schievink WI. Follow-up of intracranial aneurysms in autosomal dominant polycystic kidney disease by magnetic resonance angiography. J Am Soc Nephrol. 1996;7:2135–41.
13. Irazabal MV, Huston J III, Kubly V, et al. Extended follow-up of unruptured intracranial aneurysms detected by presymptomatic screening in patients with autosomal dominant polycystic kidney disease. Clin J Am Soc Nephrol. 2011;6:1274–85.
14. Qian Q, Younge BR, Torres VE. Retinal arterial and venous occlusions in patients with ADPKD. Nephrol Dial Transplant. 2007;22:1769–71.
15. Hossack KF, Leddy CL, Johnson AM, et al. Echocardiographic findings in autosomal dominant polycystic kidney disease. N Engl J Med. 1988;319:907–12.
16. Leier CV, Baker PB, Kilman JW, Wooley CF. Cardiovascular abnormalities associated with adult polycystic kidney disease. Ann Intern Med. 1984;100:683–8.
17. Ivy DD, Shaffer EM, Johnson AM, et al. Cardiovascular abnormalities in children with autosomal dominant polycystic kidney disease. J Am Soc Nephrol. 1995;5:2032–6.
18. Lumiaho A, Ikaheimo R, Miettinen R, et al. Mitral valve prolapse and mitral regurgitation are common in patients with polycystic kidney disease type 1. Am J Kidney Dis. 2001;38:1208–16.
19. Timio M, Monarca C, Pede S, et al. The spectrum of cardiovascular abnormalities in autosomal dominant polycystic kidney disease: a 10-year follow-up in a five-generation kindred. Clin Nephrol. 1992;37:245–51.
20. Kim K, Drummond I, Ibraghimov-Beskrovnaya O, et al. Polycystin 1 is required for the structural integrity of blood vessels. Proc Natl Acad Sci U S A. 2000;97:1731–6.
21. Ecder T, Schrier RW. Cardiovascular abnormalities in autosomal-dominant polycystic kidney disease. Nat Rev Nephrol. 2009;5:221–8.
22. Turkmen K, Oflaz H, Uslu B, et al. Coronary flow velocity reserve and carotid intima media thickness in patients with autosomal dominant polycystic kidney disease: from impaired tubules to impaired carotid and coronary arteries. Clin J Am Soc Nephrol. 2008;3:986–91.
23. Namli S, Oflaz H, Turgut F, et al. Improvement of endothelial dysfunction with simvastatin in patients with autosomal dominant polycystic kidney disease. Ren Fail. 2007;29:55–9.
24. Oflaz H, Alisir S, Buyukaydin B, et al. Biventricular diastolic dysfunction in patients with autosomal-dominant polycystic kidney disease. Kidney Int. 2005;68:2244–9.
25. Kocaman O, Oflaz H, Yekeler E, et al. Endothelial dysfunction and increased carotid intima-media thick-

ness in patients with autosomal dominant polycystic kidney disease. Am J Kidney Dis. 2004;43:854–60.
26. Turkmen K, Tufan F, Alpay N, et al. Insulin resistance and coronary flow velocity reserve in patients with autosomal dominant polycystic kidney disease. Intern Med J. 2012;42:146–53.
27. Wang D, Iversen J, Wilcox CS, Strandgaard S. Endothelial dysfunction and reduced nitric oxide in resistance arteries in autosomal-dominant polycystic kidney disease. Kidney Int. 2003;64:1381–8.
28. Nacasch N, Werner M, Golan E, Korzets Z. Arterial dissections in autosomal dominant polycystic kidney disease – chance association or part of the disease spectrum? Clin Nephrol. 2010;73:478–81.
29. Torra R, Nicolau C, Badenas C, et al. Abdominal aortic aneurysms and autosomal dominant polycystic kidney disease. J Am Soc Nephrol. 1996;7:2483–6.
30. Kato A, Takita T, Furuhashi M, et al. Abdominal aortic aneurysms in hemodialysis patients with autosomal dominant polycystic kidney disease. Nephron. 2001;88:185–6.
31. Yaghoubian A, de Virgilio C, White RA, Sarkisyan G. Increased incidence of renal cysts in patients with abdominal aortic aneurysms: a common pathogenesis? Ann Vasc Surg. 2006;20:787–91.
32. Mannik M, Striker GE. Removal of glomerular deposits of immune complexes in mice by administration of excess antigen. Lab Investig. 1980;42:483–9.
33. Ul HA, Moatasim A. Adult polycystic kidney disease: a disorder of connective tissue? Int J Clin Exp Pathol. 2008;1:84–90.
34. Ojeda JL, Ros MA, Icardo JM, Garcia-Porrero JA. Basement membrane alterations during development and regression of tubular cysts. Kidney Int. 1990;37:1270–80.
35. Calvet JP. Polycystic kidney disease: primary extracellular matrix abnormality or defective cellular differentiation? Kidney Int. 1993;43:101–8.
36. Shannon MB, Patton BL, Harvey SJ, Miner JH. A hypomorphic mutation in the mouse laminin alpha5 gene causes polycystic kidney disease. J Am Soc Nephrol. 2006;17:1913–22.
37. Gabow PA, Johnson AM, Kaehny WD, et al. Factors affecting the progression of renal disease in autosomal-dominant polycystic kidney disease. Kidney Int. 1992;41:1311–9.
38. Perrone RD, Ruthazer R, Terrin NC. Survival after end-stage renal disease in autosomal dominant polycystic kidney disease: contribution of extrarenal complications to mortality. Am J Kidney Dis. 2001;38:777–84.
39. Sharp CK, Zeligman BE, Johnson AM, et al. Evaluation of colonic diverticular disease in autosomal dominant polycystic kidney disease without end-stage renal disease. Am J Kidney Dis. 1999;34:863–8.
40. Scheff RT, Zuckerman G, Harter H, et al. Diverticular disease in patients with chronic renal failure due to polycystic kidney disease. Ann Intern Med. 1980;92:202–4.
41. McCune TR, Nylander WA, Van Buren DH, et al. Colonic screening prior to renal transplantation and its impact on post-transplant colonic complications. Clin Transpl. 1992;6:91–6.
42. Lederman ED, McCoy G, Conti DJ, Lee EC. Diverticulitis and polycystic kidney disease. Am Surg. 2000;66:200–3.
43. Andreoni KA, Pelletier RP, Elkhammas EA, et al. Increased incidence of gastrointestinal surgical complications in renal transplant recipients with polycystic kidney disease. Transplantation. 1999;67:262–6.
44. Lederman ED, Conti DJ, Lempert N, et al. Complicated diverticulitis following renal transplantation. Dis Colon Rectum. 1998;41:613–8.
45. Hadimeri H, Norden G, Friman S, Nyberg G. Autosomal dominant polycystic kidney disease in a kidney transplant population. Nephrol Dial Transplant. 1997;12:1431–6.
46. Dominguez FE, Albrecht KH, Heemann U, et al. Prevalence of diverticulosis and incidence of bowel perforation after kidney transplantation in patients with polycystic kidney disease. Transpl Int. 1998;11:28–31.
47. Gabow PA. Autosomal dominant polycystic kidney disease – more than a renal disease. Am J Kidney Dis. 1990;16:403–13.
48. Morris-Stiff G, Coles G, Moore R, et al. Abdominal wall hernia in autosomal dominant polycystic kidney disease. Br J Surg. 1997;84:615–7.
49. Li L, Szeto CC, Kwan BC, et al. Peritoneal dialysis as the first-line renal replacement therapy in patients with autosomal dominant polycystic kidney disease. Am J Kidney Dis. 2011;57:903–7.
50. Del PG, Bajo MA, Costero O, et al. Risk factors for abdominal wall complications in peritoneal dialysis patients. Perit Dial Int. 2003;23:249–54.
51. Modi KB, Grant AC, Garret A, Rodger RS. Indirect inguinal hernia in CAPD patients with polycystic kidney disease. Adv Perit Dial. 1989;5:84–6.
52. Driscoll JA, Bhalla S, Liapis H, et al. Autosomal dominant polycystic kidney disease is associated with an increased prevalence of radiographic bronchiectasis. Chest. 2008;133:1181–8.

Part IV

ADPKD: Clinical Trials and Emerging Therapies

12 Role of Renin-Angiotensin-Aldosterone System Inhibition in Autosomal Dominant Polycystic Kidney Disease

Pranav S. Garimella and Dana C. Miskulin

Introduction

Activation of the renin-angiotensin-aldosterone system (RAAS) is believed to play a role in the development of hypertension and in the structural and functional progression of kidney disease in ADPKD. Studies in animal models and humans have evaluated the utility of blocking the RAAS pathway on blood pressure control, kidney growth, and kidney function. In this chapter we review the evidence from experimental and clinical studies implicating activation of RAAS in the pathogenesis of ADPKD, as well as results of observational and randomized control trials (RCTs) testing RAAS inhibition.

Experimental Evidence for Heightened RAAS Activity in ADPKD

Early studies of nephrectomy specimens from patients with ADPKD showed stretching, compression, and obliteration of the renal vasculature from surrounding cysts [1]. Compression on the vasculature is postulated to lead to focal ischemia, with subsequent RAAS activation, which in turn leads to generation of angiotensin II and release of pro-inflammatory cytokines [2–6]. Some of these cytokines are mitogens, which stimulate cyst growth and perpetuate the cycle of focal ischemia, RAAS activation, and more cytokine release (Fig. 12.1) [7]. Several lines of evidence implicate the RAAS in ADPKD progression. Histochemical staining of human nephrectomy specimens revealed increased numbers of renin granules in the juxtamedullary apparatus, along arterioles, and within cyst walls [4]. Cystic epithelium has been demonstrated to produce ectopic renin [8], as well as all other major RAAS components including angiotensinogen, angiotensin-converting enzyme (ACE), and angiotensin II [9]. Angiotensin II and aldosterone have been shown to induce signaling cascades leading to proliferation of tubular epithelial cells [10, 11].

In addition, some [12, 13], but not all [14–16], clinical studies have found elevated plasma renin activity in ADPKD patients. In one study that matched ADPKD patients to essential hypertensives based on age, BP level, and 24 h urine sodium excretion, baseline plasma renin levels were higher, and there was a greater increase after ACE inhibition and with upright position in the ADPKD patients [12]. This same study found increased renovascular resistance, and greater renal vasodilation and reduction in filtration fraction in response to ACE inhibitors (ACE-I) as

P. S. Garimella, MD, MPH
D. C. Miskulin, MD, MS (✉)
Division of Nephrology, Department of Medicine, Tufts Medical Center, Boston, MA, USA
e-mail: pgarimella@ucsd.edu; dmiskulin@tuftsmedicalcenter.org

B. D. Cowley, Jr., J. J. Bissler (eds.), *Polycystic Kidney Disease*,
https://doi.org/10.1007/978-1-4939-7784-0_12

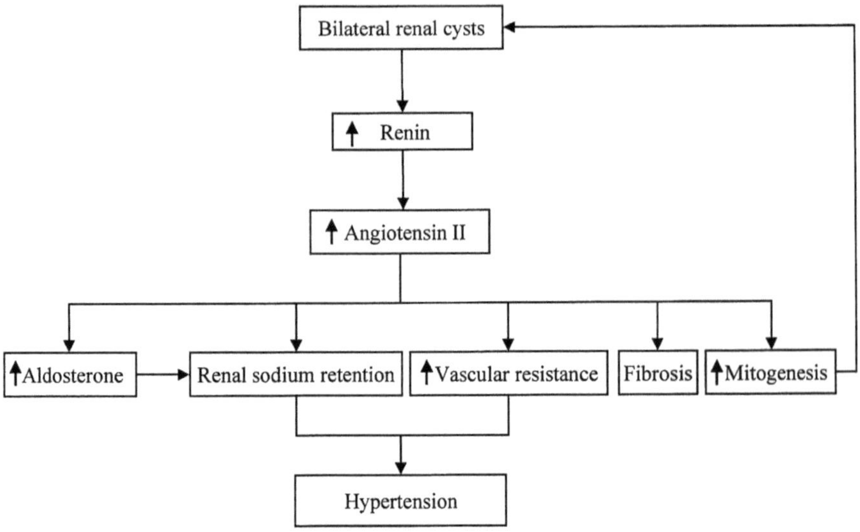

Fig. 12.1 Theoretical model: the effect of the RAAS in the development of hypertension and progression of ADPKD (Reproduced from Ecder and Schrier [7] with permission from the Journal of the American Society of Nephrology)

compared with healthy controls [17], suggesting heightened local RAAS activity. Failure to suppress plasma renin with salt loading has also been demonstrated in ADPKD [13].

In the PCK rat model, treatment with lisinopril as compared with vehicle resulted in a lower kidney weight/body weight and lower cyst volume index score [18]. In support of a role of the RAAS activity in cystogenesis, there was a reduction in proliferative signaling pathways (ERK1, ERK2, and PCNA levels) and apoptotic pathways (MAPK, SAPK/JNK) in the lisinopril as compared with vehicle-treated animals. Additional support for a link between RAAS activation and cystogenesis includes observations in several studies showing larger kidneys in hypertensive children and young adults with ADPKD and normal or near-normal kidney function, as compared with those with normotension [5, 19].

Randomized Controlled Trials Comparing ACE-I or ARB Versus Other Antihypertensive Classes in ADPKD

Randomized controlled trials (RCTs) that have compared RAAS blocker monotherapy versus other antihypertensive drug classes or placebo and that have a sample size >40 patients are shown in Table 12.1. The largest trial had fewer than 100 patients, and 2 of the 4 studies are secondary analyses of a subgroup of the full population of patients with ADPKD. Smaller studies are included in the Reference Section for completeness [3, 20, 21]. As can be seen, the evidence is very limited. In secondary analyses of the REIN trial (n = 64), which involved patients with GFR 30–60 mL/min [22], benazepril reduced the endpoint of doubling serum creatinine (sCr), ESRD, or death in patients with glomerulonephritis and diabetic kidney disease, but not in ADPKD. In an individual patient meta-analysis of the ADPKD subgroups (n = 142 patients) from eight RCTs assessing ACE-I versus placebo [23] (including the abovementioned REIN trial [22]), ACE inhibitors reduced urinary protein excretion but did not decrease doubling of sCr, reaching ESRD or death [RR = 0.73, 95% CI (0.41–1.29)] (Fig. 12.2). In addition to the major issue of limited statistical power for the composite kidney outcome, another limitation was that baseline protein excretion was >1 g/d in the ADPKD subgroup, which is unusual for ADPKD.

In a double-blind RCT comparing enalapril to atenolol in 61 hypertensive ADPKD patients with GFR >85 ml/min and enalapril to placebo in 28 normotensive ADPKD patients, there was no

Table 12.1 Summary table of RCTs (with sample size>40) comparing RAAS blockade with other antihypertensive classes in ADPKD

Study	Study population	Intervention/control	Outcomes	Results
Maschio 1996 [22]	583 with CKD, 64 in ADPKD subgroup	Benazepril ($n = 30$)	Doubling of baseline serum Cr or the need for dialysis	No difference in primary outcome in benazepril vs. placebo (8/30 vs. 9/34)
		Placebo ($n = 34$)		
Marin 2001 [51]	45 patients with ADPKD and HTN	Fosinopril ($n = 29$)	Doubling of serum creatinine or need for dialysis	11 patients in fosinopril and 8 in the nifedipine group reached primary endpoint
		Nifedipine ($n = 16$)		
Schrier 2002 [26]	72 ADPKD with HTN and LVH	Enalapril ($n = 36$)	Change in LVMI and kidney function	Those in aggressive BP control group had greater decrease in LVMI. No difference in mean BP over follow-up for enalapril vs. amlodipine. Enalapril was more effective in decreasing LVMI than amlodipine ($p < 0.01$). No difference in kidney function in those on enalapril compared to amlodipine
		Amlodipine (=36) both groups randomized to aggressive vs. regular BP control		
Van Dijk 2003 [24]	79 ADPKD, 28 with HTN	Among 51 without HTN	Progression of renal failure	In those without HTN, no difference in change in renal function in enalapril vs. placebo (−7 vs. −9 ml/min; $p = 0.4$)
		Enalapril ($n = 32$)		
		Placebo ($n = 29$)		
		Among 28 with HTN		In those with HTN, no difference in change in renal function between enalapril and atenolol
		Enalapril ($n = 13$)		
		Atenolol ($n = 15$)		
Jafar 2005 [23]	Meta-analysis of 8 RCTs	ACE-I ($n = 68$)	Decline in proteinuria, reduction in GFR, or the need for dialysis	Kidney disease progression occurred in 29% in the ACE-I group and 41% in the control group ($p = 0.14$). ACE-I reduced proteinuria from baseline greater ($p = 0.03$)
	142 in ADPKD subgroup	Control ($N = 74$)		
Zeltner 2008 [25]	46 ADPKD with HTN	Ramipril ($n = 23$)	Doubling of sCr, 50% reduction in GFR, or the need for dialysis	No differences in renal function, urinary albumin excretion, and LVMI were detected among those taking ramipril compared to metoprolol
		Metoprolol ($n = 23$)		
Stallone 2012 [28]	55 ADPKD	Ramipril ($n = 18$)	Reduction of renal, cyst volume, and rate of change of GFR	Cyst and renal volume increased in all three groups. No difference between groups. No difference in renal function at 24 months between the three study groups
		Ramipril + high-dose rapamycin ($n = 19$)		
		Ramipril + low-dose rapamycin ($n = 18$)		

CKD chronic kidney disease, *PKD* polycystic kidney disease, *Scr* serum creatinine, *CrCl* creatinine clearance, *HTN* hypertension, *BP* blood pressure, *ACE-I* angiotensin-converting enzyme inhibitor, *LVH* left ventricular hypertrophy, *LVMI* left ventricular mass index, *RAAS* renin-angiotensin-aldosterone system, *CCB* calcium channel blocker, *GFR* glomerular filtration rate

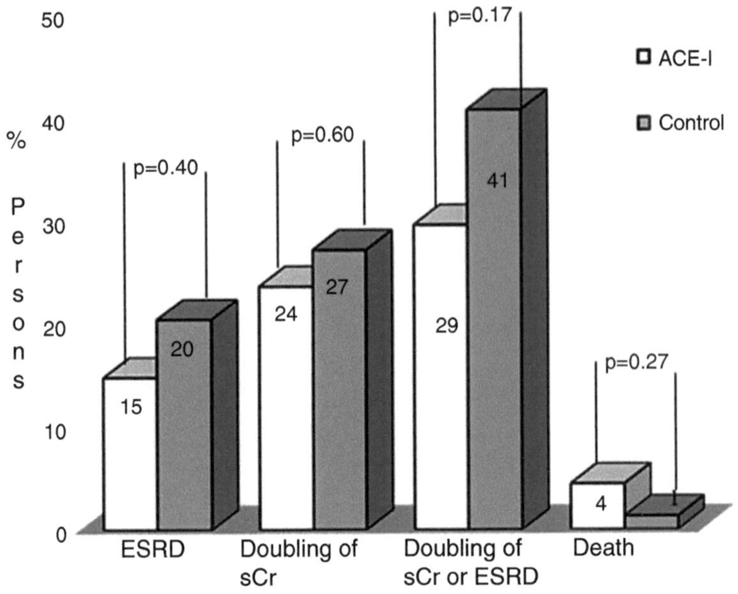

Fig. 12.2 Effects of ACE-I versus other antihypertensive classes on doubling sCr, ESRD, or death in the ADPKD subgroup of the AIPRD meta-analysis. ESRD end-stage renal disease, sCr serum creatinine, ACE-I angiotensin-converting enzyme inhibitor, RR relative risk (Created using data from Ref. [23])

difference in the rate of decline in eGFR across treatment arms for either subset [24]. In another RCT of 46 patients with hypertension, ramipril did not significantly alter the rate of decline in kidney function decline or reduce albuminuria as compared with metoprolol [25]. In a post hoc analysis, treatment to a mean arterial pressure (MAP) ≤97 mm Hg, as compared with a MAP >97 mm Hg, was associated with a greater reduction in ventricular mass index (LVMI) group (p = 0.017) independent of the antihypertensive agent used. In a 7-year RCT assessing the effects of rigorous (<120/80 mmHg) versus standard (135–140/85–90 mmHg) blood pressure control and of enalapril versus amlodipine, LVMI returned to normal range in 67% of the enalapril-treated patients versus 36% of the amlodipine-treated ($p < 0.05$), despite similar level of blood pressure control [26]. Due to the study design, the effects of enalapril versus amlodipine could only be studied in a nonrandomized manner. Rigorous blood pressure control also reduced LVMI significantly more than standard blood pressure control. Creatinine clearance, however, did not differ across comparison by BP level or lisinopril versus amlodipine treatment arms. One small RCT, comparing telmisartan with enalapril, found a similar reduction in blood pressure in both groups without appreciable changes in kidney function at 1-year follow-up [27]. Recent studies evaluating the effect of RAAS blocking agents alone or in combination with other drugs have not shown significant differences in renal function decline [21, 28–30].

To summarize, evidence, showing a benefit of RAAS blockers over other antihypertensive classes or placebo, exists only for reducing left ventricular mass and proteinuria (the latter atypical of ADPKD). The data are insufficient for conclusions to be drawn about effects of RAAS versus other antihypertensive classes or placebo on kidney function, due to the extremely small sample sizes represented in these trials. Nonetheless, RAAS blockers are the most frequently prescribed drugs in ADPKD in current practice, as reflected in the Consortium for Radiologic Imaging Studies of Polycystic Kidney Disease (CRISP) cohort where 72% of all hypertensive patients were treated with ACE-I or ARB prior to enrollment [6].

Theoretical Basis for Dual RAAS Inhibition in ADPKD

More recently, the concept of intrarenal RAAS activation has come to the forefront in understanding the pathophysiology of many forms of hypertension [31, 32]. The renoprotective effect of ACE-I or ARB monotherapy may be limited by compensatory feedback increases in renin release with continued generation of angiotensin. Dual RAAS blockade through combination of an ACE-I with an ARB, a direct renin inhibitor, or an aldosterone antagonist has been proposed as a strategy to counteract this compensatory feedback [33] Meta-analysis of trials examining BP effects of dual blockade of the RAAS in the general population suggests more BP-lowering effect, but when restricted to trials that used maximal doses of ACE-I or ARB monotherapy for comparison, there was no benefit of combination therapy [34]. Dual RAAS blockade in the ONTARGET trial, which involved patients with coronary artery or peripheral artery or cerebrovascular disease or diabetes with end-organ damage who were treated with a fixed dose combination of ramipril and telmisartan versus telmisartan alone, showed higher rates of syncope, doubling of serum creatinine, and no benefit on the composite outcome of fatal and nonfatal CV events [35].

The effects of single versus dual RAAS blockade in patients with CKD have also been studied in several trials. Irrespective of the underlying kidney disease and degree of initial proteinuria, dual RAAS blockade was associated with a greater reduction in urinary protein and better BP control but also with a greater incidence of adverse events including hyperkalemia, hypotension, and decline in eGFR [33, 36–38]. The largest study of dual versus single RAAS blockade, NEPHRON-D, which involved 1442 patients with diabetic nephropathy, >300 mg/d of albuminuria, and an eGFR of 30–89 ml/min/1.73 m^2, was terminated after 2.2 years due to safety concerns of significant increases in hyperkalemia and AKI in the losartan- and lisinopril-treated arm [39]. There was no signal of a benefit on CV events or mortality of lisinopril and losartan over losartan plus placebo at 2.2 years.

There may be a stronger rationale for the use of dual RAAS blockade in patients with ADPKD than with other forms of CKD. A study of human ADPKD nephrectomy specimens revealed intense interstitial inflammation, with high tissue concentrations of angiotensin II and an abundance of mast cells that exhibited chymase-like activity [40]. Confirming the presence of chymases, the addition of ADPKD kidney tissue extracts to angiotensin I led to generation of angiotensin II, which could be blocked by chymostatin. Chymase is an alternative enzyme for the conversion of angiotensin I to angiotensin II. Angiotensin II stimulates renal fibroblast activity [41], and studies in rats have shown that angiotensin II infusions resulted in TGF-beta 1 generation, which is the prototype fibrosis cytokine in the kidney [42]. Since both ACE-Is and ARBs reduce TGF-beta 1 and limit fibrosis in animal models, it is hypothesized that the combination may have a similar effect in humans [43, 44].

Clinical Trials Assessing Dual Blockade of the RAAS Versus Monotherapy and Level of BP Control on ADPKD Progression

The recently published HALT-PKD Studies are large, multicenter RCTs that assessed the impact of dual- versus single-level blockade of the RAAS and the effects of two different levels of BP control on ADPKD progression [45, 46]. HALT Study A was conducted in ADPKD individuals with hypertension (use of antihypertensive agents or BP >130/80 mm Hg) and early disease (defined as eGFR >60 mL/min/1.73 m^2) [45]. There was no minimum TKV requirement. The study had a 2×2 factorial design, under which, participants were randomized to each of the two interventions, which were (1) telmisartan plus lisinopril as compared with placebo plus lisinopril and (2) treatment to a standard BP goal of 120–130/70–80 mm Hg versus a low goal of <110/<70 mm Hg. The 7-day average of twice daily BPs taken at home guided antihypertensive therapy. The primary outcome was growth of total kidney volume (TKV), measured via MRI at baseline, 2, 4, and 5 years.

The comparison of ARB/ACE-I versus placebo/ACE-I revealed no difference in the percent change in TKV per year (Fig. 12.3), change in eGFR, albuminuria, left ventricular mass index (LVMI), renal vascular resistance, or renal blood flow across treatment arms. The secondary intervention, treatment to two levels of BP control, was successfully achieved, with the average difference in systolic and diastolic BP across arms

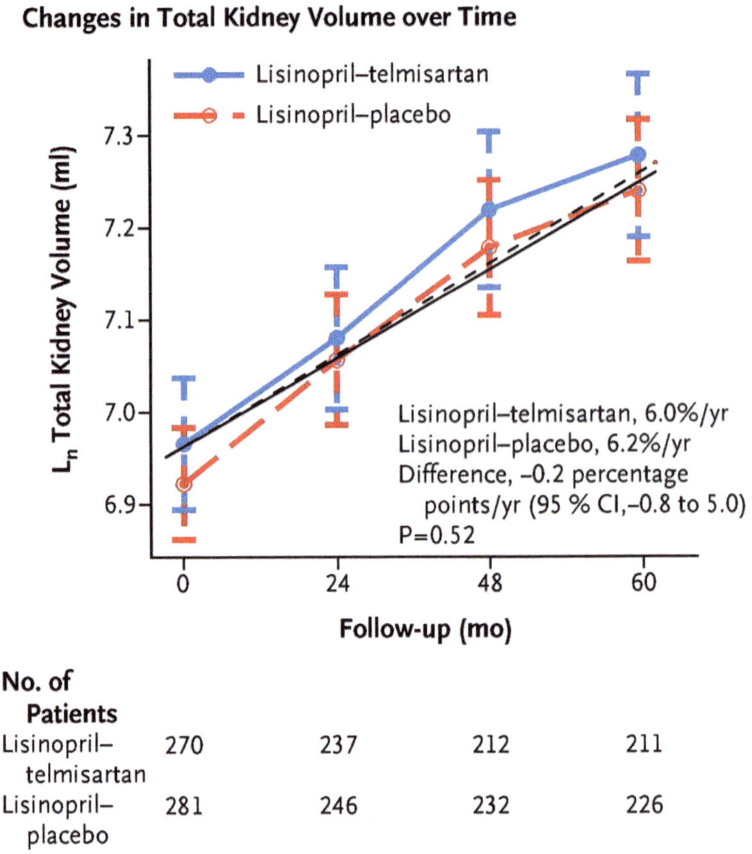

Fig. 12.3 Effects of ACE-I/ARB combination vs. ACE-I monotherapy on change in total kidney volume in ADPKD patients with baseline eGFR >60 mL/min/1.73 m^2 (From Schrier et al [45], Page 2264. Copyright © (2014) Massachusetts Medical Society. Reprinted with permission. http://www.nejm.org/doi/full/10.1056/NEJMoa1402685)

over the course of the study being 13.4 and 9.3 mm Hg, respectively. The annual rate of TKV growth in the low BP arm was 5.6% per year as compared with 6.6% per year in the standard arm, which represents a 14% slower TKV growth rate with intensive BP lowering ($p < 0.01$) (Fig. 12.4). In subgroup analyses, the benefit of the low BP goal on TKV was even greater in males, in individuals with larger TKVs, and in patients under age 30 with baseline TKV > 75th percentile. In spite of the reduction in growth of TKV with intensive BP control, the decline in eGFR was similar between the two groups (Fig. 12.4b). Changes in urinary albumin excretion (−3.77% per year versus 2.43% per year; $p < 0.001$) and LVMI (−1.17 vs −0.057 g per square meter per year; $p < 0.001$) were better with intensive BP control. RBF declined similarly across BP arms, and there was a greater increase in RVR in the standard BP arm.

Putting this into context, a 14% lower rate of TKV growth equates to 12.6 mL/year, (based on a median baseline KTV of 1264 mL) which is modest, and compares to a 40% reduction in TKV growth and a 1 mL/min/year slower decline in eGFR seen with tolvaptan treatment [47]. However, treatment to the low BP was easy to achieve, was well tolerated, does slow TKV growth, and also confers cardiovascular benefit via reducing LVMI, and for all of these reasons, patients with GFR >60 mL/min/1.73 m^2 should be treated to a BP <110/70 mm Hg. The trial was well designed and executed, but one potential limitation in design was that BP was achieved using a stepped algorithm with ACE-Is and ARBs as the first steps, and thus patients in the low BP arm were also treated with higher doses of RAAS blockers. This means that one cannot exclude the possibility that the benefit of low BP was due to more intensive RAAS blockade though the difference in the amount of RAAS blocking therapy across BP arms was much less than was present across ACE-I/ARB vs ACE-I/placebo arms, where no difference was found.

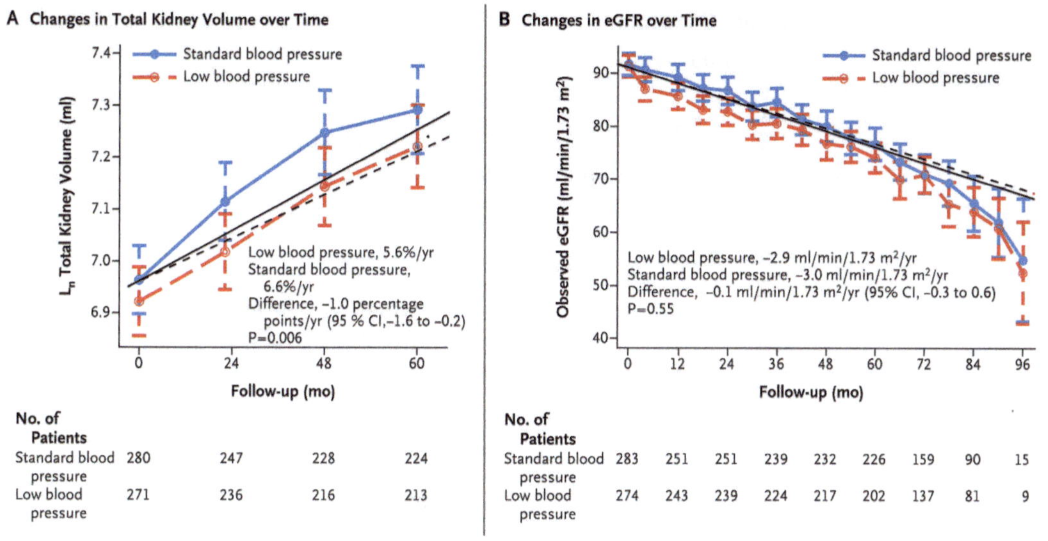

Fig. 12.4 (**a**, **b**) Effects of intensive BP control to <110/70 mmHg versus 120–130/80 mm Hg on changes in total kidney volume and eGFR in ADPKD patients with baseline eGFR >60 mL/min/1.73 m^2 (From Schrier et al. [45], Page 2261. Copyright © (2014) Massachusetts Medical Society. Reprinted with permission. http://www.nejm.org/doi/full/10.1056/NEJMoa1402685)

HALT Study B enrolled 486 patients with moderately advanced disease (eGFR 25–60 mL/min) and assessed the single intervention of combination RAAS blockade with telmisartan/lisinopril versus placebo/lisinopril on the time to 50% decline in baseline eGFR, ESRD, or death [46]. All patients were treated to a BP of ≤130/80 mm Hg. MRI of the kidneys and heart was not performed. Results showed no difference in the primary composite outcome (Fig. 12.5) or in the rate of eGFR decline (−3.91 ml/min/1.73 m^2 per year [95% CI, −3.65 to −4.17] versus −3.87 ml per minute per 1.73 m^2 per year [95% CI, −3.61 to −4.14]) between the telmisartan/lisinopril and placebo/lisinopril treatment arms. The incidence of hyperkalemia ($K > 5.6$ mEq/L) was low overall and was not different between the with ARB/ACE-I and ACE-I treatment arms, at nine versus five events, respectively, over the course of the study. AKI (sCr increase ≥0.3 mg/dL) occurred in 9% and 12.3% of the ARB/ACE-I versus ACE-I treatment arms, respectively. Combination RAAS blockade also had no effect on hospitalization for cardiovascular disorders as compared with ACE-I monotherapy (2.30 events per 100 person-years and 1.28 events per 100 person-years, respectively) nor on other secondary outcomes of pain or health-related quality of life.

An interesting observation from both trials was the small number of antihypertensive agents that was needed to control BP. An ACE-I alone or ACE-I/ARB combination controlled BP in 67% and 83% percent of Study A patients in the low or standard BP goals, respectively, while in Study B, 62 and 53% of patients in the ACE-I alone and ARB/ACE-I arms were controlled with RAAS blockers only. This compares to the CRIC study where only 15 and 25% of patients with similar GFR as Study B were treated with 1 or 2 classes of antihypertensive drugs, respectively, and only 46% of them had BP < 130/80 mm Hg [48]. One potential explanation for why BP was so much easier to control in the ADPKD patients as compared with other CKD patients is because therapy was based on home measurements which run lower than office readings, the latter used in most studies. Interestingly, the office and home readings were not far apart in the HALT Study, as can be seen in the baseline data [49]. Alternatively, the ease at which BP was controlled in the HALT Study supports the postulate that RAAS is etiologic in the hypertension of ADPKD.

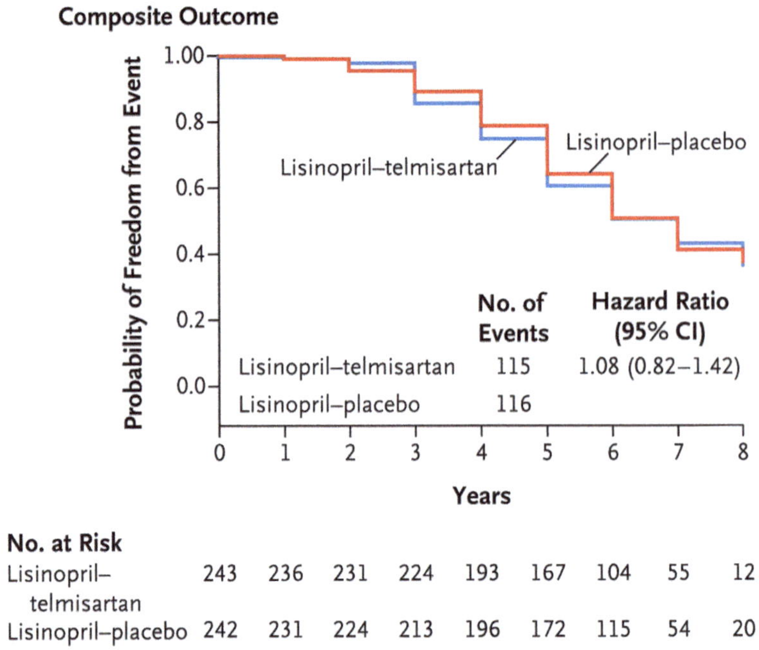

Fig. 12.5 Effects of dual RAAS blockade with ARB/ACE versus ACE-I monotherapy on time to 50% decline in eGFR, ESRD, or death in ADPKD patients with baseline eGFR 25–60 mL/min/1.73 m^2 (From The New England Journal of Medicine, Torres VE, Abebe KZ, Chapman AB, Schrier RW, Braun WE, Steinman TI, Winklhofer FT, Brosnahan G, Czarnecki PG, Hogan MC, Miskulin DC, Rahbari-Oskoui FF, Grantham JJ, Harris PC, Flessner MF, Bae KT, Moore CG, Perrone RD, Blood Pressure in Early Autosomal Dominant Polycystic Kidney Disease. Volume 371, Page 2271. Copyright © (2014) Massachusetts Medical Society. Reprinted with permission. http://www.nejm.org/doi/full/10.1056/NEJMoa1402686)

Conclusions

There are no well-designed trials that have compared RAAS blockers with other antihypertensive classes on kidney outcomes in ADPKD. However, extrapolating from other trials in CKD showing benefits in reducing progression, including relatively non-proteinuric forms of CKD [50] and the theoretical benefit of reducing the hyperfiltration injury that would be expected with declining functional nephron mass in a progressive form of CKD, plus the fact that these drugs are well tolerated and are very effective at controlling BP (as seen in the HALT Studies), it seems reasonable to use RAAS blockers as first-line agents for hypertensive treatment in ADPKD. Strong evidence from the HALT-PKD Studies shows no benefit of dual blockade of the RAAS with ACE-I/ARB in early (eGFR >60 mL/min) or late (eGFR 20–60 mL/min) disease as compared with ACE-I monotherapy on eGFR decline and no effect on TKV growth or LVMI in early disease. Because of the lack of benefit of combination ACEi/ARB therapy, and because the risks of hyperkalemia and AKI in a closely monitored clinical trial may not be representative of routine clinical practice, dual blockade of the RAAS is not recommended. Intensive BP lowering to <110/70 mm Hg as compared with 120–130/80 mm Hg in early ADPKD (eGFR >60 mL/min) was associated with a reduction in TKV growth and LVMI. Based on this evidence, ADPKD patients with GFR >60 mL/min should be treated to BP <110/70 mm Hg. Treating to the low BP goal in patients with more advanced disease is not recommended because of the potential for AKI or accelerated GFR decline as a result of severe reductions in blood flow in tortuous blood vessels that are compressed by surrounding cysts, that are characteristic in advanced ADPKD. Low BP could also cause syncope in older patients who may suffer imbalance because of abdominal distension from the massive organomegaly as well as the physical disability that accompanies late stages of CKD.

References

1. Dalgaard OZ. Bilateral polycystic disease of the kidneys: a follow-up of two hundred and eighty-four patients and their families. Acta Med Scand. 1957;328(S1):1–255.
2. Barrett BJ, Foley R, Morgan J, Hefferton D, Parfrey P. Differences in hormonal and renal vascular responses between normotensive patients with autosomal dominant polycystic kidney disease and unaffected family members. Kidney Int. 1994;46(4):1118–23.
3. Ecder T, Edelstein CL, Fick-Brosnahan GM, et al. Diuretics versus angiotensin-converting enzyme inhibitors in autosomal dominant polycystic kidney disease. Am J Nephrol. 2001;21(2):98–103.
4. Graham PC, Lindop GB. The anatomy of the renin-secreting cell in adult polycystic kidney disease. Kidney Int. 1988;33(6):1084–90.
5. Gabow PA, Chapman AB, Johnson AM, et al. Renal structure and hypertension in autosomal dominant polycystic kidney disease. Kidney Int. 1990;38:1177–80.
6. Chapman AB, Guay-Woodford LM, Grantham JJ, et al. Renal structure in early autosomal-dominant polycystic kidney disease (ADPKD): the Consortium for Radiologic Imaging Studies of Polycystic Kidney Disease (CRISP) cohort. Kidney Int. 2003;64(3):1035–45.
7. Ecder T, Schrier RW. Hypertension in autosomal-dominant polycystic kidney disease: early occurrence and unique aspects. J Am Soc Nephrol. 2001;12(1):194–200.
8. Torres VE, Donovan KA, Scicli G, et al. Synthesis of renin by tubulocystic epithelium in autosomal-dominant polycystic kidney disease. Kidney Int. 1992;42(2):364–73.
9. Loghman-Adham M, Soto CE, Inagami T, Cassis L. The intrarenal renin-angiotensin system in autosomal dominant polycystic kidney disease. Am J Physiol Ren Physiol. 2004;287(4):F775–88.
10. Thomas W, Dooley R, Harvey BJ. Aldosterone as a renal growth factor. Steroids. 2010;75:550–4.
11. Watanabe G, Lee RJ, Albanese C, Rainey WE, Batlle D, Pestell RG. Angiotensin II activation of cyclin D1-dependent kinase activity. J Biol Chem. 1996;271:22570–7.
12. Chapman AB, Johnson A, Gabow PA, Schrier RW. The renin-angiotensin-aldosterone system and autosomal dominant polycystic kidney disease. N Engl J Med. 1990;323(16):1091–6.
13. Bell PE, Hossack KF, Gabow PA, Durr JA, Johnson AM, Schrier RW. Hypertension in autosomal dominant polycystic kidney disease. Kidney Int. 1988;34(5):683–90.
14. Anderson R, Miller P, Linas S, Katz F, Holmes J. Role of the renin-angiotensin system in hypertension of polycystic kidney-disease. Mineral Electrolyte Metab. 1979;2:137–41.
15. Nash DA Jr. Hypertension in polycystic kidney disease without renal failure. Arch Intern Med. 1977;137(11):1571–5.
16. Valvo E, Gammaro L, Tessitore N, et al. Hypertension of polycystic kidney disease: mechanisms and hemodynamic alterations. Am J Nephrol. 1985;5(3):176–81.
17. Watson ML, Macnicol AM, Allan PL, Wright AF. Effects of angiotensin converting enzyme inhibition in adult polycystic kidney disease. Kidney Int. 1992;41(1):206–10.
18. Jia G, Kwon M, Liang HL, et al. Chronic treatment with lisinopril decreases proliferative and apoptotic pathways in autosomal recessive polycystic kidney disease. Pediatr Nephrol. 2010;25(6):1139–46.
19. Cadnapaphornchai MA, McFann K, Strain JD, Masoumi A, Schrier RW. Prospective change in renal volume and function in children with ADPKD. Clin J Am Soc Nephrol: CJASN. 2009;4(4):820–9.
20. Ecder T, Chapman AB, Brosnahan GM, Edelstein CL, Johnson AM, Schrier RW. Effect of antihypertensive therapy on renal function and urinary albumin excretion in hypertensive patients with autosomal dominant polycystic kidney disease. Am J Kidney Dis. 2000;35(3):427–32.
21. Mitobe M, Yoshida T, Sugiura H, et al. Clinical effects of calcium channel blockers and renin-angiotensin-aldosterone system inhibitors on changes in the estimated glomerular filtration rate in patients with polycystic kidney disease. Clin Exp Nephrol. 2010;14(6):573–7.
22. Maschio G, Alberti D, Janin G, et al. The Angiotensin-Converting-Enzyme Inhibition in Progressive Renal Insufficiency Study Group. Effect of the angiotensin-converting-enzyme inhibitor benazepril on the progression of chronic renal insufficiency. N Engl J Med. 1996;334(15):939–45.
23. Jafar TH, Stark PC, Schmid CH, et al. The effect of angiotensin-converting-enzyme inhibitors on progression of advanced polycystic kidney disease. Kidney Int. 2005;67(1):265–71.
24. van Dijk MA, Breuning MH, Duiser R, van Es LA, Westendorp RGJ. No effect of enalapril on progression in autosomal dominant polycystic kidney disease. Nephrol Dial Transpl. 2003;18(11):2314–20.
25. Zeltner R, Poliak R, Stiasny B, Schmieder RE, Schulze BD. Renal and cardiac effects of antihypertensive treatment with ramipril vs metoprolol in autosomal dominant polycystic kidney disease. Nephrol Dial Transpl. 2008;23(2):573–9.
26. Schrier R, McFann K, Johnson A, et al. Cardiac and renal effects of standard versus rigorous blood pressure control in autosomal-dominant polycystic kidney disease: results of a seven-year prospective randomized study. J Am Soc Nephrol. 2002;13(7):1733–9.
27. Nakamura T, Sato E, Fujiwara N, et al. Changes in urinary albumin excretion, inflammatory and oxidative stress markers in ADPKD patients with hypertension. Am J Med Sci. 2012;343(1):46–51.

28. Stallone G, Infante B, Grandaliano G, et al. Rapamycin for treatment of type I autosomal dominant polycystic kidney disease (RAPYD-study): a randomized, controlled study. Nephrol Dial Transpl. 2012;27(9):3560–7.
29. Soliman AR, Ismail E, Zamil S, Lotfy A. Sirolimus therapy for patients with adult polycystic kidney disease: a pilot study. Transplant Proc. 2009;41(9):3639–41.
30. Soliman A, Zamil S, Lotfy A, Ismail E. Sirolimus produced S-shaped effect on adult polycystic kidneys after 2-year treatment. Transplant Proc. 2012;44(10):2936–9.
31. Navar LG, Harrison-Bernard LM, Nishiyama A, Kobori H. Regulation of intrarenal angiotensin II in hypertension. Hypertension. 2002;39(2 Pt 2):316–22.
32. Warnock DG. Prevention, protection, and the intrarenal renin-angiotensin systems. Semin Nephrol. 2001;21(6):593–602.
33. Susantitaphong P, Sewaralthahab K, Balk EM, Eiam-ong S, Madias NE, Jaber BL. Efficacy and safety of combined vs. single renin-angiotensin-aldosterone system blockade in chronic kidney disease: a meta-analysis. Am J Hypertension. 2013;26(3):424–41.
34. Doulton TW, He FJ, MacGregor GA. Systematic review of combined angiotensin-converting enzyme inhibition and angiotensin receptor blockade in hypertension. Hypertension. 2005;45(5):880–6.
35. Yusuf S, Teo KK, Pogue J, et al. Telmisartan, ramipril, or both in patients at high risk for vascular events. N Engl J Med. 2008;358(15):1547–59.
36. Jennings DL, Kalus JS, Coleman CI, Manierski C, Yee J. Combination therapy with an ACE inhibitor and an angiotensin receptor blocker for diabetic nephropathy: a meta-analysis. Diabet Med: J Br Diabet Assoc. 2007;24(5):486–93.
37. Kunz R, Friedrich C, Wolbers M, Mann JF. Meta-analysis: effect of monotherapy and combination therapy with inhibitors of the renin angiotensin system on proteinuria in renal disease. Ann Intern Med. 2008;148(1):30–48.
38. MacKinnon M, Shurraw S, Akbari A, Knoll GA, Jaffey J, Clark HD. Combination therapy with an angiotensin receptor blocker and an ACE inhibitor in proteinuric renal disease: a systematic review of the efficacy and safety data. Am J Kidney Dis: Off J Natl Kidney Found. 2006;48(1):8–20.
39. Fried LF, Emanuele N, Zhang JH, et al. Combined angiotensin inhibition for the treatment of diabetic nephropathy. N Engl J Med. 2013;369(20):1892–903.
40. McPherson EA, Luo Z, Brown RA, et al. Chymase-like angiotensin II-generating activity in end-stage human autosomal dominant polycystic kidney disease. J Am Soc Nephrol: JASN. 2004;15(2):493–500.
41. Ruiz-Ortega M, Egido J. Angiotensin II modulates cell growth-related events and synthesis of matrix proteins in renal interstitial fibroblasts. Kidney Int. 1997;52(6):1497–510.
42. Rosenberg ME, Hostetter TH. Effect of angiotensin II and norepinephrine on early growth response genes in the rat kidney. Kidney Int. 1993;43(3):601–9.
43. Burdmann EA, Andoh TF, Nast CC, et al. Prevention of experimental cyclosporin-induced interstitial fibrosis by losartan and enalapril. Am J Phys. 1995;269(4 Pt 2):F491–9.
44. Zoja C, Donadelli R, Corna D, et al. The renoprotective properties of angiotensin-converting enzyme inhibitors in a chronic model of membranous nephropathy are solely due to the inhibition of angiotensin II: evidence based on comparative studies with a receptor antagonist. Am J Kidney Dis: Off J Natl Kidney Found. 1997;29(2):254–64.
45. Schrier RW, Abebe KZ, Perrone RD, Torres VE, Braun WE, Steinman TI, Winklhofer FT, Brosnahan G, Czarnecki PG, Hogan MC, Miskulin DC, Rahbari-Oskoui FF, Grantham JJ, Harris PC, Flessner MF, Bae KT, Moore CG, Chapman AB. Blood pressure in early autosomal dominant polycystic kidney disease. N Engl J Med. 2014;371:2255–66.
46. Torres VE, Abebe KZ, Chapman AB, Schrier RW, Braun WE, Steinman TI, Winklhofer FT, Brosnahan G, Czarnecki PG, Hogan MC, Miskulin DC, Rahbari-Oskoui FF, Grantham JJ, Harris PC, Flessner MF, Bae KT, Moore CG, Chapman AB, Perrone RD. Angiotensin blockade in late autosomal dominant polycystic kidney disease. N Engl J Med. 2014;371:2267–76.
47. Torres VE, Chapman AB, Devuyst O, et al. Tolvaptan in patients with autosomal dominant polycystic kidney disease. N Engl J Med. 2012;367:2407–18.
48. Muntner P, Anderson A, Charleston J, et al. Hypertension awareness, treatment, and control in adults with CKD: results from the Chronic Renal Insufficiency Cohort (CRIC) study. Am J Kidney Dis: Off J Natl Kidney Found. 2010;55:441–51.
49. Torres VE, Chapman AB, Perrone RD, et al. Analysis of baseline parameters in the HALT polycystic kidney disease trials. Kidney Int. 2012;81(6):577–85.
50. Wright JT, Bakris G, Greene T, et al. Effect of blood pressure lowering and antihypertensive drug class on progression of hypertensive kidney disease: results from the AASK trial. JAMA. 2002;288:2421–33.
51. Marin R, Ruilope LM, Aljama P, et al. A random comparison of fosinopril and nifedipine GITS in patients with primary renal disease. J Hypertens. 2001;19(10):1871–6.

13 Vasopressin Receptor Antagonism in PKD

Maria V. Irazabal and Vicente E. Torres

Introduction

Autosomal dominant polycystic kidney disease (ADPKD) is a systemic disorder where progressive development and enlargement of kidney cysts lead to renal complications including progression to end-stage renal disease (ESRD). Cyst development starts in utero and continues through the patients' lifetime. Most of the patients present with bilateral and diffuse involvement of the kidneys which usually maintain a reniform shape even though they can reach more than 20 times the normal kidney volume.

The *PKD1* and *PKD2* genes encode the glycoproteins polycystin-1 (PC1) and polycystin-2 (PC2), respectively. Together, both proteins form a complex that is believed to function as a transient receptor potential (TRP) channel involved in the regulation of intracellular calcium homeostasis [1, 2].

The main phenotypic changes observed in ADPKD result from the reduction in one of the polycystins (PC1 or PC2) beyond a critical level and are characterized by the inability to maintain planar cell polarity (PCP), an increase in proliferation and apoptosis, the expression of a secretory phenotype, and remodeling of the extracellular matrix. The principal signaling pathways implicated in these phenotypic changes include the intracellular deregulation of calcium homeostasis, cyclic adenosine monophosphate (cAMP) accumulation and activation of protein kinase A (PKA), activation of mitogen-activated protein kinase (MAPK) and mammalian target of rapamycin (mTOR) kinases, and canonical Wnt signaling and other intracellular signaling mechanisms [3–5].

Role of Calcium and cAMP in ADPKD

Cyclic AMP signaling has been shown to play a central role in the pathogenesis of ADPKD, and intracellular levels of cAMP have been found to be increased in many animal models, not only in the kidney but also in other tissues affected by the disease, including cholangiocytes [6], vascular smooth muscle [7], and choroid plexus [8]. The levels of cAMP are tightly regulated by the activity of soluble and G-protein-coupled receptor (GPCR)-associated adenylyl cyclases (ACs), and phosphodiesterases (PDEs). Many hypotheses have been proposed to explain the increased levels of cAMP, most of which are related to altered calcium signaling. A reduction in intracellular calcium concentration, due to the dis-

M. V. Irazabal, MD · V. E. Torres, MD, PhD (✉)
Division of Nephrology and Hypertension,
Mayo Clinic, Rochester, MN, USA
e-mail: Irazabal.maria@mayo.edu;
torres.vicente@mayo.edu

B. D. Cowley, Jr., J. J. Bissler (eds.), *Polycystic Kidney Disease*,
https://doi.org/10.1007/978-1-4939-7784-0_13

ruption of the polycystins, inhibits directly the activity of calcium-/calmodulin-dependent PDE1 and indirectly PDE3, in addition to activating membrane-bound calcium-inhibitable AC6, hence, producing a net increase in cAMP concentration. Depletion of calcium in the endoplasmic reticulum (ER) may also induce the assembly of stromal interaction molecule 1 (STIM1) and concomitant activation of AC6 [9]. Additionally, a dysfunctional ciliary protein complex (encompassing A-kinase anchoring protein 150, AC5/AC6, PC2, PDE4C, and PKA) may result in activation of AC5/AC6 (due to decreased calcium influx through PC2) and inhibition of PDE4C (due to mutations in HNF-1β), thus increasing cAMP (Fig. 13.1) [10].

The main effects of increased cAMP levels are through activation of PKA and downstream effectors. The Wnt signaling pathways are required for normal epithelial tubulogenesis. At early stages, the canonical Wnt/β-catenin pathway is required for metanephric mesenchymal to epithelial transition; however, noncanonical Wnt/PCP signaling is required later to establish and maintain the normal tubules [11]. PKA is known to enhance Wnt/β-catenin signaling, and this sustained activation interferes with nephrogenesis and results in disorganized epithelial clusters and dilated renal tubules. Under normal conditions, PKA signaling inhibits cellular proliferation through inhibition of MAPK signaling. However, when intracellular calcium levels are reduced such as in PKD, PKA activates MAPK kinase (MEK) in a Src, Ras, and B-raf-dependent manner. Successively, MEK phosphorylates and activates MAPK, also known as extracellular signal-regulated kinase (ERK) [12, 13]. Furthermore, PKA has been shown to activate mTOR [14, 15] (via ERK-mediated phosphorylation of tuberin), which regulates a variety of cellular processes involved with growth, proliferation, and autophagy [16]. In addition, PKA mediates upregulation of cAMP response element-binding protein (CREB) [17], paired box gene 2 (Pax2) [18], and signal transducer and activator of transcription 3 (STAT3) [3, 19], all likely contributors to the proliferative phenotype of the cystic epithelium.

Once renal cysts reach a diameter of approximately 2 mm, they detach from the original tubular segment, and additional growth is dependent on transepithelial fluid secretion. Studies have shown that cAMP signaling contributes to the hypersecretory phenotype observed in PKD. Fluid secretion was induced by treatment with forskolin, in intact cysts excised from patients with ADPKD [20]. The bulk of this fluid secretion is driven by the active transport of chloride into the lumen of the cyst [21, 22], which is drawn across the basolateral membrane epithelium by the combined activity of the Na^+K^+ATPase and the $Na^+K^+Cl^-$ cotransporter. PKA phosphorylates the cystic fibrosis transmembrane conductance regulator (CFTR), inducing the opening of its channel which allows chloride ions to flow down the electrochemical gradient and into the cyst [23]. The role of CFTR channels in PKD has been supported by the observation that pathogenic mutations of the CFTR in the context of PKD attenuate cyst growth by preventing fluid accumulation within the cyst lumen [24] and patients concomitantly affected with cystic fibrosis and ADPKD present a milder cystic phenotype [25, 26].

Vasopressin and Vasopressin Receptors in ADPKD

The antidiuretic hormone, arginine vasopressin (AVP), is a small 9 amino acid peptide secreted by the posterior pituitary gland in response to increased plasma osmolality but also a decrease in plasma volume. The precursor of AVP is a 164 amino acid peptide synthesized in the hypothalamus and cleaved into three peptides, mature AVP, neurophysin, and copeptin, during its descent along the axons of the pituitary stalk.

The effects of AVP occur through the stimulation of G-protein-coupled receptors (GPCRs) present on different cell types. The V1a and V1b receptors are coupled to Gαq proteins and activate a calcium signaling pathway, while the AVP V2 receptors (V2R) are coupled to Gαs proteins and activate a cAMP pathway.

The V1a receptors are present in several organs (Fig. 13.2) including the kidney (vasa recta, medullary interstitial cells). The binding of AVP to V1a results in a decrease in blood

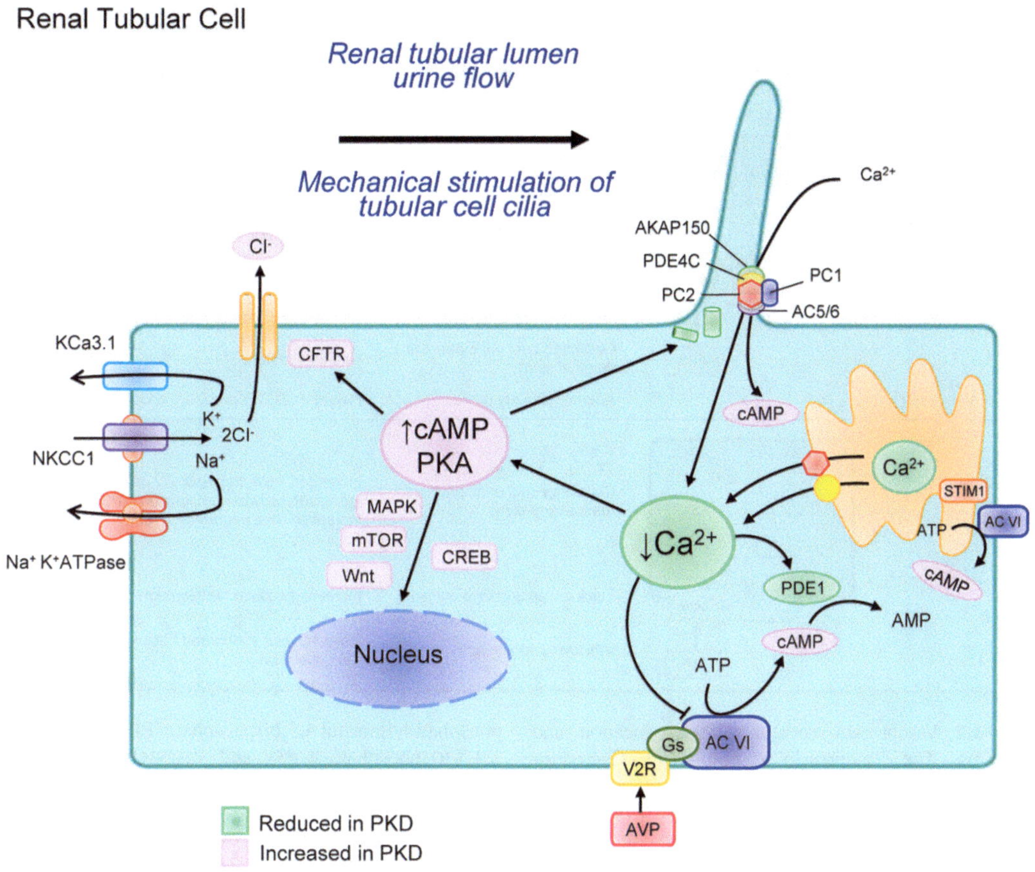

Fig. 13.1 Diagram depicting the central role of reduced intracellular calcium and increased cAMP signaling in PKD. Increased levels of cAMP may be explained as follows: (1) a reduction in intracellular calcium inhibits directly the activity of calcium-/calmodulin-dependent PDE1 and indirectly cGMP-inhibitable PDE3, in addition to activating membrane-bound calcium-inhibitable AC6, producing a net increase in cAMP concentration. (2) A dysfunctional ciliary protein complex (encompassing A-kinase anchoring protein 150, AC5/AC6, PC2, PDE4C, and PKA) may result in activation of AC5/AC6 (due to decreased calcium influx through PC2) and inhibition of PDE4C (due to mutations in HNF-1β). (3) Depletion of calcium in the endoplasmic reticulum may also induce the assembly of stromal interaction molecule 1 (STIM1) and concomitant activation of AC6. Increased cAMP levels results in hyperactivation of cAMP/PKA signaling leading to disruption in tubulogenesis (enhanced Wnt/b-catenin signaling); stimulation of chloride and fluid secretion (CFTR phosphorylation); activation of proliferative signaling pathways, including mitogen-activated protein kinase/extracellularly regulated kinase (MAPK/ERK), mTOR, and b-catenin signaling; and activation of many transcription factors, such as cAMP response element-binding protein (CREB), paired box gene 2 (Pax2), and signal transducer and activator of transcription 3 (STAT3)

flow to the inner medulla and stimulation of prostaglandin synthesis. The V1b receptor stimulates the release of adrenocorticotropin from the anterior pituitary. The V2R is expressed in the kidney tubule, predominantly in the thick ascending limb of Henle (TALH) and collecting ducts (CD), where its primary function in response to AVP is to concentrate the urine. The binding of AVP to the V2R stimulates membrane-bound AC6, increasing the levels of cAMP which in turn activates PKA leading to the phosphorylation of several proteins including aquaporin-2 (AQP2). Subsequently, AQP2 accumulates in the apical plasma membrane of CD principal cells, increasing transepithelial water permeability and facilitating osmotically driven water reabsorption.

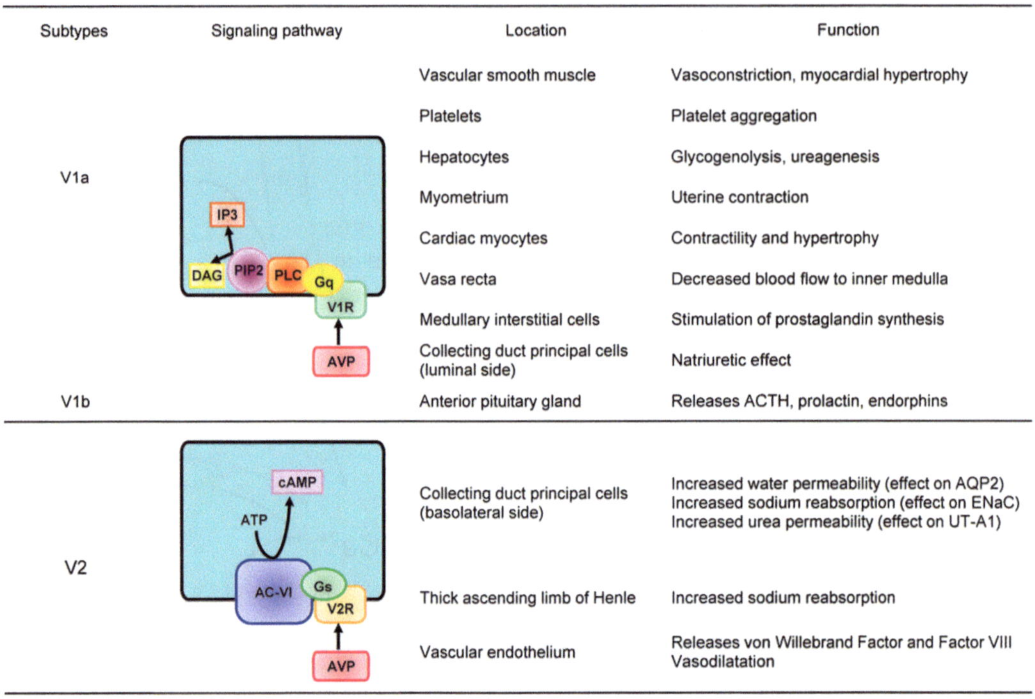

Fig. 13.2 Vasopressin receptor subtypes, location, and functions. The vasopressin receptors are G-protein-coupled receptors (GPCRs) with unique tissue distributions and functions. The binding of AVP to V1a and V1b stimulates phospholipase C (PLC), hydrolyzing phosphatidylinositol 4,5-bisphosphate (PIP2) into inositol 1,4,5-trisphosphate (IP3) and diacylglycerol (DAG), while activation of V2 stimulates membrane-bound AC6, increasing the levels of cAMP

The presence of impaired urinary concentrating capacity is common among patients with ADPKD even at a young age, and the severity has been shown to correlate with kidney volume [27]. A distortion in the renal architecture due to cysts, causing a defective medullary osmotic gradient, thus reducing the ability to reabsorb water, has been the most common mechanism proposed for this [27]. However, previous studies in rodents [28] and children with ADPKD [29] have shown that the urinary concentrating defect may precede renal cyst development, suggesting other possible mechanisms.

The urinary concentrating defect and elevated vasopressin levels contribute to cystogenesis. Recently, plasma copeptin levels, co-secreted in equimolar amounts with AVP, have been associated with disease severity in a cross-sectional analysis of 102 ADPKD (CKD 1–4) subjects [30] and with renal enlargement and GFR decline in a 3-year longitudinal study of 241 ADPKD (CKD 1–2) subjects [31].

Vasopressin Receptor Antagonism in the Treatment of ADPKD

Cysts in ARPKD and ADPKD derive predominantly from CD and distal nephron, which express V2R and are sensitive to AVP. AVP acting on V2R is the main AC agonist in CD. The important role of AVP through its secondary messenger cAMP and further activation of PKA in the pathogenesis of PKD provide an opportunity as therapeutic targets.

Two different approaches can be considered in order to reduce the detrimental effects of circulating AVP. One is to centrally modulate its secretion, which could be achieved by increasing water intake and continuously maintaining the osmolality of the urine <250–300 mOsm/kg H_2O. A study in the PCK rat (ARPKD model) showed that suppression of AVP secretion by increasing water intake (3.5-fold increase in urine output) attenuated PKD progression [32, 33]. Moreover, almost complete inhibition of cystogenesis was observed in PCK rats lacking circulating AVP (generated by crossing PCK and Brattleboro rats), and a fully rescued cystic phenotype was achieved with the administration of V2R agonist 1-desamino-8-d-arginine-vasopressin (DDAVP) [34]. However, patients with ADPKD may find increasing water intake a difficult prescription with which to comply in the long term and may increase the risk for hyponatremia.

Another option is to pharmacologically block the V2R. The almost exclusive localization of V2R to the distal nephron and CD provides opportunities for treatment with relative safety and may be more effective than suppressing AVP secretion by increasing water ingestion. Preclinical studies supported further investigation of V2R antagonism as a potential therapy for PKD.

V2R antagonists mozavaptan and tolvaptan attenuated PKD progression in rodent models of nephronophthisis (pcy mouse), ARPKD (PCK rat), PKD2 (*Pkd2*$^{WS25/-}$-mouse), and PKD1 (when treatment started shortly after induction of *Pkd1* knockout) [35–39]. Satavaptan blocked tubular expression of sFRP4, a secreted frizzled-related protein that affects Wnt signaling, is overexpressed in polycystic kidneys, and promotes cystogenesis of zebrafish pronephros [40]. Further, tolvaptan inhibited AVP-induced chloride secretion and cyst growth of human ADPKD cells in collagen matrices [41].

Clinical Trials Evaluating V2R Antagonists in ADPKD

Tolvaptan is an orally effective, highly potent, and selective AVP V2R antagonist, inducing free water clearance. It is currently approved by the US Food and Drug Administration (FDA) for the treatment of hypervolemic or euvolemic hyponatremia (≤125 mEq/L or symptomatic and resistant) in the syndrome of inappropriate secretion of antidiuretic hormone (SIADH) and heart failure, by the European Medicines Agency (EMA) for hyponatremia associated with SIADH and by the Pharmaceuticals and Medical Devices Agency (PMDA) in Japan for the treatment of volume overload resistant to diuretics in heart failure and of fluid retention resistant to diuretics in hepatic cirrhosis.

Preliminary dosing studies in patients with ADPKD showed that split-dose administration of tolvaptan was more effective, compared to a single dose, in achieving sustained suppression of vasopressin action, evidenced by 24-h urine osmolality decrease to <300 mOsm/L.

Two phase 2, open-label, multicenter clinical trials, in North America and Japan, were conducted to determine the long-term safety, tolerability, and efficacy of split-dose tolvaptan over 3 years. Forty-six patients in the United States were randomized to either 45/15 (n = 22) or 60/30 (n = 24) mg daily, split doses of tolvaptan, after an initial 2-month titration phase to determine efficacy (Uosm persistently <300 mOsm/kg in 70% and 77% of patients, respectively) and self-reported tolerability (for the rest of life in 96% and 61% of patients, respectively). Seventeen patients in Japan received a 15/15-mg split dose. Patient safety was assessed by regular monitoring of adverse events (AEs), directed physical examinations, vital signs, laboratory tests, and electrocardiogram measurements. AEs were mainly related to the aquaretic effect of tolvaptan and natural history of ADPKD. Twelve patients (19%) withdrew from the study, and AE was the reason in half of those cases. Efficacy was assessed by changes in total kidney volume (TKV) and eGFR and compared to historical control patients from the CRISP and MDRD studies that were matched by gender, hypertension, age, and baseline TKV or eGFR. Baseline TKV (controls 1422, tolvaptan 1635 mL) and eGFR (both 62 mL/min/1.73 m^2) were similar. The long-term treatment of patients with tolvaptan was associated with a slower increase in TKV (1.7% vs. 5.8% per year, $p < 0.001$) and slower decrease in eGFR (−0.71 vs. −2.1 ml/min/1.73 m^2 per year, $p = 0.01$) when compared with historical control ADPKD patients [42].

Transient increases in serum creatinine and uric acid observed during the phase 2 clinical trials prompted further investigation of the possible mechanisms of these changes by studying renal hemodynamics and function. A study involving 20 patients with ADPKD and estimated creatinine clearances by the Cockcroft–Gault equation ≥30 ml/min was conducted to determine the short-term effects of tolvaptan on renal function, when administered at a daily split dose of 45/15-mg for 1 week. Tolvaptan-induced aquaresis was accompanied by an 8.6% reduction in iothalamate clearance and by a 13% increase in serum uric acid without a significant change in renal blood flow as measured by para-aminohippurate clearance or MRI. A blinded post hoc analysis of renal MRIs showed that tolvaptan significantly reduced TKV by 3.1% ($p < 0.001$) and individual cyst volume by 1.6% ($p < 0.001$), likely due to its antisecretory action and more noticeably in patients with GFR ≥60 ml/min per 1.73 m^2 [43]. More recently, a study including 27 patients with ADPKD and CKD stages 1 through 4 studied the effects of tolvaptan at 90/30 mg split dose daily for 3 weeks on renal function. The study showed a significant decrease in GFR (7.8 and 4.3 ml/min per 1.73 m^2, $p < 0.05$) in patients with baseline GFR >60 and 30–60 ml/min per 1.73 m^2, respectively, without a significant change in those subjects with baseline eGFR <30 ml/min per 1.73 m^2 (0.7 ml/min per 1.73 m^2). These changes were reversible after withdrawal of tolvaptan. Changes in effective renal plasma flow and filtration fraction were not different between patients with lower compared to higher baseline GFR [44]. Further analysis on efficacy parameters showed a significant ($p < 0.001$) decrease in TKV by 3.7% after 3 weeks treatment. Only TKV remained slightly but significantly lower than the baseline value (1.7%, $p = 0.006$) 3 weeks after withdrawal of tolvaptan. The changes in urine volume, free water clearance, urine osmolality, and TKV were less pronounced in participants with lower baseline GFRs [45].

The largest clinical study conducted in patients with ADPKD to date is the Tolvaptan Efficacy and Safety in Management of ADPKD and its Outcomes (TEMPO) 3:4. This study was a phase 3, multicenter, randomized, double-blinded, placebo-controlled, parallel-group clinical study, designed to assess the impact of tolvaptan therapy on the progression of ADPKD [46]. One thousand four hundred and forty five patients with ADPKD, between 18 and 50 years old, with a baseline TKV >750 mL and CrCL>60 mL/min, were enrolled in the study between January 2007 and January 2009, across 129 sites worldwide. Patients were randomized 2:1 to tolvaptan or placebo ($n = 961$ and $n = 483$; one withdrawal pretreatment) with a daily split dose of 45/15 mg titrated at weekly intervals to 60/30 and 90/30 mg, and the maximally tolerated dose was maintained for 3 years. MRIs were acquired yearly, whereas serum creatinine and other laboratory parameters were measured every 4 months. One thousand one hundred and fifty seven patients completed all 3 years of the trial, corresponding to 77% and 86.2% of the tolvaptan and placebo group, respectively. Fifteen percent of the subjects withdrawing in the tolvaptan group was due to adverse events (including aquaresis-related symptoms in 8%), compared to 5% of the subjects treated with placebo (including aquaresis-related symptoms in 0.4%). In the tolvaptan group, therapy consisted of either a high dose (90/30 mg/day, $n = 404$), medium dose (60/30 mg/day, $n = 157$), or low dose (45/15 mg/day, $n = 179$), with high rates of self-reported adherence in the majority of patients. For the primary efficacy analysis, 1307 patients having at least one follow-up MRI were included, while all 1445 patients were included for the secondary safety analysis.

Results showed a reduction in the rate of kidney growth by 49% with tolvaptan during the 3-year trial; TKV increased an average of 2.8% per year in patients treated with tolvaptan versus 5.5% per year growth rate in the placebo group ($p < 0.001$). Treatment effect was greatest from baseline to year 1 but continued to be significant from year 1 to year 2 and from year 2 to year 3. Prespecified subgroup analysis, including stratification by sex, age, diagnosis of hypertension, baseline TKV, and baseline creatinine clearance, showed that tolvaptan had a beneficial effect on TKV in all subgroups. However, this effect was nominally greater in patients 35 years of age or older and those with hypertension and/

or a TKV of greater or equal to 1500 mL. The administration of tolvaptan was also associated with a reduction in the rate of renal function decline measured by the slope of the reciprocal of serum creatinine from −3.81 (mg per milliliter)$^{-1}$ per year on placebo to −2.61 (mg per milliliter)$^{-1}$ per year on tolvaptan ($p < 0.001$) and by the change in the average serum creatinine from pretreatment to posttreatment after discontinuation of the study drug (1.04–1.27 mg/dL in the placebo compared to 1.05–1.21 mg/dL in the tolvaptan-treated patients, $p < 0.001$). The analysis of a secondary composite endpoint showed fewer ADPKD-related events per 100 person-years of follow-up with tolvaptan than placebo (hazard ratio 0.87, 95% CI. 0.78–0.97, $p = 0.01$). This result was driven by fewer events of renal function decline and kidney pain, but no effect of treatment was detected on hypertension or albuminuria events.

Aquaresis-related adverse events (thirst, polyuria, nocturia, and polydipsia) were more frequent in the tolvaptan group, whereas ADPKD-related adverse events (kidney pain, hematuria, urinary tract infection, and back pain) were more frequent in the placebo group. Elevations of serum sodium and uric acid were observed more frequently in the patients treated with tolvaptan, but these were not considered to be severe. Elevations of alanine aminotransferase of potential clinical significance were also observed more frequently in the patients treated with tolvaptan than in those receiving placebo (4.9% vs. 1.2%). Two patients in the tolvaptan group had concurrent elevations in the alanine aminotransferase or aspartate aminotransferase level (>3 times the upper limit of the normal range) and of the bilirubin level (>2 times the upper limit of the normal range) which resolved after discontinuation of the drug.

Based on these results, tolvaptan has been approved in Japan, Canada, and Europe as a therapy for ADPKD with CKD stages 1–3 and rapidly progressive disease. In the United States, tolvaptan is not currently approved as a therapy for ADPKD and should not be administered outside of an approved research study.

References

1. Vassilev PM, Guo L, Chen XZ, Segal Y, Peng JB, Basora N, et al. Polycystin-2 is a novel cation channel implicated in defective intracellular Ca(2+) homeostasis in polycystic kidney disease. Biochem Biophys Res Commun. 2001;282(1):341–50.
2. Anyatonwu GI, Ehrlich BE. Organic cation permeation through the channel formed by polycystin-2. J Biol Chem. 2005;280(33):29488–93.
3. Torres VE, Harris PC. Strategies targeting cAMP signaling in the treatment of polycystic kidney disease. J Am Soc Nephrol. 2014;25:18–32.
4. Yamaguchi T, Hempson SJ, Reif GA, Hedge AM, Wallace DP. Calcium restores a normal proliferation phenotype in human polycystic kidney disease epithelial cells. J Am Soc Nephrol. 2006;17(1):178–87.
5. Paavola J, Schliffke S, Rossetti S, Kuo IY, Yuan S, Sun Z, et al. Polycystin-2 mutations lead to impaired calcium cycling in the heart and predispose to dilated cardiomyopathy. J Mol Cell Cardiol. 2013;58:199–208.
6. Masyuk TV, Masyuk AI, Torres VE, Harris PC, Larusso NF. Octreotide inhibits hepatic cystogenesis in a rodent model of polycystic liver disease by reducing cholangiocyte adenosine 3′,5′-cyclic monophosphate. Gastroenterology. 2007;132(3):1104–16.
7. Kip SN, Hunter LW, Ren Q, Harris PC, Somlo S, Torres VE, et al. [Ca2+]i reduction increases cellular proliferation and apoptosis in vascular smooth muscle cells: relevance to the ADPKD phenotype. Circ Res. 2005;96(8):873–80.
8. Banizs B, Komlosi P, Bevensee MO, Schwiebert EM, Bell PD, Yoder BK. Altered pH(i) regulation and Na(+)/HCO3(−) transporter activity in choroid plexus of cilia-defective Tg737(orpk) mutant mouse. Am J Physiol Cell Physiol. 2007;292(4):C1409–16.
9. Spirli C, Locatelli L, Fiorotto R, Morell CM, Fabris L, Pozzan T, et al. Altered store operated calcium entry increases cyclic 3′,5′-adenosine monophosphate production and extracellular signal-regulated kinases 1 and 2 phosphorylation in polycystin-2-defective cholangiocytes. Hepatology. [Research Support, N.I.H., Extramural Research Support, Non-U.S. Gov't]. 2012;55(3):856–68.
10. Choi YH, Suzuki A, Hajarnis S, Ma Z, Chapin HC, Caplan MJ, et al. Polycystin-2 and phosphodiesterase 4C are components of a ciliary A-kinase anchoring protein complex that is disrupted in cystic kidney diseases. Proc Natl Acad Sci U S A. 2011;108(26):10679–84.
11. Carroll TJ, Das A. Planar cell polarity in kidney development and disease. Organogenesis. [Research Support, N.I.H., Extramural Research Support, Non--U.S. Gov't Review]. 2011;7(3):180–90.
12. Hanaoka K, Guggino WB. cAMP regulates cell proliferation and cyst formation in autosomal polycystic kidney disease cells. J Am Soc Nephrol. 2000;11(7):1179–87.

13. Yamaguchi T, Pelling JC, Ramaswamy NT, Eppler JW, Wallace DP, Nagao S, et al. cAMP stimulates the in vitro proliferation of renal cyst epithelial cells by activating the extracellular signal-regulated kinase pathway. Kidney Int. 2000;57(4):1460–71.
14. Distefano G, Boca M, Rowe I, Wodarczyk C, Ma L, Piontek KB, et al. Polycystin-1 regulates extracellular signal-regulated kinase-dependent phosphorylation of tuberin to control cell size through mTOR and its downstream effectors S6K and 4EBP1. Mol Cell Biol. 2009;29(9):2359–71.
15. Spirli C, Okolicsanyi S, Fiorotto R, Fabris L, Cadamuro M, Lecchi S, et al. ERK1/2-dependent vascular endothelial growth factor signaling sustains cyst growth in polycystin-2 defective mice. Gastroenterology. [Research Support, N.I.H., Extramural Research Support, Non-U.S. Gov't]. 2010;138(1):360–71 e7.
16. Betz C, Hall MN. Where is mTOR and what is it doing there? J Cell Biol. 2013;203(4):563–74.
17. Aguiari G, Bizzarri F, Bonon A, Mangolini A, Magri E, Pedriali M, et al. Polycystin-1 regulates amphiregulin expression through CREB and AP1 signalling: implications in ADPKD cell proliferation. J Mol Med (Berl Germany). 2012;90(11):1267–82.
18. Qin S, Taglienti M, Cai L, Zhou J, Kreidberg JA. c-Met and NF-kappaB-dependent overexpression of Wnt7a and -7b and Pax2 promotes cystogenesis in polycystic kidney disease. J Am Soc Nephrol. 2012;23(8):1309–18.
19. Talbot JJ, Song X, Wang X, Rinschen MM, Doerr N, Lariviere WB, et al. The cleaved cytoplasmic tail of polycystin-1 regulates Src-dependent STAT3 activation. J Am Soc Nephrol. 2014;25:1737–48.
20. Ye M, Grantham JJ. The secretion of fluid by renal cysts from patients with autosomal dominant polycystic kidney disease. N Engl J Med. 1993;329(5):310–3.
21. Veizis IE, Cotton CU. Role of kidney chloride channels in health and disease. Pediatr Nephrol (Berl Germany). 2007;22(6):770–7.
22. Grantham JJ. Mechanisms of progression in autosomal dominant polycystic kidney disease. Kidney Int Suppl. 1997;63:S93–7.
23. Sullivan LP, Wallace DP, Grantham JJ. Epithelial transport in polycystic kidney disease. Physiol Rev. 1998;78(4):1165–91.
24. Li H, Yang W, Mendes F, Amaral MD, Sheppard DN. Impact of the cystic fibrosis mutation F508del-CFTR on renal cyst formation and growth. Am J Physiol Ren Physiol. 2012;303:F1176–86.
25. O'Sullivan DA, Torres VE, Gabow PA, Thibodeau SN, King BF, Bergstralh EJ. Cystic fibrosis and the phenotypic expression of autosomal dominant polycystic kidney disease. Am J Kidney Dis. 1998;32(6):976–83.
26. Xu N, Glockner JF, Rossetti S, Babovich-Vuksanovic D, Harris PC, Torres VE. Autosomal dominant polycystic kidney disease coexisting with cystic fibrosis. J Nephrol. 2006;19(4):529–34.
27. Gabow PA, Kaehny WD, Johnson AM, Duley IT, Manco-Johnson M, Lezotte DC, et al. The clinical utility of renal concentrating capacity in polycystic kidney disease. Kidney Int. 1989;35(2):675–80.
28. Carone FA, Ozono S, Samma S, Kanwar YS, Oyasu R. Renal functional changes in experimental cystic disease are tubular in origin. Kidney Int. [Research Support, U.S. Gov't, P.H.S.]. 1988;33(1):8–13.
29. Seeman T, Dusek J, Vondrak K, Blahova K, Simkova E, Kreisinger J, et al. Renal concentrating capacity is linked to blood pressure in children with autosomal dominant polycystic kidney disease. Physiol Res Acad Sci Bohemoslovaca. [Clinical Trial Research Support, Non-U.S. Gov't]. 2004;53(6):629–34.
30. Meijer E, Bakker SJ, van der Jagt EJ, Navis G, de Jong PE, Struck J, et al. Copeptin, a surrogate marker of vasopressin, is associated with disease severity in autosomal dominant polycystic kidney disease. Clin J Am Soc Nephrol. 2011;6(2):361–8.
31. Boertien WE, Meijer E, Zittema D, van Dijk MA, Rabelink TJ, Breuning MH, et al. Copeptin, a surrogate marker for vasopressin, is associated with kidney function decline in subjects with autosomal dominant polycystic kidney disease. Nephrol Dial Transplant Off Publ Eur Dial Transplant Assoc Eur Ren Assoc. 2012;27(11):4131–7.
32. Nagao S, Nishii K, Katsuyama M, Kurahashi H, Marunouchi T, Takahashi H, et al. Increased water intake decreases progression of polycystic kidney disease in the PCK rat. J Am Soc Nephrol. 2006;17(8):2220–7.
33. Hopp K, Wang X, Ye H, Irazabal MV, Harris PC, Torres VE. Effects of hydration in rats and mice with polycystic kidney disease. Am J Physiol Ren Physiol. [Research Support, N.I.H., Extramural Research Support, Non-U.S. Gov't]. 2015;308(3):F261–6.
34. Wang X, Wu Y, Ward CJ, Harris PC, Torres VE. Vasopressin directly regulates cyst growth in polycystic kidney disease. J Am Soc Nephrol. 2008;19(1):102–8.
35. Gattone VH 2nd, Maser RL, Tian C, Rosenberg JM, Branden MG. Developmental expression of urine concentration-associated genes and their altered expression in murine infantile-type polycystic kidney disease. Dev Genet. 1999;24(3–4):309–18.
36. Gattone VH 2nd, Wang X, Harris PC, Torres VE. Inhibition of renal cystic disease development and progression by a vasopressin V2 receptor antagonist. Nat Med. 2003;9(10):1323–6.
37. Torres VE, Wang X, Qian Q, Somlo S, Harris PC, Gattone VH 2nd. Effective treatment of an orthologous model of autosomal dominant polycystic kidney disease. Nat Med. 2004;10(4):363–4.
38. Wang X, Gattone V 2nd, Harris PC, Torres VE. Effectiveness of vasopressin V2 receptor antagonists OPC-31260 and OPC-41061 on polycystic kidney disease development in the PCK rat. J Am Soc Nephrol. 2005;16(4):846–51.
39. Meijer E, Gansevoort RT, de Jong PE, van der Wal AM, Leonhard WN, de Krey SR, et al. Therapeutic potential of vasopressin V2 receptor antagonist in a mouse model for autosomal dominant polycystic kidney disease: optimal timing and dosing of the drug. Nephrol Dial Transplant. 2011;26(8):2445–53.

40. Romaker D, Puetz M, Teschner S, Donauer J, Geyer M, Gerke P, et al. Increased expression of secreted frizzled-related protein 4 in polycystic kidneys. J Am Soc Nephrol JASN. [Research Support, Non--U.S. Gov't]. 2009;20(1):48–56.
41. Reif GA, Yamaguchi T, Nivens E, Fujiki H, Pinto CS, Wallace DP. Tolvaptan inhibits ERK-dependent cell proliferation, Cl(−) secretion, and in vitro cyst growth of human ADPKD cells stimulated by vasopressin. Am J Physiol Ren Physiol. [Research Support, N.I.H., Extramural Research Support, Non-U.S. Gov't]. 2011;301(5):F1005–13.
42. Higashihara E, Torres VE, Chapman AB, Grantham JJ, Bae K, Watnick TJ, et al. Tolvaptan in autosomal dominant polycystic kidney disease: three years' experience. Clin J Am Soc Nephrol. 2011;6:2499–507.
43. Irazabal MV, Torres VE, Hogan MC, Glockner J, King BF, Ofstie TG, et al. Short-term effects of tolvaptan on renal function and volume in patients with autosomal dominant polycystic kidney disease. Kidney Int. 2011;80(3):295–301.
44. Boertien WE, Meijer E, de Jong PE, Bakker SJ, Czerwiec FS, Struck J, et al. Short-term renal hemodynamic effects of tolvaptan in subjects with autosomal dominant polycystic kidney disease at various stages of chronic kidney disease. Kidney Int. [Clinical Trial Research Support, Non-U.S. Gov't]. 2013;84(6):1278–86.
45. Boertien WE, Meijer E, de Jong PE, Ter Horst GJ, Renken RJ, van der Jagt EJ, et al. Short-term effects of tolvaptan in individuals with autosomal dominant polycystic kidney disease at various levels of kidney function. Am J Kidney Dis Off J Natl Kidney Found. 2015;65:833–41.
46. Torres VE, Chapman AB, Devuyst O, Gansevoort RT, Grantham JJ, Higashihara E, et al. Tolvaptan in patients with autosomal dominant polycystic kidney disease. N Engl J Med. 2012;367(25):2407–18.

14 End-Stage Renal Disease in Patients with Autosomal Dominant Polycystic Kidney Disease

Ahd Al Khunaizi and Ahsan Alam

Incidence and Prevalence of End-Stage Renal Disease

The incident number of individuals with cystic kidney disease reaching end-stage renal disease (ESRD) in the USA has more than doubled from under 1000 in the early 1980s to over 2000 by the early 2000s [1]. Despite this rising number over the past three decades, the proportion of ESRD attributable to ADPKD has been outpaced by the rise in diabetic kidney disease. Thus the overall proportion of ESRD attributable to PKD has steadily declined from 8% in 1980 to slightly under 3% in 2011.

Data from the Danish National Registry reported on 693 patients that reached ESRD with ADPKD between 1990 and 2007. In this population there was an increase in the incidence of ESRD, with 6.45 per million people (pmp) between 1990 and 1995, 7.39 pmp between 1996 and 2001, and 7.59 pmp between 2002 and 2007. In addition, the prevalence of patients with ESRD due to ADPKD also increased across the same time periods, with 55.9, 58.5, and 60.6 pmp, respectively. The age of ESRD onset also increased from 55.9 years in the 1990–1995 cohort to 60.6 years in the 2002–2007 cohort. This suggests that over time, older people with ADPKD were more often being classified with ESRD or initiated renal replacement therapy. It may also suggest that chronic kidney disease care for those with ADPKD has improved over the time, leading to a delay in the onset of ESRD [2]. The male-to-female ratio for the onset of ESRD fell from 1.6 to 1.1, suggesting that male gender was playing less of a role as a prognostic risk factor for progression to ESRD [2].

Survival on dialysis has improved in patients with ADPKD, as compared to non-ADPKD patients [2, 3]. Whether this relates to improved hypertension control, a greater use of angiotensin blocking agents, or other advances in medical management in those with ADPKD remains unclear. Patients with ADPKD have favorable survival on renal replacement therapy compared to similarly matched nondiabetic patients with ESRD [4] (Fig. 14.1). This may be in part due to comorbidities found in patients with ESRD due to hypertension that may not exist in patients that develop ESRD due to a genetic mutation causing ADPKD or because of earlier treatment of hypertension in the ADPKD patient population.

A. Al Khunaizi, MD
McGill University Health Centre, Montreal, QC, Canada

A. Alam, MD, MS, FRCPC (✉)
Division of Nephrology, Department of Medicine, McGill University Health Centre, Royal Victoria Hospital, Montreal, QC, Canada
e-mail: ahsan.alam@mcgill.ca

B. D. Cowley, Jr., J. J. Bissler (eds.), *Polycystic Kidney Disease*,
https://doi.org/10.1007/978-1-4939-7784-0_14

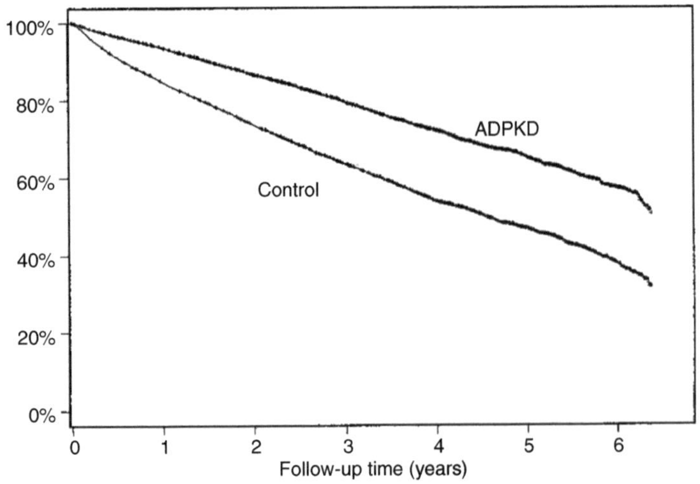

Fig. 14.1 The survival of 9435patients with ADPKD following ESRD, compared with 206,989 age, gender, and year of ESRD-matched nondiabetic controls from USRDS (log rank test $p = 0.0001$) (From Perrone et al. [4]. Reprinted with permission from Elsevier via STM Permissions Guidelines)

Choice of Renal Replacement Therapy

The best choice for renal replacement modality for those with ADPKD is extrapolated from patient outcomes in the general ESRD population. Currently the optimal therapy remains kidney transplantation, and ideally from a living kidney donor, if available [5]. Although kidney transplantation should be recommended as first-line therapy, the patient's preferences, risk profile for infection and malignancy, comorbidities, urgency to initiate renal replacement therapy, social support, and the patient's comprehension of their disease and risks must be kept in perspective.

Despite current efforts to slow cyst growth and GFR decline, almost half of patients with ADPKD reach ESRD by age 60 [6]. Some patients with ADPKD may need to initiate dialysis before kidney transplantation is possible, while some may be ineligible for a transplant. Options for these patients include both hemodialysis (HD, in-center or home-based) and peritoneal dialysis (PD).

Peritoneal Dialysis

Peritoneal dialysis offers a potentially more lifestyle-friendly mode of renal replacement therapy; however, several concerns regarding peritoneal dialysis in ADPKD patients have been raised. The extrarenal manifestations of abdominal wall hernias and leaks are prevalent in those with ADPKD, which would complicate the administration of PD fluid. Another theoretical concern is the higher prevalence of colonic diverticulosis or diverticulitis in patients with ADPKD, which could lead to increased rates of peritonitis. Finally, enlarged polycystic kidneys could restrict the available space to instill PD fluid or restrict the area for peritoneal exchange. Restrictions on the volume of PD fluid infused can result in suboptimal dialysis clearance or patient discomfort with larger volumes. Additionally, there may be an increased concern for hydrothorax with PD. While nephrectomy can offer a possible solution to the lack of intra-abdominal space, the loss of residual kidney function may be a greater concern, as it is known that preserving residual kidney function confers a survival advantage in ESRD patients on PD [7].

Outcomes on PD for patients with ADPKD have been evaluated by several observational and registry studies [8–10]. The US National CAPD Registry reported a median time to peritonitis of 8.2 months in patients with ADPKD, compared to 6.3–7.4 months in other subgroups of kidney failure [11]. Several observational studies comparing patients with ADPKD with matched patients with other causes of ESRD have shown little difference in technique survival or peritonitis rates [8–10, 12, 13]. In many of these studies, the reported rate of hernias was higher in the ADPKD group.

Registry and cohort studies inherently are at risk of bias, particularly selection bias as patients with ADPKD are directed to PD or HD based on several factors that may be judged to be associated with better success using a particular modality. This is highlighted by examining the competing risks of patients on PD with and without ADPKD. In the French RDPLF peritoneal dialysis registry, 344 patients with ADPKD were compared to 3818 nondiabetic and non-ADPKD patients [12]. The most common outcome for non-ADPKD patients was death, followed by transfer to hemodialysis, and then kidney transplantation. However, in those with ADPKD, the most common outcome was transplantation followed by transfer to hemodialysis and death.

Clinical trials randomizing ADPKD patients to hemodialysis or peritoneal dialysis are unlikely to be conducted. To overcome some of the selection bias of observational studies, a study reported out of Hong Kong is helpful to describe the natural outcomes of ADPKD patients initiated with PD [14]. In Hong Kong, all ESRD patients were assigned to PD first and only switched to HD if there was ultrafiltration or technique failure. Using this mostly unselected population of 42 patients with ADPKD and 84 matched nondiabetic controls, they found no differences in technique or patient survival between the two groups. There was also no significant difference in the transition of patients to hemodialysis. Two urgent surgical hernia repairs did occur in the ADPKD cohort, but all patients resumed PD after recovery with no recurrent hernias.

To date, there is no evidence that specifically correlates total kidney or liver volume with PD success or clinical outcomes in patients with ADPKD. Given the preponderance of clinical studies and reports, it appears that patients with ADPKD can safely and effectively be treated with PD when they reach end-stage renal disease, keeping in mind the potential limitations of this modality.

Hemodialysis

Initiating hemodialysis for ADPKD is generally similar to non-ADPKD patients. Nonetheless, there are some unique issues to be considered in the surveillance and management of patients with ADPKD on hemodialysis.

Renal and Extrarenal Complications

There are limited studies that examine renal and extrarenal complications of ADPKD after initiation of hemodialysis, and most of these come from single-center reports rather than large prospective registries. Renal complications such as pain, hematuria, and renal cyst infections can still occur after ESRD. In cohort studies, symptoms related to these complications vary considerably. After 5 years on hemodialysis, over 50% of patients with ADPKD will experience at least one episode of kidney pain or gross hematuria, while cyst infections will occur in 12% [15]. Although the risk of renal cell carcinoma has not been shown to be increased once on hemodialysis, it is prudent to evaluate cases of gross hematuria, as acquired cystic disease is still a clinical issue in any patient on hemodialysis. Recurrent episodes of hematuria may prompt cessation of heparin anticoagulation on dialysis, addressing coagulopathies, including uremic platelet dysfunction, and finally, when refractory bleeding persists, embolization or nephrectomy of the involved kidney may be a last resort.

Most extrarenal complications have not been reported to be increased after starting dialysis. Cardiac valvular disease, congestive heart failure, valve replacement, and endocarditis are not known to be increased in ADPKD compared to other dialysis patients [15]. An analysis of Medicare patients in the United States Renal Data System (USRDS) showed that the incidence of intracranial hemorrhage was almost threefold higher in those with ADPKD as compared to non-ADPKD, after accounting for competing risks. The absolute risk remained low at 10.9 per 1000 patient-years in those with ADPKD, compared to 7.5 per 1000 patient-years in those with ESRD due to other causes. Nonetheless, in those with an aneurysm rupture, the death rate was significantly higher. This study could not examine the potential influence of family history or PKD genetics [16].

Anemia Management

It has been hypothesized that expanding cysts within the renal parenchyma leads to pericystic hypoxia, the stimulation of hypoxia-inducible factor-alpha, and eventually resulting in higher endogenous erythropoietin production [17]. Data from nephrectomized ADPKD kidneys have also shown erythropoietin levels to be elevated independent of oxygen tension. Moreover, patients with ADPKD may also start dialysis with more residual kidney function, and thus endogenous erythropoietin production may be higher than for other causes of kidney failure.

Relatively higher hemoglobin values have been frequently observed in ADPKD patients, and this finding may persist even after reaching end-stage renal disease [18]. Moreover, the absence of erythropoiesis-stimulating agent (ESA) therapy is more than five times higher in patients with ADPKD than non-ADPKD patients [19]. In general, ADPKD patients that maintain a higher hemoglobin level do not appear to be at any increased mortality risk, and phlebotomy is not indicated when hemoglobin levels are above the conventional target range for patients treated with ESAs [19].

Hypertension

Hypertension is a common early finding in ADPKD, occurring in 50–70% of cases before any significant reduction in glomerular filtration rate [20]. The stimulation of the renin-angiotensin-aldosterone system, a result of renal parenchymal ischemia caused by cyst expansion, likely plays an integral role in the development of hypertension. As a result, angiotensin-converting enzyme inhibitors and angiotensin receptor blockers are the mainstay of treatment in these patients [21, 22]. For ADPKD patients specifically on dialysis, there is no further recommendation regarding the preferred antihypertensive agent(s) which should be used.

Among hemodialysis patients, those with ADPKD display a similar U-shaped blood pressure and mortality relationship as those without ADPKD. Despite this hypertension "paradox," which showed that lower blood pressure was associated with higher mortality as compared with normal and higher blood pressure, what is still evident is that the survival in any blood pressure category remained higher for those with ADPKD, as compared to those with other causes of ESRD [23]. Randomized clinical trials are needed to define optimal blood pressure targets in the hemodialysis population.

Mineral Bone Disease

The presence of ADPKD does not appear to modify the association between mineral bone disease markers and mortality in hemodialysis patients. Nonetheless, ADPKD patients with higher levels of mineral bone disease biomarkers still have superior survival to non-ADPKD patients with similar markers [24].

Anticoagulation

Patients with ADPKD on dialysis continue to be at risk for macroscopic hematuria, cyst bleeding, and intracranial aneurysms. However, there are no specific recommendations for modifying the use of systemic anticoagulants for hemodialysis. Should severe or persistent cyst bleeding or macrohematuria occur, it would be prudent to stop systemic anticoagulants and investigate for the underlying cause to guide management.

Kidney Transplantation

Similar to other ESRD patients, the optimal renal replacement therapy option for patients with ADPKD is kidney transplantation. A preemptive kidney transplant, when available, should be the preferred approach. Nonetheless, issues related to the selection of a living donor from the same family, the indications for native nephrectomy, the choice of immunosuppression, and the elevated risk of certain posttransplant complications should be recognized.

Rates and Prevalence of Kidney Transplantation

Patients with ADPKD represent less than 5% of the total US ESRD population. Similarly, the absolute number of deceased and living donor kidney transplants is also small. However, the rate of kidney transplantation in the USA for those with cystic kidney disease is much higher than any other renal disease (Fig. 14.2). The rate of deceased donor kidney transplantation is approximately 6.4 transplants per 100 dialysis patient-years, compared with 3.7, 2.0, and 2.0 for glomerulonephritis, diabetes, and hypertension, respectively. For living kidney donation, the rate is 4.1 transplants per 100 dialysis patient-years, compared to 2.1, 0.7, and 0.9 for glomerulonephritis, diabetes, and hypertension, respectively. There has been little change in these rates over the past decade in the USA [1].

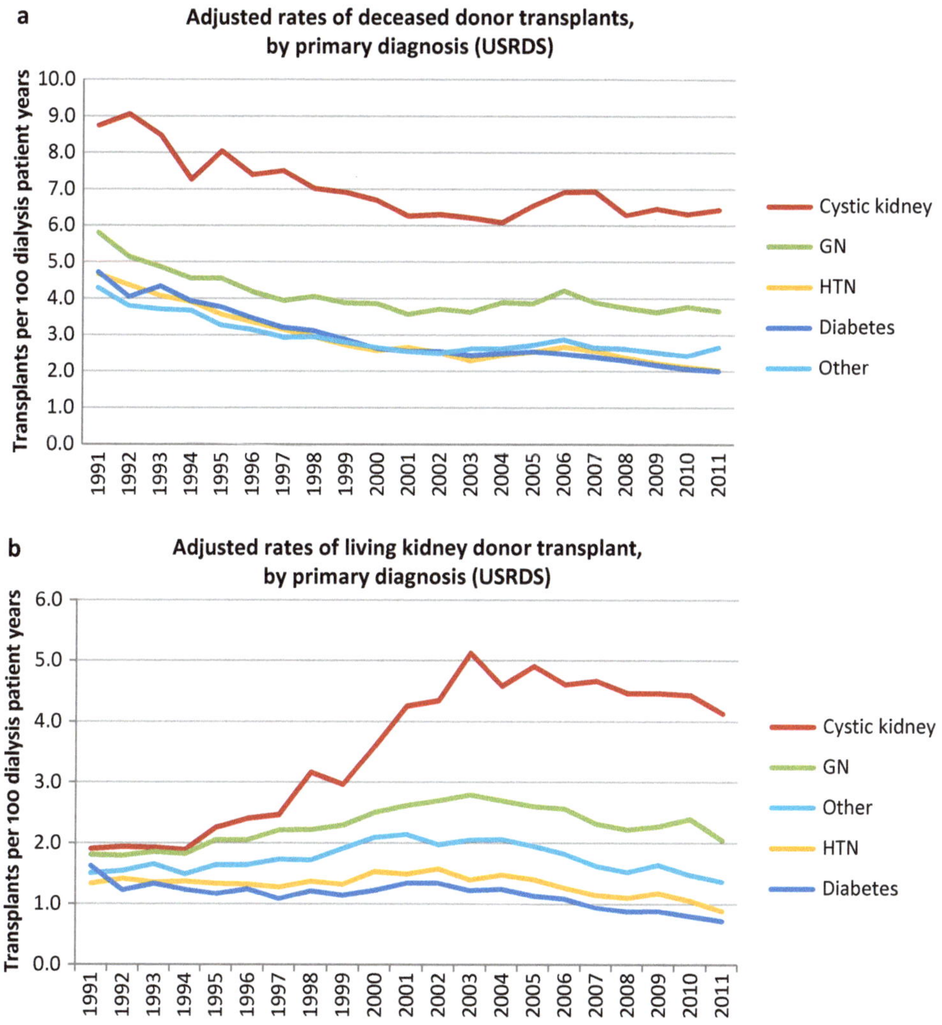

Fig. 14.2 The adjusted rate of kidney transplantation for those with cystic versus other primary diagnoses (**a**) deceased and (**b**) living donors. Adapted from USRDS (Data from United States Renal Data System, 2013 Annual Data Report: Epidemiology of Kidney Disease in the United States. National Institutes of Health, National Institute of Diabetes and Digestive and Kidney Diseases, Bethesda, MD, 2014)

The incidence of kidney transplantation in the first year after initiating dialysis is 5% for the total US ESRD population. In those with ADPKD, their incidence of kidney transplantation is as high as 25% in the first year after starting dialysis [25].

Pretransplant Considerations

Alloimmunization

Sensitization to human leukocyte antigen (HLA) can be induced by blood transfusion, prior organ transplantation, and pregnancy. The presence of such HLA antibodies can delay or prevent kidney transplantation [26].

Individuals with ADPKD may manifest gross hematuria from cyst bleeding or rupture, but their need for blood transfusions in this context is extremely uncommon. On the other hand, native nephrectomy of massively enlarged or recurrently bleeding and infected ADPKD kidneys may significantly raise the risk of requiring a blood transfusion. In addition, declining GFR is associated with anemia, yet this appears to be less of an issue in those with ADPKD, and management is driven mainly by erythropoiesis-stimulating agents and iron supplementation.

To minimize alloimmunization, the avoidance of blood transfusions should be encouraged, similar to non-ADPKD patients. Specifically, the benefits of native nephrectomy should be balanced with risks, including that of sensitization from transfusion. The use of blood transfusions should be limited to urgent and lifesaving indications.

Aneurysm Screening

The rupture of an intracranial aneurysm portends a severe prognosis. As kidney transplantation involves the use of a scarce and precious resource, namely, a kidney from a deceased or living donor, some transplant centers advocate for screening of ADPKD patients for occult intracranial aneurysms. The rationale is that this approach would allow for preemptive management of unruptured aneurysms, which would avoid rupture and thus improve morbidity and premature mortality of the transplant recipient and maximize the use of the allograft. There are, however, no studies that specifically examine the utility of screening asymptomatic patients with ADPKD for intracranial aneurysms prior to kidney transplantation. Screening for intracranial aneurysms is traditionally indicated for those with symptoms compatible with an aneurysm or in the context of a family history of ruptured aneurysm, subarachnoid hemorrhage, unexplained stroke, or premature death. Widespread screening of asymptomatic patients with ADPKD is not supported [27].

Living Kidney Donation

Kidney transplantation from a living donor allows for several potential advantages: eliminating the need for dialysis (preemptive transplantation), providing the recipient the opportunity to plan for the transplant as an elective procedure, offering improved short-term and long-term graft survival, and shortening the wait time for patients on the deceased donor wait-list.

A clear challenge for patients with ADPKD is finding a kidney donor among family members, given the genetic nature of the disease. An autosomal dominant disease implies that statistically there is a 50% chance that each sibling or child of that potential recipient also carries the genetic mutation, thus excluding any affected family members and reducing the available donor pool. With multiple potential recipients in a family, this further raises the demands on any healthy donors.

In potential donors from ADPKD families where there may be no apparent evidence of cystic disease by ultrasonography, the exclusion of the disease may be reliably concluded in those above age 40 [28]. In younger potential donors, the diagnosis is more difficult to exclude with sufficient certainty. In this setting, further evaluation with higher resolution imaging of cysts (i.e., MRI) or genetic testing is appropriate [29] (see also Chaps. 1 and 7). If a mutation in the recipient has been characterized, a familial mutation analysis may be performed. When no mutation in the family has been identified, the alternative is to perform full gene sequencing of both *PKD1* and *PKD2* genes in the potential donor to help exclude the disease.

Eligible candidates that are blood type or cross-match incompatible with their intended recipient may still have the opportunity to enter into a living donor paired-exchange program, if available in their country or region. These programs increase the chance of recipients finding a compatible kidney donor and can match two pairs, or they may create a chain of many donor-recipient pairs. Patients with ADPKD can be informed of this potential approach, as it still offers all the advantages of living kidney donation.

Native Nephrectomy

As total kidney volume increases with disease progression, patients may develop more and increasingly severe symptoms. The indications for native kidney nephrectomy are driven by symptoms: chronic pain, early satiety symptoms, chronic or refractory cyst infections, recurrent hematuria or suspicion of malignancy, recurrent nephrolithiasis, and, rarely, refractory hypertension. As previously mentioned, the decision to intervene with nephrectomy should be balanced by the risks for transfusion requirements in a potential kidney transplant candidate.

Prior to kidney transplantation, the presence of massively enlarged polycystic kidneys may provide another indication for ipsilateral native nephrectomy. This would be to provide adequate space for the surgical implantation of the renal allograft.

Several approaches are available for the removal of native kidneys peri-transplant and each with its own potential advantages and disadvantages. Nephrectomy can be performed using laparoscopic techniques. Bilateral nephrectomy pretransplant may be indicated in extreme circumstances and would preclude avoiding dialysis. This approach would also lead to the complete loss of urine output (residual kidney function), which is valuable for those on dialysis. Finally, the more extensive and complicated the surgery, the more risk of requiring a blood transfusion. However, the removal of the native kidneys allows for adequate space for the allograft and no concern for future kidney surgery in an immunosuppressed patient.

For asymptomatic patients, a simultaneous ipsilateral nephrectomy is sometimes performed to allow for space for the transplant allograft. This technique allows for a single surgery, which is associated with shorter cumulative hospital stays and better patient satisfaction. The combined nephrectomy and transplant surgery does lead to a longer and more complicated procedure, with the potential for a longer cold ischemia time in deceased donor transplants. There have also been reports of greater transfusion requirements. Published reports have not shown any significant differences in allograft function when comparing staged or simultaneous nephrectomy and those without.

Finally, a staged nephrectomy (also known as deferred or sandwich nephrectomy) begins with a simultaneous nephrectomy, and once the transplant is successful, a contralateral nephrectomy is performed. This does require an additional surgery but allows for the kidney function and immunosuppression to stabilize posttransplant.

Several studies have reported on their success of pretransplant and simultaneous nephrectomy compared to transplant without nephrectomy and unilateral versus bilateral nephrectomy. The majority of these reports are retrospective reviews involving single centers and often with individual surgeons [30, 31]. A comparison of transplant compared to transplant with ipsilateral nephrectomy showed no difference in intraoperative or postoperative complications, including no increased length of stay or blood loss. The largest report involved the routine approach of simultaneous nephrectomy in all ADPKD transplant patients [32]. In 100 consecutive kidney transplant recipients, 22 surgical complications were documented, with 12 complications attributed to the additional nephrectomy: 4 lymphocele, 4 wound dehiscence or hernia, and 4 postoperative hematomas or bleeding. Of these 100 patients, 22 had previously undergone a contralateral nephrectomy. Of the remaining 78 patients, 20 underwent contralateral nephrectomy subsequent to their transplant. The overall 1- and 5-year patient survival was 97% and 93%, and 1- and 5-year graft survival was 96% and 80% [32]. As there were no concomitant controls available at this center, it is unclear how these result compare to alternative strategies, and the indication for nephrectomy was not based on clinical indications as demonstrated by the fact that some kidneys were as small as 500 g in weight.

Separate studies comparing simultaneous with staged nephrectomy showed a longer cumulative operative time, greater blood loss and transfusion requirements, and longer hospital stay in those with the staged bilateral nephrectomy; however postoperative short-term graft function and 5-year graft and patient survival were similar in both groups [31, 33, 34].

Overall, it is difficult to conclude the true impact of native nephrectomy in asymptomatic ADPKD patients, as the data is based on case series, and there are no randomized trials. In the hands of experienced transplant centers and surgeons with the appropriate expertise, the outcomes of native nephrectomy, whether unilateral or bilateral, may not impact intermediate-term graft and patient outcomes. However, keeping the native kidneys in situ, if possible, would avoid the inherent complexity of performing any additional surgery, and thus minimize the risk for blood transfusion and sensitization, and maintaining residual renal function, which could simplify fluid management and preserve erythropoietin production [35]. There is insufficient evidence to support routine nephrectomy, and it should probably be restricted to centers with experience in performing the procedure safely.

Posttransplant Considerations

What happens to symptom evolution and total kidney volume after transplantation is not clearly understood. Data examining 33 patients that were followed by CT imaging at the time of transplant and then 1, 3, and 5 years posttransplant reported on the rate of kidney volume change [36]. In this cohort, the mean bilateral kidney volume at the time of transplant was 3100 mL, all but one had basiliximab induction, all patients received calcineurin inhibitors and prednisone, and over 85% received mycophenolate mofetil. All but one patient experienced a decrease in kidney volume after transplantation, with an average decrease of 37.7% at 1 year and 40.6% at 3 years. Interestingly, the majority of the decline was observed in the first year after transplant. Also, in 16 of 18 patients with a polycystic liver, there was an increase in liver volume. These results provide an argument against pretransplant nephrectomy in the absence of infection, bleeding, malignancy, or inadequate room for the allograft. It does highlight the possibility of increasing liver-related symptoms after transplant.

Choice of Immunosuppression

In animal models of ADPKD, the inhibition of the mammalian target of rapamycin (mTOR) was shown to slow disease progression [37, 38]. This observation was further supported in retrospective studies of transplanted patients with ADPKD. A retrospective review of kidney transplants for ADPKD at the Cleveland Clinic identified seven patients with CT scans in the pre- and posttransplant period and classified these into sirolimus and non-sirolimus treatment [39]. It was determined that the total kidney volume change was −24.8 ± 9.7% (−1.4% per month) in those on sirolimus and −8.6 ± 11.2% (−0.3% per month) in the non-sirolimus treatment group. A similar phenomenon was described with polycystic liver volume [40]. In 16 patients with abdominal imaging studies within 11 months before and 7 months after transplantation, sirolimus was associated with a 11.9% decrease in liver volume, while there was a 14.1% increase for those treated with tacrolimus.

Since these observations, randomized clinical trials in non-transplant patients with ADPKD have not demonstrated slowing of kidney volume progression or slowing of renal impairment in those treated with mTOR inhibitors [41, 42]. In addition, there is also the possibility that native cyst growth may slow simply from the fibrosis associated with calcineurin inhibitors.

Currently, no specific recommendations can be made that relate to the choice of immunosuppression in patients with ADPKD. As with any transplant recipient, the primary objectives should be to prevent graft rejection and avoid complications of over-immunosuppression to ensure optimal long-term graft and patient survival.

Liver and Kidney Transplantation

Liver involvement is one of the most common extrarenal manifestations in ADPKD. The majority of ADPKD patients do not develop symptoms related to liver cystic disease. Occasionally, congenital hepatic fibrosis and biliary tract dilatation can manifest, but most commonly symptoms relate to progressive enlargement of a polycystic liver. Hepatocellular function, however, most often remains preserved. Women are more likely to develop cystic liver involvement, and the number of cysts has been correlated to estrogen use and number of pregnancies [43]. A massively enlarged polycystic liver can result in chronic symptoms of abdominal fullness and pain. Early satiety and dyspnea can result from mechanical compression and displacement of the adjacent organs. Eventually the chronic liver enlargement can become physically disabling and even lead to malnutrition and severely impaired quality of life.

Orthotopic liver transplantation has been performed in patients with ADPKD in the absence of renal dysfunction. When surgical liver resection is unsuccessful or not feasible, liver transplantation can be considered in the context of disabling symptoms, portal hypertension, or liver dysfunction and optimally before physical function significantly deteriorates. One-year mortality following liver or liver-kidney transplantation in patients with ADPKD has been estimated to be 18% [44].

Similar to patients without ADPKD, isolated liver transplantation has been associated with an early decline in GFR. Summarizing data from various case series, it is reported that the mean GFR decline is 15 ml/min per year. This rate of GFR decline is faster than that expected from ADPKD alone and is likely a result of the use of calcineurin inhibitors. Regardless, a strategy of combined liver-kidney transplantation prior to kidney failure is not supported, and the monitoring of kidney allograft GFR and rejection are generally confounded when residual native kidney function is still present [44].

Posttransplant Complications

Certain complications are increased in those with ADPKD compared to non-ADPKD controls posttransplant, and there is significant heterogeneity in the reports from different case series and longitudinal studies. Urinary tract infections have been reported to be increased as much as twofold in ADPKD patients, although some longitudinal studies find little evidence of any increased infection risk [45, 46]. Similarly, colonic diverticulitis has also been reported to be more prevalent and rarely associated with life-threatening bowel perforation.

In all kidney transplant recipients, cardiovascular disease remains the major complication affecting patient outcomes. Preventing or treating factors that elevate cardiovascular risk should be an important objective in transplant patient care. The largest multicenter longitudinal cohort study (DIVAT) followed 534 ADPKD patients for 15 years after kidney transplant. Hypertension (49.7% vs. 42.3%) and hyperlipidemia (49.7% vs. 39.3%) were significantly more prevalent in patients with ADPKD. New-onset diabetes after transplant was also more likely (12.4% vs 9.6%, $p = 0.06$). Nevertheless, patient survival and the incidence of stroke were no different in those with and without ADPKD [46].

Another potential concern has been the incidence of cerebrovascular and thromboembolic disease. Several longitudinal cohort studies, examining cerebrovascular events among ADPKD patients following kidney transplant, have not shown any increased risk of stroke. Although there was an increase in hemorrhagic bleeds in univariate analysis, this was subsequently accounted for by underlying risk factors in multivariate analyses [45–47]. The Assessment of Lescol in Renal Transplantation (ALERT) study was a randomized, double blind clinical trial examining fluvastatin in kidney transplant recipients [48]. Of the 2102 patients included in the analysis of cerebrovascular disease and mortality, 321 had ADPKD as their primary cause of kidney failure. This study showed that 8.8% of the population experienced a cerebrovascular event over the 6.7-year median follow-up (i.e., incidence rate of 1.3% events per year), and ADPKD was an independent risk factor for hemorrhagic stroke, but not ischemic stroke, with over a fourfold increase in hazard ratio [48]. With respect to venous thromboembolic disease, the DIVAT study was a multicenter cohort study in France, which demonstrated an incidence of thromboembolic disease of 8.6% in those ADPKD compared to 5.8% in the control population ($p = 0.009$) [46].

Posttransplant malignancy has not been found to be increased in patients with ADPKD [49]. Specifically, renal cell cancers and other solid organ tumors do not appear to be more prevalent compared to other transplant recipients [46, 50]. Since malignancy risk may be increased in general for kidney transplant recipients and kidney cancer is increased for those with prolonged dialysis duration, attention to periodic cancer screening and general preventative measures should be no different in those with ADPKD. The largest registry study using data from the Scientific Registry of Transplant Recipients (SRTR) found that the adjusted cancer risk was 16% lower in ADPKD patients when compared to the general population. Specifically, renal cell carcinomas showed no increased incidence rate (89.2 vs. 106.0 per 100,000 person-years) [51].

ADPKD in a Transplanted Kidney

Recurrence of cystic disease in a transplanted kidney is never observed. However, kidneys have been transplanted from ADPKD donors. Progression of cyst and total kidney volume expansion has been demonstrated in these kidneys; however, these allografts can still last for many years with adequate GFR [52]. The question of whether kidneys from deceased ADPKD donors with acceptable kidney function and normal size may be appropriate for transplantation requires the full consent of the potential recipient, but may be considered by some programs.

Patient and Graft Survival

Kidney transplantation in patients with ADPKD yields favorable patient outcomes that are comparable to similar (nondiabetic) ESRD patient populations and are likely better than those with diabetic kidney disease [4, 50]. The DIVAT study also found that death-censored graft survival was higher in ADPKD patients. This was in spite of the ADPKD patients in their registry receiving kidneys from older donors with a higher prevalence of cardiovascular disease, having a lower proportion of living kidney donors, and having longer cold ischemia time [46]. The largest study of ADPKD patients posttransplant ($N = 3170$) compared to nondiabetic controls ($N = 1554$) found a difference in the overall survival between the groups [4] (Fig. 14.3).

Conclusion

Autosomal dominant PKD leads to kidney failure in many affected individuals. Their management after reaching ESRD remains challenging, particularly given the lack of disease-specific management options. Nonetheless, the outcomes of these individuals are favorable both on dialysis and with kidney transplantation.

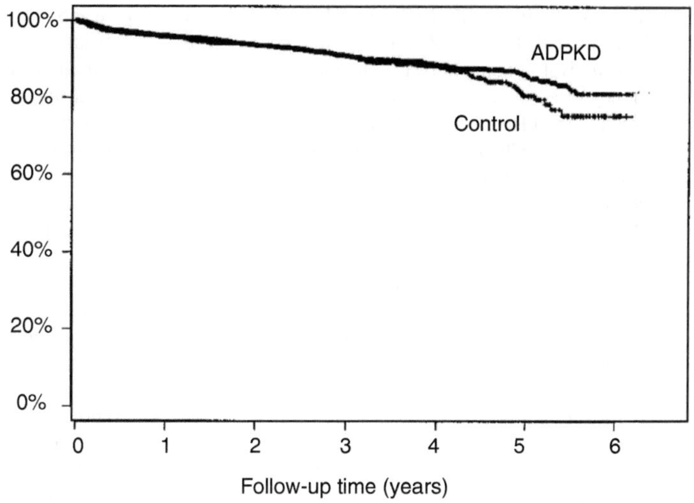

Fig. 14.3 The survival of 3170 patients with ADPKD following kidney transplantation, compared with 1554 nondiabetic controls from USRDS (log rank test $p = 0.23$) (From Perrone et al. [4]. Reprinted with permission from Elsevier via STM Permissions Guidelines)

References

1. Collins AJ, Foley RN, Herzog C, et al. US renal data system 2012 annual data report. Am J Kidney Dis. 2013;61(A7):e1–476.
2. Orskov B, Romming Sorensen V, Feldt-Rasmussen B, Strandgaard S. Improved prognosis in patients with autosomal dominant polycystic kidney disease in Denmark. Clin J Am Soc Nephrol. 2010;5:2034–9.
3. Haynes R, Kheradmand F, Winearls CG. Survival after starting renal replacement treatment in patients with autosomal dominant polycystic kidney disease: a single-centre 40-year study. Nephron Clin Pract. 2012;120:c42–7.
4. Perrone R, Ruthazer R, Terrin N. Survival after end-stage renal disease in autosomal dominant polycystic kidney disease: contribution of extrarenal complications to mortality. Am J Kidney Dis. 2001;38:777–84.
5. Wolfe R, Ashby V, Milford E, et al. Comparison of mortality in all patients on dialysis, patients on dialysis awaiting transplantation, and recipients of a first cadaveric transplant. New Eng J Med. 1999;341:1725–30.
6. Hateboer N, v Dijk MA, Bogdanova N, et al. Comparison of phenotypes of polycystic kidney disease types 1 and 2. European PKD1-PKD2 study group. Lancet. 1999;353:103–7.
7. Perl J, Bargman JM. The importance of residual kidney function for patients on dialysis: a critical review. Am J Kidney Dis. 2009;53:1068–81.
8. Pandya BK, Friede T, Williams JD. A comparison of peritonitis in polycystic and non-polycystic patients on peritoneal dialysis. Perit Dial Int. 2004;24:79–81.
9. Hadimeri H, Johansson AC, Haraldsson B, Nyberg G. CAPD in patients with autosomal dominant polycystic kidney disease. Perit Dial Int. 1998;18:429–32.
10. Kumar S, Fan SL, Raftery MJ, Yaqoob MM. Long term outcome of patients with autosomal dominant polycystic kidney diseases receiving peritoneal dialysis. Kidney Int. 2008;74:946–51.
11. Nolph KD, Cutler SJ, Steinberg SM, Novak JW. Continuous ambulatory peritoneal dialysis in the United States: a three-year study. Kidney Int. 1985;28:198–205.
12. Lobbedez T, Touam M, Evans D, Ryckelynck JP, Knebelman B, Verger C. Peritoneal dialysis in polycystic kidney disease patients. Report from the French peritoneal dialysis registry (RDPLF). Nephrol Dial Transplant. 2011;26:2332–9.
13. Portoles JM, Tato AM, Lopez-Sanchez P. Peritoneal dialysis for patients with polycystic kidney disease in Spain. Am J Kidney Dis. 2011;58:493. author reply 4
14. Li L, Szeto CC, Kwan BC, Chow KM, Leung CB, Kam-Tao LP. Peritoneal dialysis as the first-line renal replacement therapy in patients with autosomal dominant polycystic kidney disease. Am J Kidney Dis. 2011;57:903–7.
15. Christophe JL, van Ypersele de Strihou C, Pirson Y. Complications of autosomal dominant polycystic kidney disease in 50 haemodialysed patients. A case-control study. The U.C.L. collaborative group. Nephrol Dial Transplant. 1996;11:1271–6.
16. Yoo DJ, Agodoa L, Yuan CM, Abbott KC, Nee R. Risk of intracranial hemorrhage associated with autosomal dominant polycystic kidney disease in patients with end stage renal disease. BMC Nephrol. 2014;15:39.
17. Eckardt K, Mollmann M, Neumann R, et al. Erythropoietin in polycystic kidneys. J Clin Invest. 1989;84:1160–6.
18. Abbott KC, Agodoa LY. Polycystic kidney disease in patients on the renal transplant waiting list: trends in hematocrit and survival. BMC Nephrol. 2002;3:7.

19. Shah A, Molnar MZ, Lukowsky LR, Zaritsky JJ, Kovesdy CP, Kalantar-Zadeh K. Hemoglobin level and survival in hemodialysis patients with polycystic kidney disease and the role of administered erythropoietin. Am J Hematol. 2012;87:833–6.
20. Gabow PA, Chapman AB, Johnson AM, et al. Renal structure and hypertension in autosomal dominant polycystic kidney disease. Kidney Int. 1990;38:1177–80.
21. Schrier RW, Abebe KZ, Perrone RD, et al. Blood pressure in early autosomal dominant polycystic kidney disease. N Engl J Med. 2014;371:2255–66.
22. Torres VE, Abebe KZ, Chapman AB, et al. Angiotensin blockade in late autosomal dominant polycystic kidney disease. N Engl J Med. 2014;371:2267–76.
23. Molnar MZ, Lukowsky LR, Streja E, et al. Blood pressure and survival in long-term hemodialysis patients with and without polycystic kidney disease. J Hypertens. 2010;28:2475–84.
24. Lukowsky LR, Molnar MZ, Zaritsky JJ, et al. Mineral and bone disorders and survival in hemodialysis patients with and without polycystic kidney disease. Nephrol Dial Transplant. 2012;27:2899–907.
25. U.S. Renal Data System. USRDS 2008 annual data report: atlas of chronic kidney disease and end-stage renal disease in the United States. National Institutes of Health, National Institute of Diabetes and Digestive and Kidney Diseases 2008; Bethesda.
26. Yabu JM, Anderson MW, Kim D, et al. Sensitization from transfusion in patients awaiting primary kidney transplant. Nephrol Dial Transplant. 2013;28:2908–18.
27. Irazabal MV, Huston J 3rd, Kubly V, et al. Extended follow-up of unruptured intracranial aneurysms detected by presymptomatic screening in patients with autosomal dominant polycystic kidney disease. Clin J Am Soc Nephrol. 2011;6:1274–85.
28. Pei Y, Hwang YH, Conklin J, et al. Imaging-based diagnosis of autosomal dominant polycystic kidney disease. J Am Soc Nephrol JASN. 2015;26:746–53.
29. Kanaan N, Devuyst O, Pirson Y. Renal transplantation in autosomal dominant polycystic kidney disease. Nat Rev Nephrol. 2014;10:455–65.
30. Patel P, Horsfield C, Compton F, Taylor J, Koffman G, Olsburgh J. Native nephrectomy in transplant patients with autosomal dominant polycystic kidney disease. Ann R Coll Surg Engl. 2011;93:391–5.
31. Martin AD, Mekeel KL, Castle EP, et al. Laparoscopic bilateral native nephrectomies with simultaneous kidney transplantation. BJU Int. 2012;110:E1003–7.
32. Neeff HP, Pisarski P, Tittelbach-Helmrich D, et al. One hundred consecutive kidney transplantations with simultaneous ipsilateral nephrectomy in patients with autosomal dominant polycystic kidney disease. Nephrol Dial Transplant. 2013;28:466–71.
33. Lucas SM, Mofunanya TC, Goggins WC, Sundaram CP. Staged nephrectomy versus bilateral laparoscopic nephrectomy in patients with autosomal dominant polycystic kidney disease. J Urol. 2010;184:2054–9.
34. Skauby MH, Oyen O, Hartman A, Leivestad T, Wadstrom J. Kidney transplantation with and without simultaneous bilateral native nephrectomy in patients with polycystic kidney disease: a comparative retrospective study. Transplantation. 2012;94:383–8.
35. Bennett WM. Peritransplant management of retained native kidneys in autosomal dominant polycystic kidney disease. Nephrol Dial Transplant. 2013;28:245–6.
36. Yamamoto T, Watarai Y, Kobayashi T, et al. Kidney volume changes in patients with autosomal dominant polycystic kidney disease after renal transplantation. Transplantation. 2012;93:794–8.
37. Tao Y, Kim J, Schrier RW, Edelstein CL. Rapamycin markedly slows disease progression in a rat model of polycystic kidney disease. J Am Soc Nephrol: JASN. 2005;16:46–51.
38. Wahl PR, Serra AL, Le Hir M, Molle KD, Hall MN, Wuthrich RP. Inhibition of mTOR with sirolimus slows disease progression in Han:SPRD rats with autosomal dominant polycystic kidney disease (ADPKD). Nephrol Dial Transplant. 2006;21:598–604.
39. Shillingford JM, Murcia NS, Larson CH, et al. The mTOR pathway is regulated by polycystin-1, and its inhibition reverses renal cystogenesis in polycystic kidney disease. Proc Natl Acad Sci U S A. 2006;103:5466–71.
40. Qian Q, Du H, King BF, et al. Sirolimus reduces polycystic liver volume in ADPKD patients. J Am Soc Nephrol: JASN. 2008;19:631–8.
41. Serra AL, Poster D, Kistler AD, et al. Sirolimus and kidney growth in autosomal dominant polycystic kidney disease. N Engl J Med. 2010;363:820–9.
42. Walz G, Budde K, Mannaa M, et al. Everolimus in patients with autosomal dominant polycystic kidney disease. N Engl J Med. 2010;363:830–40.
43. Sherstha R, McKinley C, Russ P, et al. Postmenopausal estrogen therapy selectively stimulates hepatic enlargement in women with autosomal dominant polycystic kidney disease. Hepatology. 1997;26:1282–6.
44. Chauveau D, Fakhouri F, Grunfeld JP. Liver involvement in autosomal-dominant polycystic kidney disease: therapeutic dilemma. J Am Soc Nephrol: JASN. 2000;11:1767–75.
45. Hadimeri H, Norden G, Friman S, Nyberg G. Autosomal dominant polycystic kidney disease in a kidney transplant population. Nephrol Dial Transplant. 1997;12:1431–6.
46. Jacquet A, Pallet N, Kessler M, et al. Outcomes of renal transplantation in patients with autosomal dominant polycystic kidney disease: a nationwide longitudinal study. Transpl Int: Off J Eur Soc Organ Transplant. 2011;24:582–7.
47. Oliveras A, Roquer J, Puig JM, et al. Stroke in renal transplant recipients: epidemiology, predictive risk factors and outcome. Clin Transpl. 2003;17:1–8.
48. Abedini S, Holme I, Fellstrom B, et al. Cerebrovascular events in renal transplant recipients. Transplantation. 2009;87:112–7.

49. Niemczyk M, Niemczyk S, Paczek L. Autosomal dominant polycystic kidney disease and transplantation. Ann Transplant: Q Pol Transplant Soc. 2009;14:86–90.
50. Stiasny B, Ziebell D, Graf S, Hauser IA, Schulze BD. Clinical aspects of renal transplantation in polycystic kidney disease. Clin Nephrol. 2002;58:16–24.
51. Wetmore JB, Calvet JP, Yu AS, et al. Polycystic kidney disease and cancer after renal transplantation. J Am Soc Nephrol: JASN. 2014;25:2335–41.
52. Vichot AA, Geller DS, Perazella MA. Progression of polycystic kidney disease in a kidney transplant. Kidney Int. 2013;83:533.

Management of ADPKD Today

15

Ronald D. Perrone and Osama W. Amro

Until recently, no disease-modifying treatment has been widely approved for the treatment of ADPKD. The vasopressin V2 receptor blocker tolvaptan has been demonstrated to slow the rate of kidney volume growth and decline in eGFR when GFR is well preserved [1] and to slow the decline in eGFR in more advanced disease [2]. See Chap. 13 for full details [1, 2]. Additional novel therapeutic strategies are currently being explored with promising results [3]. It is anticipated that the management of ADPKD will undergo a revolution in the future with the translation of new treatments into routine clinical practice.

In addition to specific treatments, the management of patients with ADPKD relies on general measures, such as blood pressure control, dietary modification, and treatment of dyslipidemia, which may reduce cardiovascular complications of the disease. In addition, supportive therapy, including pain control, treatment of infection, and renal replacement therapy when needed are cornerstones of therapy. Should additional specific treatments for ADPKD become available in the future, the treatment should be combined with these therapeutic approaches to maximize the benefit, further slow or halt the disease progression, and address disease complications. A framework for classifying ADPKD into stages of progression is shown in Fig. 15.1.

Subclinical, early, late, and advanced stages are descriptively characterized. There is no hard and fast cutoff between the stages, and much overlap would be expected to exist. Nonetheless, we find this framework to be useful to understand the onset of different complications during the course of the disease. It is important to recognize that ADPKD progression is highly variable among families and among individuals within families and that the kidney manifestations and progression are primarily the result of changes in kidney size resulting from the growth of multiple cysts within the kidneys. Early in the disease, when cysts are small or undetectable, most patients are asymptomatic. As cysts expand, complications ensue. Early complications include impaired concentrating ability, resulting potentially in polyuria or nocturia. Cyst rupture, and hematuria, nephrolithiasis, and the development of hypertension follow as kidneys expand. GFR declines rapidly (4.3 ml/min/1.73 m^2 per year) when kidneys exceed 1500 ml in size or somewhat more slowly with a htTKV of 600 cc/m [4]. The development of complications appears to be related to kidney enlargement, although there is a

R. D. Perrone, MD (✉)
CTRC, Tufts University CTSI, Tufts University School of Medicine, Boston, MA, USA

Division of Nephrology, Department of Medicine, Tufts Medical Center, Boston, MA, USA
e-mail: rperrone@tuftsmedicalcenter.org

O. W. Amro, MD, MS
Swedish Center for Comprehensive Care, Swedish Medical Center, Seattle, WA, USA

B. D. Cowley, Jr., J. J. Bissler (eds.), *Polycystic Kidney Disease*,
https://doi.org/10.1007/978-1-4939-7784-0_15

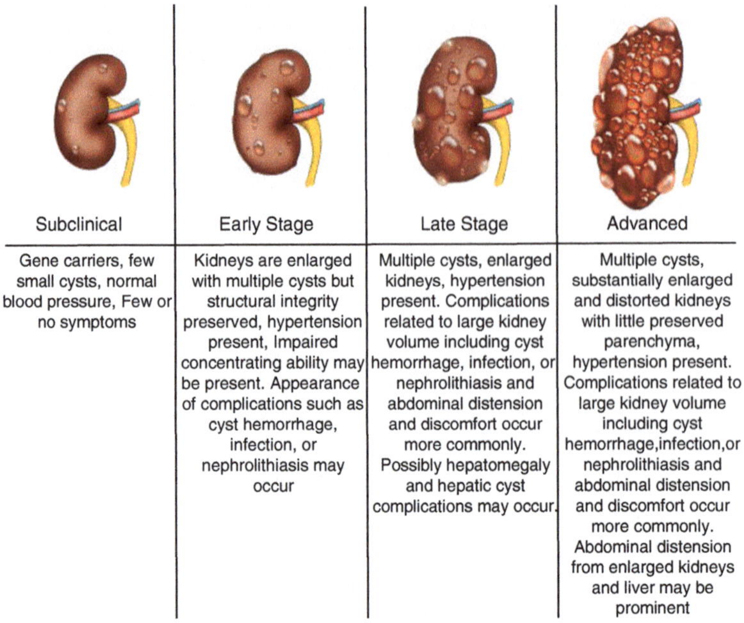

Fig. 15.1 Clinical stages of ADPKD

poor correlation of pain with TKV [5]. We present management strategies that are associated with these early and late clinical stages of ADPKD (Fig. 15.1).

Subclinical and Early Stage Management

The management of patients in these early clinical stages relies on counseling and risk factor modification.

Risk Factor Modifications

Management of Hypertension in ADPKD

Hypertension is an early and frequent finding of ADPKD, occurring in approximately 60% of the patients prior to deterioration in kidney function [6]. Hypertension is associated with increased kidney size and loss of kidney function and is an important risk factor for cardiovascular death, the most frequent cause of mortality in ADPKD patients [7–9].

Hypertension in patients with ADPKD is believed to be mediated by increased activity of the renin-angiotensin system (RAS) [10] and to a lesser degree by extracellular volume expansion [11]. It has been suggested that cyst expansion, leading to focal areas of renal ischemia and enhanced renin release, is responsible for RAS activation [12].

Blood Pressure Goal

The optimal blood pressure goal for patients with ADPKD is not known; however, new research suggests that rigorous blood pressure control is beneficial in early ADPKD. The HALT PKD study, a 7-year randomized placebo-controlled interventional trial, showed benefits of rigorous blood pressure control (blood pressure target of <110/70 mm Hg) on kidney volume progression rate, left ventricular mass index, and urinary albumin excretion in patients with early ADPKD [13]. This low blood pressure goal was well tolerated and easy to achieve. This study may change our current treatment strategies for younger patients with early ADPKD (eGFR>60 ml/min) to target a blood pressure of <110/70 mm Hg.

For patients with more advanced ADPKD (eGFR<60 ml/min) or older individuals, it is reasonable to target a blood pressure of 130/80 or below especially in the presence of proteinuria.

Choice of Antihypertensive Agent

The early and effective treatment of hypertension regardless of antihypertensive medication use should delay the onset of ESRD [14]. However, a careful selection of antihypertensive medication might provide extra advantage.

Lifestyle modification with salt restriction, weight management, and encouragement of regular exercise should be the mainstay of treatment in all patients with hypertension. If lifestyle modification is not successful in achieving blood pressure goal, pharmacotherapy should be initiated.

Given what we know about the mechanism of hypertension in patients with ADPKD, an angiotensin-converting enzyme (ACE) inhibitor or angiotensin II receptor blocker (ARB) should be the drug of choice. This is particularly important for patients with proteinuria, as studies suggest a benefit of ACE inhibitors in patients with ADPKD and proteinuria in slowing disease progression [15]. An extra potential advantage of this class of medications is the possible protection they provide against secondary glomerular injury by reducing intraglomerular pressure.

Dyslipidemia

Although no studies have specifically looked at control of dyslipidemia in patients with ADPKD, evidence from the general population and in CKD appears to support the use of lipid-lowering agents, in particular statins.

Compelling evidence has shown favorable outcomes and significant reduction in the incidence of major atherosclerotic events in patients with advanced chronic kidney disease treated with statins [16]. As this study included patients with ADPKD, it may be reasonable to expect these results to apply also to ADPKD patients. Dyslipidemia may also accelerate and perpetuate the rate of GFR decline. However, the supportive data for this notion are largely derived from post hoc analyses of several large trials, which may be limited by unmeasured confounders [17, 18].

Screening for Dyslipidemia

Due to the prevalence of cardiovascular risk factors in the ADPKD population [19], a lipid profile (total cholesterol, LDL cholesterol (LDL-C), HDL cholesterol, and triglycerides) should be obtained for newly identified ADPKD patients. Initial evaluation of the lipid profile mainly serves to establish the diagnosis of severe hypercholesterolemia and/or hypertriglyceridemia.

Dyslipidemia Management

Therapeutic lifestyle measures to reduce serum cholesterol should be encouraged in all patients with ADPKD. Many of these measures, including adoption of a reduced fat diet and regular exercise, may improve general health independent of any effect on the lipid profile.

Previous guidelines have emphasized the potential value of LDL-C as an indication for pharmacological treatment with lipid-lowering agents [20]. This approach is no longer recommended given the lack of data to support targeting LDL-C in populations with and without CKD [21], the substantial within-person variability in LDL-C measurements [22], and the potential for medication-related toxicity. The current evidence suggests that patients with chronic kidney disease and significant risk factors for coronary artery disease should be prescribed a lipid-lowering agent (2013 KDIGO). Given the paucity of data that can guide dyslipidemia treatment in patients with ADPKD, it is reasonable to extrapolate our management approach based on the data for chronic kidney disease in general.

Since higher cardiovascular risk and not elevated LDL-C are now the primary indications to initiate lipid-lowering treatment in CKD patients, we favor starting lipid-lowering agents in all patients with ADPKD with any risk factor for coronary artery disease as this population is clearly at high risk to develop cardiovascular disease. Statins are the drug of choice as they may have other potential favorable outcomes in patients with ADPKD. In one study, simvastatin was shown to have a beneficial effect on inflammatory markers, renal blood flow, and endothelial function in a group of patients with ADPKD [23].

Furthermore, in a randomized controlled trial [24], pravastatin was shown to be effective in slowing the progression of kidney volume in children with ADPKD. The mechanisms underlying the effect of pravastatin on ADPKD are believed to be independent of lipid-lowering effects of the medication. It is proposed that the inhibition of the conversion of hepatic hydroxymethylglutaryl-CoA to mevalonate can alter posttranslational modification of proteins, including Ras and Rho, which may alter signal transduction, cell proliferation, and possibly kidney cyst enlargement in ADPKD. Despite the promising results of pravastatin use in children with ADPKD, further validation and careful consideration of risks versus potential benefits are needed prior to routine use of statin in children with ADPKD who have no dyslipidemia or clear risk factors for coronary artery disease.

Monitoring Response to Treatment

As detailed earlier, clinical practice guidelines are used to emphasize the use of targets for LDL-C (e.g., 70 or 100 mg/dl) in managing dyslipidemia [20, 25]. This requires repeated measurements of LDL-C and treatment escalation with higher doses of statin or initiation of combination with lipid-lowering therapy ("treat-to-target" strategy); this approach is no longer recommended (2013 KDIGO). The rationale behind this change in recommendations was based on the fact that treat-to-target strategy has never been proven beneficial in any clinical trial and higher doses of statins have not been proven to be safe in the setting of CKD. An alternative "fire-and-forget" strategy for patients with CKD is being proposed. This implies that repeat cholesterol testing is not necessary in most patients.

Diet and Fluid Intake in ADPKD

The optimal diet for ADPKD is yet to be identified. Prior studies have shown only marginal benefit of a low-protein diet (0.28 g of protein for every kilogram of body weight per day) in ADPKD patients with low eGFR [26]. We generally recommend moderate protein restriction (0.8 g of protein for every kilogram of body weight per day); this protein intake is consistent with the Recommended Dietary Allowance (RDA) for healthy men and women that is based on analyses of available nitrogen balance studies [27].

A high-protein diet is believed to contribute to protein-induced hyperfiltration. An increase in the filtered load of amino acids may enhance proximal sodium reabsorption via sodium-amino acid cotransporters in the proximal tubule. The decrease in sodium chloride delivery to the macula densa may then activate tubuloglomerular feedback, leading to an elevation in glomerular filtration rate in an attempt to restore macula densa delivery back to normal [28, 29].

Another potential harmful effect of high-protein intake on ADPKD is the stimulation of vasopressin secretion associated with high-osmolar daily load in the context of fixed water ingestion. Moderate protein restriction of 0.8 g protein per kilogram of patient weight for patients not on dialysis is usually well tolerated by patients and is not known to be associated with malnourishment or other harmful effects. Caffeine intake may contribute to ADPKD disease progression; this is primary based on in vitro studies examining the relationship between caffeine and cyst epithelial cells. Phosphodiesterase inhibition by caffeine increases the accumulation of adenosine 3′,5′-cyclic monophosphate (cAMP), and through this mechanism, it activates the extracellular signal-regulated kinase (ERK) pathway to stimulate cellular proliferation and increases transepithelial fluid secretion by ADPKD cystic epithelium [30]. Ingestion of one to three cups of coffee could lead to plasma caffeine levels in a range that increases cAMP levels and potentiates the effect of vasopressin to increase cAMP [30]. One observational study, however, demonstrated no impact of coffee intake on TKV growth or GFR progression in 151 patients with ADPKD followed by the SUISSE PKD cohort [31]. Despite the lack of human clinical trial data to support this effect, we still believe that consuming less caffeine might be beneficial in patients with ADPKD. We generally advise patients to limit their caffeine intake. Patients should be educated about the common sources of caffeine in food and drinks as many patients might be consuming far more caffeine than they believe they do. Food or drinks other than brewed coffee, such as carbonated beverages, tea, chocolates, and energy drinks, contain significant levels of caffeine.

Herb and natural supplement use is widespread in the US adult population based on data from the National Center for Health Statistics [32]. Herbal manufacturing processes frequently lack standardization and are not regulated as drugs by the US Food and Drug Administration (FDA). Toxic contaminants have been repeatedly found in herbal supplements available for consumers. We generally discourage the use of herbal supplements in patients with ADPKD; one particular compound that might carry exceptional risk for patients with ADPKD is forskolin. Forskolin is synthesized by the plant *Coleus forskohlii* and is sold for weight management and as a cardiovascular tonic agent. Forskolin, a widely known, potent adenylyl cyclase agonist, has been isolated and identified within the cyst fluid of patients with polycystic kidney disease [33]. Forskolin may have a role in promoting the enlargement of cysts in ADPKD patients. Patients should avoid preparations that contain this compound.

Fluid Intake

It has been long established that patients with ADPKD have impaired urine-concentrating ability and higher levels of arginine vasopressin (AVP) than healthy controls [34]. AVP is a potent activator of adenylyl cyclase in collecting duct cells; most of the cysts in ADPKD are of collecting duct origin. It has been shown that AVP is a key player in the progression of polycystic kidney disease [35, 36].

High water intake has been proposed as a physiological approach to decrease vasopressin secretion in patients with ADPKD. In an animal model of polycystic kidney disease where cysts originated from the distal nephron, high water intake suppressed plasma levels of AVP and slowed cyst progression [37]. A pilot study evaluated the effects of acute and chronic water ingestion on urine osmolality and cAMP concentrations in 13 subjects with ADPKD and 10 healthy controls [38]. Chronic water loading of around 3 l per day increased urine volume and decreased urine osmolality in ADPKD subjects. The 24-h cAMP excretion did not change with chronic water loading, although it did with acute water loading.

Given all of the above, patients with ADPKD are advised to consume 2–3 l of fluid daily [39]. However, adherence to high fluid intake is difficult in clinical practice [40, 41]. Part of the difficulty in sustaining high daily water ingestion enough to suppress AVP is the consumption of a diet that generates abundant osmoles; a high-osmolar load stimulates vasopressin secretion to maintain water homeostasis. Studies are needed to determine the optimum water and daily osmolar intake for patients with ADPKD. A fluid intake that is tailored to individual patients based on their AVP level has been identified. Amro and colleagues demonstrated that reduction of osmolar intake (largely salt and protein) allowed a significant reduction in water requirements (0.6 L) yet still resulted in suppression of vasopressin, as reflected in plasma copeptin levels [42].

In addition to reduced protein diet and high water intake, patients with ADPKD with hypertension should restrict salt intake. It is not known if a low-salt diet in normotensive ADPKD patients is clinically beneficial. However, higher sodium intake in subjects participating both in the CRISP and HALT cohorts was associated with more rapid progression of the disease [43, 44]. These observations suggests that control of dietary sodium may be important for the control not only of blood pressure but also of cystic disease progression. A high salt intake stimulates vasopressin secretion to maintain water homeostasis. Clinical studies are needed to determine the optimum salt intake for patients with ADPKD. It is reasonable to advise all patients with ADPKD to limit sodium intake to 1500–2000 mg (65–88 mEq) per day, but this level of sodium restriction is difficult to achieve, even in highly motivated individuals. For example, subjects followed in the Consortium for Radiologic Imaging Studies of Polycystic Kidney Disease (CRISP) observational cohort had mean sodium intake of 190–200 mEq/day despite being followed in academic clinics with substantial expertise in the treatment of ADPKD [43].

Management of Late Clinical Stage

Patients at this stage experience complications related to enlarged cystic kidneys and potentially enlarged cystic livers. In addition to continued risk factor modification, early identification and treatment of kidney volume-related complications are important to preserve kidney function and improve patient's quality of life.

Complications Related to Enlarged Cystic Kidneys

The kidneys can reach an enormous size in patients with ADPKD. This can create a range of symptoms and complications that contribute to the patients' morbidity and even mortality.

Data from the Consortium for Radiologic Imaging Studies of Polycystic Kidney Disease (CRISP) suggest that the decline in GFR correlates with increasing kidney size and cyst volume [45]. A height-adjusted kidney size of 600 cc/m is highly predictive of the development of stage 3 CKD within 8 years [4].

Acute and chronic pain, cyst infection, hematuria, nephrolithiasis, and progressive decline in kidney function are all consequences of progressive enlargement of cystic kidneys.

Pain in ADPKD

Over 60% of patients with ADPKD experience abdominal and flank pain [46]. Abdominal pain is frequently related to the kidney cysts but may also be related to liver cysts. Pain may be acute or chronic.

Acute Pain in ADPKD

It is important to investigate any episode of new flank pain or any significant change in chronic pain in patients with ADPKD. Patients might develop cyst infection or rupture that requires treatment in a timely manner. It is also important to remember that patients with ADPKD are at risk for developing abdominal pain not related to their kidney disease. Careful history and physical examination are usually revealing. Cyst hemorrhage, urinary tract infection, and nephrolithiasis are common causes of acute pain in ADPKD. The frequency of cyst hemorrhage, gross hematuria, and nephrolithiasis is associated with increased kidney volume [47].

Chronic Pain in ADPKD

Chronic flank and back pain are fairly common in patients with advanced ADPKD. In a cross-sectional study that examined quality of life in patients with ADPKD [5], back pain was present in 51% of patients, of whom 30% experienced it sometimes and 21% experienced it often or always. The pain is usually related to a combination of enlarged cysts causing stretching of the kidney capsule and an exaggerated lumbar lordosis causing mechanical pain. Symptoms related to abdominal fullness and pain are greater in patients with large kidney volume and decreased kidney function (eGFR <45 ml/min) [5]. Management of chronic pain is very important as pain might become severe impacting the patient's quality of life and overall well-being. A non-pharmacological approach should be started first. Wearing supporting garments or a corset, avoiding high heels, and having physical therapy, acupuncture, and heat pads can all be beneficial in pain management. Management of posture using the Alexander Technique has also been proposed [48].

If non-pharmacological methods fail, a non-narcotic analgesic should be tried. This includes acetaminophen, tramadol, or gabapentin. Nonsteroidal anti-inflammatory drugs, although effective, should be avoided in patients with reduced GFR. If pain persists in spite of the above, narcotics should be used sparingly.

When used appropriately, opioids can lead to significant pain reduction and improvement in patient function [49]. Referral to a pain clinic for chronic pain management can be helpful. In severe cases, surgical interventions such as decortication, cyst marsupialization, or even nephrectomy are required to control intractable

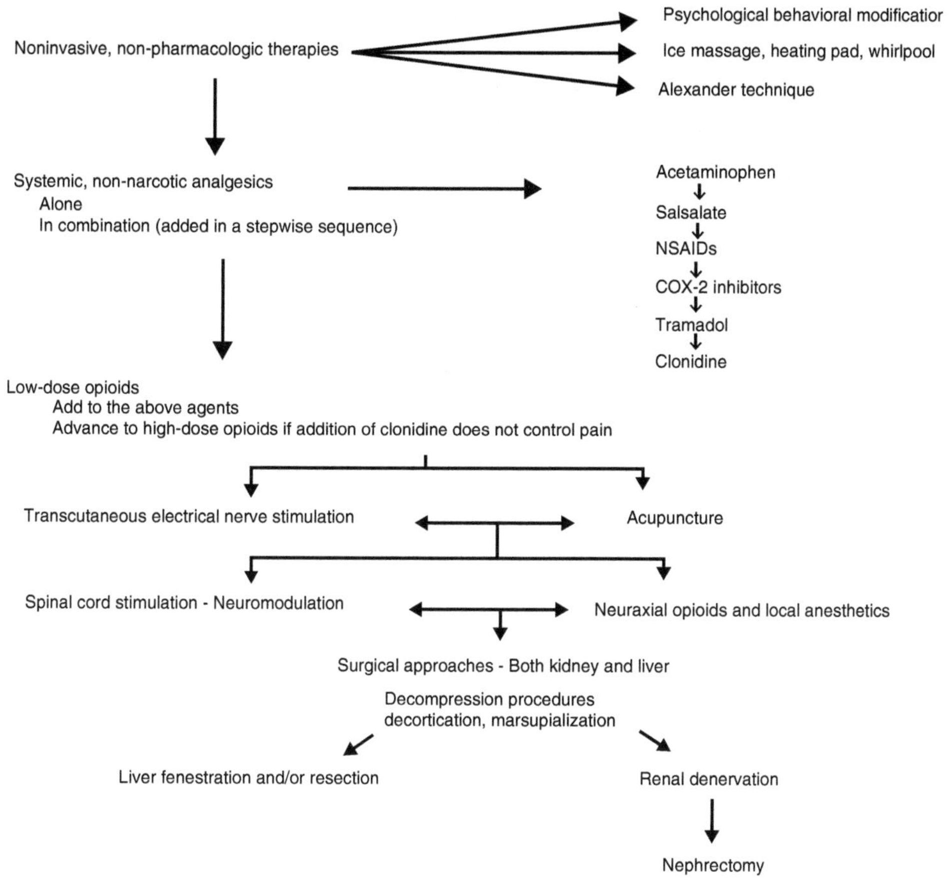

Fig. 15.2 Pain management in ADPKD. Pain management in polycystic kidney disease patients should follow a sequential approach, starting with measures that are noninvasive and simple and have relatively few side effects, and then slowly progress toward more complex and invasive measures (Reprinted from Ref. [48] with permission from Elsevier via STM Permissions Guidelines)

chronic pain. Laparoscopic renal denervation may yield favorable results for pain control in patients with refractory chronic pain [50]. The various options for an effective combined and sequential chronic pain management in ADPKD are noted in Fig. 15.2 [51].

Urinary Tract and Cyst Infection

Cyst infection and acute pyelonephritis are the most common kidney infections in ADPKD patients. Approximately 30–50% of patients will have a urinary tract infection during their lifetime. Cyst infections that require hospitalization occur in approximately 9% of ADPKD patients [52].

Clinical Presentation

ADPKD patients with kidney infection usually present with fever, flank pain, nausea, and vomiting [53]. Distinguishing between acute pyelonephritis and an infected cyst is often difficult bearing in mind that both types of infection can occur simultaneously. Certain characteristics may help differentiate between pyelonephritis and cyst infection [54].

With pyelonephritis, the manifestations are acute with features similar to any patient without ADPKD. In contrast, patients with a cyst infection frequently have a more insidious presentation, and cyst infection may present with pyuria and absence of bacteriuria [55]; blood cultures may also be positive [56]. Patients with an infected cyst may have a new area of discrete tenderness on exam, whereas pyelonephritis tends to be associated with diffuse flank pain and costovertebral angle tenderness. The presence of white cell casts is suggestive of acute pyelonephritis, and the urine culture is usually positive. In contrast, the sediment may be bland, and the urine culture may be negative in case of an infected cyst, since cysts may not be in contact with the renal collecting system [55]. However, pyuria is found in up to 45% of uninfected patients with ADPKD [57]. Therefore, interpretation of laboratory results should be done with consideration of the clinical context.

Diagnosis

Establishing the diagnosis of kidney infection in a patient with ADPKD requires a similar approach for a patient without the disease. Thorough history, physical examination, urinalysis, urine culture, and blood culture are important steps in establishing the diagnosis as detailed above. However, imaging studies might provide additional information in certain patients.

Imaging Studies

In general, imaging studies are reserved for atypical or severe presentations or with bacteremia, if renal abscess is suspected, and to localize an infected cyst for drainage in case of refractory infection. Conventional radiological imaging with computed tomography or ultrasonography has low sensitivity and specificity in diagnosing cyst infection due to anatomic distortion. However, gallium or indium scanning is positive in about one-half of cases [58]. Sufficient resolution for identification of an infected cyst for drainage is rarely obtained with the above imaging modalities, unless the infected cyst is large, thick-walled, with surrounding inflammation. In limited case series, 18F-fluorodeoxyglucose positron emission tomography-computed tomography (FDG)-PET/CT scan identified renal and hepatic cyst infections with high sensitivity and specificity [59].

Choice of Antibiotics

Kidney infections in ADPKD are most commonly caused by gram-negative enteric organisms. In a retrospective study of patients with ADPKD presenting with cyst infection [52], *Escherichia coli* accounted for 74% of all retrieved bacterial strains. Clinical efficacy of initial antibiotic treatment was noted in 71% of episodes. Antibiotic treatment modification was more frequently required for patients who were receiving initial monotherapy compared with those who were receiving combination therapy. Infected cysts larger than 5 cm frequently require drainage.

Fluoroquinolones remain the preferred antibiotic of choice for cyst infections in patients with ADPKD. Drugs that can be detected in cysts are lipid soluble and secreted through tubules or have high pKa values. These include erythromycin, vancomycin, cefotaxime, ampicillin, and trimethoprim-sulfamethoxazole [60]. Drugs active against anaerobes such as metronidazole and clindamycin also achieve therapeutic concentrations in cysts [61].

Hematuria

Gross hematuria occurs in approximately 35–50% of patients with ADPKD and is more likely to occur among individuals with large kidneys [62]. Hematuria could be related to cyst infection, hemorrhage into cysts, or nephrolithiasis.

The first episode of hematuria usually causes significant anxiety and fear to patients and their families. Many times hematuria is preceded by trauma or cyst infection, but spontaneous hematuria is not uncommon.

Hematuria usually resolves spontaneously within a few days. Patients become, with time, familiar with those episodes and the pattern of its resolution. If an infection is the preceding event, antibiotic treatment along with hydration is the mainstay of management. If hematuria is related to cyst rupture, bed rest is advisable in addition to hydration. Discontinuation of antiplatelet or other anticoagulant medications may be necessary. In very rare occasions, hematuria can lead to hemodynamic instability and might require arterial embolization or even nephrectomy.

Recurrent hematuria is associated with more rapid decline in kidney function [63]. Hence, avoidance of trauma is important. Patients should avoid contact sports such as martial arts and football, particularly those with large kidneys.

Patients with ADPKD may require chronic anticoagulation for conditions not related to ADKPD such as deep vein thrombosis or atrial fibrillation. Cautious monitoring of hematuria frequency and severity is needed. Data to guide anticoagulation in patients with ADPKD are limited; therefore, careful evaluation of risks and benefits prior to initiation of anticoagulation medication is advisable [64].

Nephrolithiasis

Increased kidney size may be a risk factor for nephrolithiasis in patients with ADPKD. In one study, kidney volume was greater in 35 patients with ADPKD and nephrolithiasis compared with those patients who had ADPKD but no nephrolithiasis [65]. This finding is different from what was seen in the CRISP study [45], as there was no association observed between nephrolithiasis and kidney volume. Other factors that might predispose patients with ADPKD to nephrolithiasis include low urine volume, low urinary citrate, hyperuricosuria, and hypercalciuria [66, 67].

When nephrolithiasis is suspected based on clinical presentation, non-contrast spiral CT is effective in establishing the diagnosis. CT is also useful to exclude hydronephrosis. The treatment for nephrolithiasis in ADPKD patients is the same as in other patients. Distortion of the urinary tract by large cysts may make treatment less effective due to difficulties in instrumentation or passage of stones or stone fragments. Preventive measures should be introduced based on stone analysis, including urine alkalization and dilution, along with correction of metabolic abnormalities, if present, such as hypocitraturia or hypercalciuria. Extracorporeal shock wave lithotripsy (ESWL) and percutaneous nephrostolithotomy may be required.

A retrospective study was conducted to evaluate available options for the management of nephrolithiasis in patients with ADPKD. Among 452 cases of ADPKD, 19 patients were managed for nephrolithiasis [68]. The mean stone size was 115 mm^2 (range 36–980 mm^2). The majority of the stones were calyceal, and nine patients required intervention, while the rest were treated conservatively. Treatment offered included open nephrectomy for nonfunctioning infected kidney, extracorporeal shock wave lithotripsy (ESWL), ureterorenoscopy (URS), and percutaneous nephrolithotomy (PCNL). All patients who underwent URS and PCNL had complete clearance, while those who underwent ESWL had a residual stone. This suggests a greater degree of retained stone fragments after ESWL in ADPKD patients.

Renal Cancer

The prevalence of renal cancer is not different than the general population. In spite of that, when renal cell carcinoma occurs in patients with ADPKD it is more often concurrently bilateral (12 versus 1–5%), multicentric (28 versus 6%), and sarcomatoid in type (33 versus 1–5%) than in the general population [69]. This information suggests either a malignant potential restricted to a small subset of patients with ADPKD or an alteration in the biologic behavior of renal cell carcinoma when it develops in the setting of ADPKD.

Diagnosis

No routine surveillance is needed for asymptomatic patients; however, due to overlap between symptoms of ADPKD such as pain and hematuria with renal cell cancer symptoms, low threshold for imaging studies should be used especially if hematuria or pain doesn't follow the usual pattern that the patient had in the past.

Imaging techniques including unenhanced CT and MRI can be of limited value in diagnosis of malignancy or cyst infection. This is so because the kidneys are replaced by multiple cysts of various sizes and appearances; complex cysts resulting from cyst hemorrhage or inflammation are frequently observed. Single and multidetector CT have helped refine the diagnostic work-up by allowing image acquisition in various phases of renal enhancement after intravenous administration of contrast [70]. Contrast-enhanced MRI is also useful for specific diagnosis of complex cysts or malignancy. Treatment of renal cell carcinoma if identified in ADPKD patients doesn't differ from other populations.

Advanced Stage

The advanced stage of ADPKD is defined by the presence of multiple cysts, substantially enlarged and distorted kidneys with little preserved parenchyma, and the presence of hypertension. Complications related to large kidney volume including cyst hemorrhage, infection, or nephrolithiasis and abdominal distension and discomfort occur more commonly. Abdominal distension from enlarged kidneys and liver may be prominent.

Nephrectomy

Native nephrectomy in ADPKD is a major undertaking associated with significant morbidity [71]. Nephrectomy should be avoided whenever possible. Rarely, patients will require nephrectomy of one or both kidneys in order to better accommodate kidney transplant. Other indications for nephrectomy include recurrent urinary tract infection, intractable chronic pain, renal cell carcinoma, or chronic severe hematuria requiring ongoing transfusions. The development of the hand-assisted laparoscopic approach for nephrectomy made both unilateral and bilateral nephrectomy feasible with acceptable morbidity provided there is careful selection of patients [72].

Timing of Nephrectomy in Relation to Kidney Transplant

In the absence of a compelling indication, nephrectomy done in preparation for renal transplant should be avoided; the procedure should only be performed when very large kidneys truly interfere with graft implantation [73] or if other indications for nephrectomy exist as discussed earlier, including recurrent kidney/cyst infection. It is also important to know that the volume of native kidneys can significantly decrease after renal transplantation. In a retrospective study, the volume of native kidneys was analyzed in 33 patients with ADPKD, who underwent renal transplantation. Kidney volumes significantly decreased in all but one patient after renal transplantation; the kidney(s) volume decreased by 38% and 40% at 1 and 3 years, respectively [74].

In selected cases, nephrectomy can be safely performed either as pretransplant, simultaneous, or deferred (staged) native nephrectomy [75]. The procedure is relatively safe in terms of postoperative patient morbidity and graft function. In a retrospective study [76], 32 ADPKD patients who received a kidney transplant at the University of California, San Francisco, and underwent either pretransplant, concomitant, or posttransplant native nephrectomy were evaluated. The three groups had comparable outcome. There was no difference in intraoperative time, blood loss, postoperative complications, and mean serum creatinine 3 months following surgery.

End-Stage Renal Disease

Patients with ADPKD who progress to end-stage renal disease require renal replacement therapy. People with ADPKD on hemodialysis appear to survive longer than people with end-stage renal disease from other etiologies [77].

Peritoneal dialysis is a feasible treatment option for most patients with ADPKD [78]. However, it is less commonly performed due to the presence of the enlarged kidneys and a higher risk of abdominal wall hernia. Peritoneal dialysis should be considered on an individual basis. The prognosis after kidney transplantation is usually excellent.

Management of Extrarenal Manifestations of ADPKD

Extrarenal manifestations of the disease can occur in any clinical stage although liver cyst burden correlates roughly with the kidney disease progression.

Cerebral Aneurysm

The prevalence of cerebral aneurysms in adult patients with ADPKD is approximately 10% [79]; however, familial clustering does occur with higher prevalence in patients with family history of intracranial aneurysm. Fortunately, the great majority of such aneurysms is small and rarely present in patients younger than 30 years of age.

Screening

Asymptomatic patients older than 30 years of age with family history of cerebral aneurysm, hemorrhagic stroke, or unexplained death should be screened for the presence of cerebral aneurysm [80]. Screening should also be offered to other high-risk groups such as patients with high-risk occupations in which loss of consciousness would place them or place others at extreme danger (pilots, heavy machinery operators, etc.). ADPKD patients who are being evaluated for kidney transplant are screened for aneurysms in some but not all transplant programs although there is no evidence to suggest better outcome.

Non-contrast MRA is the preferred screening method given the lack of radiation exposure and high sensitivity. Patients with contraindication to MRA can be screened by CTA with comparable results [81].

Immediate diagnostic studies are needed for patients with symptoms suggestive of subarachnoid hemorrhage. Symptoms related to growth or changes in intracranial aneurysms are important to recognize. Sentinel bleed that often precedes aneurysmal rupture is usually accompanied by a severe headache. However, it is important to note that headache frequency is not increased in patients with ADPKD. In a survey of 184 patients with ADPKD, the frequency of headaches was found to be the same as in the general population [48].

Repeat Imaging

In the absence of a family history of intracranial aneurysm (ICA) or subarachnoid hemorrhage (SAH), repeat imaging is not needed for patients with negative initial screening after the age of 30. In a prospective 10-year follow-up study, a group of patients with ADPKD that had a negative intracranial aneurysm screening study had repeat imaging approximately 10 years after the initial study [82]. Of the 76 subjects who had negative initial imaging studies, only 2 demonstrated intracranial aneurysm. The initial imaging study of one of these subjects was retrospectively thought to be positive. Given the extremely low likelihood of developing a clinically significant intracranial aneurysm following negative study, repeat surveillance in those without a family history is not thought to be warranted.

Repeat imaging every 5–10 years in those with a positive family history of ICA or SAH is generally recommended, although there is limited study of this population.

Management

The indications for surgical or endovascular intervention for asymptomatic cerebral aneurysm are the same for patients with ADPKD as for the non-ADPKD population. Traditionally, aneurysms more than 7 mm in diameter warrant consideration for treatment [83]. More recent studies suggest utilizing a combination of size, shape and location to predict risk of rupture and need for intervention [84].

Valvular Heart Disease

With a higher prevalence of asymptomatic mitral valve prolapse, mitral and aortic valve incompetence is found in patients with ADPKD [85]. The clinical significance of those abnormalities is not clear. Screening echocardiogram is not indicated for asymptomatic patients given the lack of evidence for improved outcome with screening.

Hepatic Cysts

Almost all patients with ADPKD develop liver cysts during their lifetime [86]. However, most patients are asymptomatic and require no intervention. Liver cystic disease appears to be worsened by age, female gender, pregnancy, exposure to female hormones, severity of the renal lesion, and kidney function [87].

Complications Related to Enlarged Cystic Liver

In a minority of patients, polycystic liver disease creates significant symptoms from the compressive effects of enlarged cysts. Symptoms include pain, gastric fullness, and shortness of breath. In patients with symptomatic disease, a variety of percutaneous and surgical options exist. These include aspiration with sclerotherapy of a dominant cyst, fenestration, segmental hepatic resection, and in extreme cases even liver transplantation. Careful evaluation and appropriate referral to interventional radiology or surgery should be considered if the symptoms are disabling.

Somatostatin analogues (octreotide, lanreotide) have been shown to decrease liver volume growth and reduce symptoms related to hepatomegaly in patients with severe PLD. Nonetheless, study of these agents is limited and potential complications including diarrhea, hyperglycemia, and hepatic cyst infection would dictate their use only by experienced clinicians with expertise in PLD [88, 89].

Surgical therapy for symptomatic polycystic liver disease is more effective than minimally invasive options but has substantial mortality and morbidity [90]. Therefore, the use of the least invasive method possible for symptomatic liver cystic disease treatment is preferred [91].

In contrast to progressive deterioration of kidney function, liver function remains generally unaffected regardless of the liver size. This is attributed to the preservation of liver parenchyma. Rarely, very advanced cystic liver disease can lead to liver failure [92, 93], possibly due to compression of the portal vein by enlarging cysts. This in turn would lead to portal hypertension and its complications [94]. If liver failure occurs, isolated or combined liver and kidney transplantation can be done [95]. Liver transplant may be required on rare occasions for very severe liver cystic disease that results in massive abdominal bulk, disabling pain, and malnutrition due to compression of the gastrointestinal tract.

Cystic Liver and Hormonal Replacement Therapy

Liver cysts are usually larger in women than in men, and accelerated cyst growth in women may be due to an underlying sensitivity of the cysts to estrogen. Consistent with this observation is the fact that postmenopausal estrogen treatment is associated with selective enlargement of hepatic cysts [96]. Thus, hormonal replacement therapy should be avoided in women with ADPKD who have extensive liver cysts. In patients with mild cystic liver disease in whom hormonal replacement therapy is planned, the lowest effective dose should be used. Transdermal route is preferred as it may exert a different biological effect on liver cysts by avoidance of the first-pass effect [97]. Cysts should be monitored periodically when estrogen is being used.

Cyst Infection

Liver cysts can rarely become infected, and establishing the diagnosis is particularly challenging given the complexity of cyst appearance commonly seen in patients with advanced liver involvement. Combination of enhanced CT abdomen and 18F-fluorodeoxyglucose-positron emission tomography scanning may be helpful to establish the diagnosis [98]. MRI is a reasonable alternative for enhanced CT if IV contrast cannot be used due to poor kidney function or iodine allergy. Carbohydrate antigen 19-9 (CA 19-9), secreted by the biliary epithelium lining the cysts, might be overproduced in the case of cyst infection [99]; however, the clinical utility of CA 19-9 in diagnosing or monitoring liver cyst infection has not been established.

Treating suspected liver cyst infection should include broad-spectrum antibiotics; preference should be given to antibiotics with proven cyst penetration, such as ciprofloxacin, amikacin, and possibly ceftriaxone, which are concentrated in the bile. Drainage is often not indicated for small cysts (generally less than 5 cm), but if conservative treatment fails, percutaneous drainage or hepatic resection should be considered [100].

Quality of Life

ADPKD takes a heavy psychological toll on the patient it affects. Anxiety and depression have a high prevalence in people with chronic kidney disease in general and in ADPKD patients in particular [101]. One source of anxiety that is unique to patients with ADPKD is the issue of uncertainty. Uncertainty rises from the inability to accurately predict the disease trajectory early in the disease course. It is common for parents with ADPKD to feel guilty about passing on the disease to their children. Children in the other hand may feel frightened and resentful about the possibility of inheriting ADPKD [102]. At this time, ADPKD is not a curable disease; therefore, chronic anxiety and depression are to be expected. This makes it extremely important for nephrologists taking care of patients with ADPKD to be aware and mindful of the burden that the disease places on patients and families alike. The overarching approach to care for patients with ADPKD involves continuous education and counseling along with establishing rapport with the patient. Education should include facts as well as areas of uncertainty. Extensive counseling for patients and families should be initiated prior to and after obtaining any screening studies for family members.

Given that quality of life is a subjective feeling, the physician should explore patient's perceptions of their quality of life during routine clinic visits. Clinicians should focus on determining the specific sources of stress for patients with ADPKD. Many studies find that dietary restrictions, changes in social and family relationships, loss of image, and economic factors account for most of the concerns raised by patients [103]. Unfortunately, studies have shown that standard questionnaires used for quality of life assessment (such as the Short Form-36 (SF-36)) do not provide the sensitivity necessary to detect clinically relevant dissatisfaction with the quality of life in ADPKD patients [104]. This means that the clinician has to be proactive in detecting and addressing sources of stress in patients with ADPKD.

Antidepressant medications or anxiolytics may be needed along with non-pharmacological measures to manage anxiety and depression. In theory, the use of selective serotonin reuptake inhibitors (SSRIs) carries the risk of increasing vasopressin secretion which might lead to kidney cyst progression. This has not been studied in humans, and hence we don't recommend against the use of SSRI, but it is reasonable to use the medications sparingly. If SSRIs are to be used, frequent monitoring of serum sodium level is needed as patients with ADPKD are at risk of hyponatremia due to urine-concentrating defect [34] especially with advanced kidney disease.

Fertility and Pregnancy in ADPKD

Fertility seems not to differ from the general population in women with early ADPKD; however, as the disease progresses and kidney function declines, patients will likely have decreased fertility and a reduced conception rate similar to what is observed in patients with advanced kidney disease from other etiologies. On the other hand, several abnormalities related to male infertility were found in men with ADPKD. Those abnormalities include necrospermia (low sperm motility with a high proportion of dead sperm), seminal vesicle cysts, and ejaculatory duct cysts [105].

Seminal vesicle cysts are relatively common in patients with ADPKD; studies show a prevalence of 39–60% by ultrasound examination. However, given apparently normal fertility in males with ADPKD, the significance of this finding is not clear. The mechanism of cyst development is thought to be related to pathological dilatation of the normally tortuous vesicles. This was suggested by radiographic studies performed after injection of radiopaque dye in six patients with seminal vesicle cysts and ADPKD [106].

The infertility rate in males with ADPKD is not known, but it's presumed to be rare but higher than the general population. A database of 4108 men who were infertile was reviewed for necrospermia. Twenty-nine men were found with necrospermia unrelated to spinal cord

Table 15.1 Reproductive issues seen in patients with ADPKD

Reproductive issues in autosomal dominant polycystic kidney disease	
Male fertility	Necrospermia, ultrastructural flagellar defect, immotile sperm, seminal vesicle cysts, ejaculatory duct cysts
Female fertility	Increased risk of hypertension and preeclampsia, poor renal function predating
Pregnancy complications	Pregnancy associated with worse maternal and fetal outcomes
Fetal findings on prenatal sonogram	Enlarged hyperechogenic kidneys (if affected)
Preimplantation and prenatal diagnosis	Requires molecular testing of affected parent but clinically available. Managed care insurance generally covers the cost of testing

Adapted with permission from Vora et al. [105]

injury. Six of the 29 men (20.7%) had ADPKD [107]. We suggest that ADPKD males with complaints of infertility be referred to a fertility clinic and follow the standard approach for fertility evaluation. Screening for asymptomatic patients should be discouraged as it might lead to unnecessary anxiety and has low yield. Table 15.1 summarizes reproductive issues seen in patients with ADPKD [105].

Due to the heritable nature of ADPKD and the long-term risk of end-stage renal disease, the evaluation and counseling of couples with the disease who are pregnant or considering pregnancy should include a discussion of the modes of inheritance, natural history, available prenatal diagnostic options, and pregnancy risks.

Pregnancy carries particular risks in women with ADPKD. Careful planning and close follow-up are needed to achieve a favorable outcome.

Risks associated with pregnancy could be divided into two categories:

1. Risks related to kidney size

   Kidneys can reach a large size in patients with ADPKD; this can impose a particular challenge to women who become or plan to be become pregnant, as the product of conception normally reaches an average weight of 12–15 Kg. It is expected that patients will have exaggeration of pregnancy-related back lordosis. This might lead to worsening of back pain and significant physical stress. Orthopnea and striae gravidarum might also be encountered. However, as mentioned earlier, patients who have a large kidney size are likely to have poor kidney function and low fertility rate.

2. Risks related to kidney function and extrarenal manifestations of the disease

   New-onset hypertension and preeclampsia are fairly common in women with ADPKD. Milutinovic et al. [108] examined short-term and long-term pregnancy outcomes in women with ADPKD. 16% developed new-onset hypertension, hypertensive complications occurred in 25%, and 11% developed preeclampsia.

In general, older age and the preexistence of hypertension are associated with increased fetal prematurity rate and maternal complications. Ectopic pregnancy seems to be slightly higher in women with ADPKD with around a threefold increase in risk compared to the general population. This increase is believed to be secondary to cilia dysfunction in the fallopian tubes. Marked oligohydramnios from severe fetal polycystic kidney disease has been reported; in many cases, this will eventually lead to termination of pregnancy [109].

The relationship between pregnancy and disease progression in terms of kidney function and kidney size is poorly understood; however, it seems that most of the acute kidney injury reported in pregnant women with ADPKD is attributed to preeclampsia and worsening of hypertension. Worse long-term kidney function outcomes have been reported in women who have had 4 or more prgnancies [109].

We generally don't advise against pregnancy in women with ADPKD, but we encourage planning at an early age (before 30 years) when kidney function is preserved and kidney size not substantially increased. Close monitoring of proteinuria, blood pressure, and fetal well-being is necessary. Pregnancy in patients with large kidney size, poor kidney function (eGFR below 60 ml/min), and advanced maternal age should be considered high-risk pregnancy and should be treated as such. Continuous counseling and family support are usually needed during pregnancy.

Prenatal Genetic Diagnosis

Since ADPKD is a multisystem disorder that can lead to significant morbidity, some couples may wish to have the option of prenatal diagnosis. Chorionic villus sampling, amniocentesis, and preimplantation genetic diagnosis are available to diagnose ADPKD. By first finding the specific DNA mutation that the affected parent carries, it is possible to identify whether the fetus is affected; genetic testing has become more reliable and less expensive in recent years.

Prior to offering prenatal diagnosis, an understanding of the patient's attitude toward prenatal diagnosis is important. In a survey done in patients with ADPKD between the ages of 18 and 40, only 50% of individuals would consider the use of prenatal testing, and only 4% would terminate a pregnancy for positive results [110].

Given all of the above, we do not routinely recommend prenatal genetic testing; this approach might change in the future if a definite specific treatment could be safely offered to patients with ADPKD. If prenatal testing is to be performed, clinicians should ensure adequate family education and counseling before and after the test is performed. Preimplantation genetic diagnosis is possible only if a definitive disease mutation has been identified in the affected parent.

Monitoring Disease Progression and Patient Follow-Up

Kidney volume progression in ADPKD is the major factor determining clinical outcomes [47]. MRI is utilized for accurate estimation of total kidney volume (TKV) [43]; ultrasound and CAT scan are also useful but less accurate than MRI in estimating total kidney volume. Measurements of total kidney volume have been utilized primarily in research and are not routinely available for clinical imaging. However, assessment of total kidney volume in clinical practice may provide insights into the rate of progression [47]. Irazabal and colleagues from the CRISP consortium have developed a useful methodology for assessing prognosis in patients with typical ADPKD (cysts scattered throughout the kidney parenchyma). Using the ellipsoid formula and an online calculator, clinicians can estimate the total kidney volume from measurements of length, width and depth from standard DICOM MRI (and CT) images. The rationale of this tool is that large kidneys presenting at younger ages have grown at a more rapid rapid rate. This rapid rate of growth is associated with a worse long-term prognosis as regarding GFR decline. While this tool was developed as a research tool, clinicians with interest in ADPKD could use it to help with discussions about prognosis.

Patients with ADPKD should be followed on a regular basis. The frequency of clinic visits varies based on the disease stage, risk factors, and kidney function. Early-stage, stable patients could be followed up regularly by general practitioners or internists; referral to a nephrologist for an initial visit for ADPKD education should be done for all patients. Regular nephrology follow-up should be arranged if the patient has significant proteinuria, poorly controlled blood pressure, and frequent episodes of hematuria or if glomerular filtration rate is below 60 ml/min.

Patient Education and Support Groups

Patients should be made aware of the support foundations and groups available in their local communities. The support groups not only provide valuable education and teaching material; they help patients identify other members of the community with similar illness. Studies show that belonging to a peer support group enhances the quality of life and adherence rate in patients with advanced untreatable conditions [111]. By measures of peer support and motivated contributors, patients feel that they are actively participating in the management of their disease. The PKD foundation (http://www.pkdcure.org/) is the leading organization in the USA for supporting and educating patients with ADPKD.

References

1. Torres VE, Chapman AB, Devuyst O, Gansevoort RT, Grantham JJ, Higashihara E, Perrone RD, Krasa HB, Ouyang J, Czerwiec FS, TEMPO 3:4 Trial Investigators. Tolvaptan in patients with Autosomal Dominant Polycystic Kidney Disease. N Engl J Med. 2012;367:2407–18. PMID:23121377; PMCID:PMC3760207.
2. Torres VE, Chapman AB, Devuyst O, Gansevoort RT, Perrone RD, Koch G, Ouyang J, McQuade RD, Blais JD, Czerwiec FS, Sergeyeva O, REPRISE Trial Investigators. Tolvaptan in later-stage autosomal dominant polycystic kidney disease. N Engl J Med. 2017. https://doi.org/10.1056/NEJMoa1710030. PMID:29105594.
3. Chang MY, Ong AC. New treatments for autosomal dominant polycystic kidney disease. Br J Clin Pharmacol. 2013;76(4):524–35.
4. Chapman AB, Bost JE, Torres VE, Guay-Woodford L, Bae KT, Landsittel D, et al. Kidney volume and functional outcomes in autosomal dominant polycystic kidney disease. Clin J Am Soc Nephrol CJASN. 2012;7(3):479–86.
5. Miskulin DC, Abebe KZ, Chapman AB, Perrone RD, Steinman TI, Torres VE, et al. Health-related quality of life in patients with autosomal dominant polycystic kidney disease and CKD stages 1–4: a cross-sectional study. Am J Kidney Dis. 2013;63:214.
6. Bell PE, Hossack KF, Gabow PA, Durr JA, Johnson AM, Schrier RW. Hypertension in autosomal dominant polycystic kidney disease. Kidney Int. 1988;34(5):683–90.
7. Fick-Brosnahan GM, Belz MM, McFann KK, Johnson AM, Schrier RW. Relationship between renal volume growth and renal function in autosomal dominant polycystic kidney disease: a longitudinal study. Am J Kidney Dis Off J Natl Kidney Found. 2002;39(6):1127–34.
8. Gabow PA, Chapman AB, Johnson AM, Tangel DJ, Duley IT, Kaehny WD, et al. Renal structure and hypertension in autosomal dominant polycystic kidney disease. Kidney Int. 1990;38(6):1177–80.
9. Fick GM, Johnson AM, Hammond WS, Gabow PA. Causes of death in autosomal dominant polycystic kidney disease. J Am Soc Nephrol JASN. 1995;5(12):2048–56.
10. Barrett BJ, Foley R, Morgan J, Hefferton D, Parfrey P. Differences in hormonal and renal vascular responses between normotensive patients with autosomal dominant polycystic kidney disease and unaffected family members. Kidney Int. 1994;46(4):1118–23.
11. Danielsen H, Pedersen EB, Nielsen AH, Herlevsen P, Kornerup HJ, Posborg V. Expansion of extracellular volume in early polycystic kidney disease. Acta Med Scand. 1986;219(4):399–405.
12. Ecder T, Schrier RW. Hypertension in autosomal-dominant polycystic kidney disease: early occurrence and unique aspects. J Am Soc Nephrol: JASN. 2001;12(1):194–200.
13. Schrier RW, Abebe KZ, Perrone RD, Torres VE, Braun WE, Steinman TI, et al. Blood pressure in early autosomal dominant polycystic kidney disease. N Engl J Med. 2014;371(24):2255–66.
14. Ecder T, Chapman AB, Brosnahan GM, Edelstein CL, Johnson AM, Schrier RW. Effect of antihypertensive therapy on renal function and urinary albumin excretion in hypertensive patients with autosomal dominant polycystic kidney disease. Am J Kidney Dis Off J Natl Kidney Found. 2000;35(3):427–32.
15. Jafar TH, Stark PC, Schmid CH, Strandgaard S, Kamper AL, Maschio G, et al. The effect of angiotensin-converting-enzyme inhibitors on progression of advanced polycystic kidney disease. Kidney Int. 2005;67(1):265–71.
16. Baigent C, Landray MJ, Reith C, Emberson J, Wheeler DC, Tomson C, et al. The effects of lowering LDL cholesterol with simvastatin plus ezetimibe in patients with chronic kidney disease (study of heart and renal protection): a randomised placebo-controlled trial. Lancet. 2011;377(9784):2181–92.
17. Manttari M, Tiula E, Alikoski T, Manninen V. Effects of hypertension and dyslipidemia on the decline in renal function. Hypertension. 1995;26(4):670–5.
18. Schaeffner ES, Kurth T, Curhan GC, Glynn RJ, Rexrode KM, Baigent C, et al. Cholesterol and the risk of renal dysfunction in apparently healthy men. J Am Soc Nephrol JASN. 2003;14(8):2084–91.
19. Helal I, Reed B, Mettler P, Mc Fann K, Tkachenko O, Yan XD, et al. Prevalence of cardiovascular events in patients with autosomal dominant polycystic kidney disease. Am J Nephrol. 2012;36(4):362–70.
20. Kidney Disease Outcomes Quality Initiative (K/DOQI) Group. K/DOQI clinical practice guidelines for management of dyslipidemias in patients with kidney disease. Am J Kidney Dis: Off J Natl Kidney Found. 2003;41(4 Suppl 3):I–IV, S1–91
21. Hayward RA, Krumholz HM. Three reasons to abandon low-density lipoprotein targets: an open letter to the adult treatment panel IV of the National Institutes of Health. Circ Cardiovasc Qual Outcomes. 2012;5(1):2–5.
22. Takahashi O, Glasziou PP, Perera R, Shimbo T, Suwa J, Hiramatsu S, et al. Lipid re-screening: what is the best measure and interval? Heart. 2010;96(6):448–52.
23. Namli S, Oflaz H, Turgut F, Alisir S, Tufan F, Ucar A, et al. Improvement of endothelial dysfunction with simvastatin in patients with autosomal

dominant polycystic kidney disease. Ren Fail. 2007;29(1):55–9.
24. Cadnapaphornchai MA, George DM, McFann K, Wang W, Gitomer B, Strain JD, et al. Effect of pravastatin on total kidney volume, left ventricular mass index, and microalbuminuria in pediatric autosomal dominant polycystic kidney disease. Clin J Am Soc Nephrol CJASN. 2014;9(5):889–96.
25. Warnick GR, Wood PD. National Cholesterol Education Program recommendations for measurement of high-density lipoprotein cholesterol: executive summary. The National Cholesterol Education Program Working Group on lipoprotein measurement. Clin Chem. 1995;41(10):1427–33.
26. Klahr S, Breyer JA, Beck GJ, Dennis VW, Hartman JA, Roth D, et al. Dietary protein restriction, blood pressure control, and the progression of polycystic kidney disease. Modification of diet in renal disease study group. J Am Soc Nephrol JASN. 1995;5(12):2037–47.
27. Trumbo P, Schlicker S, Yates AA, Poos M. Food, Nutrition Board of the Institute of Medicine TNA. Dietary reference intakes for energy, carbohydrate, fiber, fat, fatty acids, cholesterol, protein and amino acids. J Am Diet Assoc. 2002;102(11):1621–30.
28. Woods LL. Mechanisms of renal hemodynamic regulation in response to protein feeding. Kidney Int. 1993;44(4):659–75.
29. King AJ, Levey AS. Dietary protein and renal function. J Am Soc Nephrol JASN. 1993;3(11):1723–37.
30. Belibi FA, Wallace DP, Yamaguchi T, Christensen M, Reif G, Grantham JJ. The effect of caffeine on renal epithelial cells from patients with autosomal dominant polycystic kidney disease. J Am Soc Nephrol JASN. 2002;13(11):2723–9.
31. Milo A. Puhan Julia Braun, Andreas L. Serra Long-term effect of coffee consumption on autosomal dominant polycystic kidneys disease progression: results from the Suisse ADPKD, a Prospective Longitudinal Cohort Study Laura Girardat-Rotar. J Nephrol DOI https://doi.org/10.1007/s40620-017-0396-8
32. Kennedy J. Herb and supplement use in the US adult population. Clin Ther. 2005;27(11):1847–58.
33. Putnam WC, Swenson SM, Reif GA, Wallace DP, Helmkamp GM Jr, Grantham JJ. Identification of a forskolin-like molecule in human renal cysts. J Am Soc Nephrol JASN. 2007;18(3):934–43.
34. Gabow PA, Kaehny WD, Johnson AM, Duley IT, Manco-Johnson M, Lezotte DC, et al. The clinical utility of renal concentrating capacity in polycystic kidney disease. Kidney Int. 1989;35(2):675–80.
35. Gattone VH 2nd, Maser RL, Tian C, Rosenberg JM, Branden MG. Developmental expression of urine concentration-associated genes and their altered expression in murine infantile-type polycystic kidney disease. Dev Genet. 1999;24(3–4):309–18.
36. Wang X, Wu Y, Ward CJ, Harris PC, Torres VE. Vasopressin directly regulates cyst growth in polycystic kidney disease. J Am Soc Nephrol JASN. 2008;19(1):102–8.
37. Nagao S, Nishii K, Katsuyama M, Kurahashi H, Marunouchi T, Takahashi H, et al. Increased water intake decreases progression of polycystic kidney disease in the PCK rat. J Am Soc Nephrol JASN. 2006;17(8):2220–7.
38. Barash I, Ponda MP, Goldfarb DS, Skolnik EY. A pilot clinical study to evaluate changes in urine osmolality and urine cAMP in response to acute and chronic water loading in autosomal dominant polycystic kidney disease. Clin J Am Soc Nephrol CJASN. 2010;5(4):693–7.
39. Torres VE, Bankir L, Grantham JJ. A case for water in the treatment of polycystic kidney disease. Clin J Am Soc Nephrol CJASN. 2009;4(6):1140–50.
40. Borghi L, Meschi T, Amato F, Briganti A, Novarini A, Giannini A. Urinary volume, water and recurrences in idiopathic calcium nephrolithiasis: a 5-year randomized prospective study. J Urol. 1996;155(3):839–43.
41. Wang CJ, Grantham JJ, Wetmore JB. The medicinal use of water in renal disease. Kidney Int. 2013;84(1):45–53.
42. Amro OW, Paulus JK, Noubary F, Perrone RD. Low-osmolar diet and adjusted water intake for vasopressin reduction in autosomal dominant polycystic kidney disease. Am J Kidney Dis. 2016;68:882–91. Epub 2016 Sep 20; PMID:27663039.
43. Torres VE, King BF, Chapman AB, Brummer ME, Bae KT, Glockner JF, et al. Magnetic resonance measurements of renal blood flow and disease progression in autosomal dominant polycystic kidney disease. Clin J Am Soc Nephrol CJASN. 2007;2(1):112–20.
44. Torres VE, Abebe KZ, Schrier RW, Perrone RD, Chapman AB, Yu AS, Braun WE, Steinman TI, Brosnahan G, Hogan MC, Rahbari FF, Grantham JJ, Bae KT, Moore CG, Flessner MF. Dietary salt restriction is beneficial to the management of autosomal dominant polycystic kidney disease. Kidney Int. 2017;91:493–500. PMID:27993381.
45. Chapman AB, Guay-Woodford LM, Grantham JJ, Torres VE, Bae KT, Baumgarten DA, et al. Renal structure in early autosomal-dominant polycystic kidney disease (ADPKD): the Consortium for Radiologic Imaging Studies of Polycystic kidney disease (CRISP) cohort. Kidney Int. 2003;64(3):1035–45.
46. Gabow PA. Autosomal dominant polycystic kidney disease–more than a renal disease. Am J Kidney Dis. 1990;16(5):403–13.
47. Grantham JJ, Chapman AB, Torres VE. Volume progression in autosomal dominant polycystic kidney disease: the major factor determining clinical outcomes. Clin J Am Soc Nephrol CJASN. 2006;1(1):148–57.
48. Bajwa ZH, Gupta S, Warfield CA, Steinman TI. Pain management in polycystic kidney disease. Kidney Int. 2001;60(5):1631–44.
49. Trescot AM, Glaser SE, Hansen H, Benyamin R, Patel S, Manchikanti L. Effectiveness of opioids

in the treatment of chronic non-cancer pain. Pain Physician. 2008;11(2 Suppl):S181–200.
50. Hogan MC, Norby SM. Evaluation and management of pain in autosomal dominant polycystic kidney disease. Adv Chronic Kidney Dis. 2010;17(3):e1–e16.
51. Steinman TI. Pain management in polycystic kidney disease. Am J Kidney Dis. 2000;35(4):770–2.
52. Sallee M, Rafat C, Zahar JR, Paulmier B, Grunfeld JP, Knebelmann B, et al. Cyst infections in patients with autosomal dominant polycystic kidney disease. Clin J Am Soc Nephrol CJASN. 2009;4(7):1183–9.
53. Rizk D, Chapman AB. Cystic and inherited kidney diseases. Am J Kidney Dis. 2003;42(6):1305–17.
54. Hwang JH, Park HC, Jeong JC, Ha Baek S, Han MY, Bang K, et al. Chronic asymptomatic pyuria precedes overt urinary tract infection and deterioration of renal function in autosomal dominant polycystic kidney disease. BMC Nephrol. 2013;14:1.
55. Schwab SJ, Bander SJ, Klahr S. Renal infection in autosomal dominant polycystic kidney disease. Am J Med. 1987;82(4):714–8.
56. Chapman AB, Thickman D, Gabow PA. Percutaneous cyst puncture in the treatment of cyst infection in autosomal dominant polycystic kidney disease. Am J Kidney Dis Off J Natl Kidney Found. 1990;16(3):252–5.
57. Sklar AH, Caruana RJ, Lammers JE, Strauser GD. Renal infections in autosomal dominant polycystic kidney disease. Am J Kidney Dis Off J Natl Kidney Found. 1987;10(2):81–8.
58. Gabow PA, Bennett WM. Renal manifestations: complication management and long-term outcome of autosomal dominant polycystic kidney disease. Semin Nephrol. 1991;11(6):643–52.
59. Bleeker-Rovers CP, de Sevaux RG, van Hamersvelt HW, Corstens FH, Oyen WJ. Diagnosis of renal and hepatic cyst infections by 18-F-fluorodeoxyglucose positron emission tomography in autosomal dominant polycystic kidney disease. Am J Kidney Dis Off J Natl Kidney Found. 2003;41(6):E18–21.
60. Qiang Z, Adams C. Potentiometric determination of acid dissociation constants (pKa) for human and veterinary antibiotics. Water Res. 2004;38(12):2874–90.
61. Bennett WM, Elzinga L, Pulliam JP, Rashad AL, Barry JM. Cyst fluid antibiotic concentrations in autosomal-dominant polycystic kidney disease. Am J Kidney Dis Off J Natl Kidney Found. 1985;6(6):400–4.
62. Gabow PA, Duley I, Johnson AM. Clinical profiles of gross hematuria in autosomal dominant polycystic kidney disease. Am J Kidney Dis Off J Natl Kidney Found. 1992;20(2):140–3.
63. Johnson AM, Gabow PA. Identification of patients with autosomal dominant polycystic kidney disease at highest risk for end-stage renal disease. J Am Soc Nephrol JASN. 1997;8(10):1560–7.
64. Balci NC, Sirvanci M, Tufek I, Onat L, Duran C. Spontaneous retroperitoneal hemorrhage secondary to subcapsular renal hematoma: MRI findings. Magn Reson Imaging. 2001;19(8):1145–8.
65. Nishiura JL, Neves RF, Eloi SR, Cintra SM, Ajzen SA, Heilberg IP. Evaluation of nephrolithiasis in autosomal dominant polycystic kidney disease patients. Clin J Am Soc Nephrol CJASN. 2009;4(4):838–44.
66. Zeier M, Fehrenbach P, Geberth S, Mohring K, Waldherr R, Ritz E. Renal histology in polycystic kidney disease with incipient and advanced renal failure. Kidney Int. 1992;42(5):1259–65.
67. Grampsas SA, Chandhoke PS, Fan J, Glass MA, Townsend R, Johnson AM, et al. Anatomic and metabolic risk factors for nephrolithiasis in patients with autosomal dominant polycystic kidney disease. Am J Kidney Dis Off J Natl Kidney Found. 2000;36(1):53–7.
68. Baishya R, Dhawan DR, Kurien A, Ganpule A, Sabnis RB, Desai MR. Management of nephrolithiasis in autosomal dominant polycystic kidney disease – a single center experience. Urol Ann. 2012;4(1):29–33.
69. Keith DS, Torres VE, King BF, Zincki H, Farrow GM. Renal cell carcinoma in autosomal dominant polycystic kidney disease. J Am Soc Nephrol JASN. 1994;4(9):1661–9.
70. Sheth S, Scatarige JC, Horton KM, Corl FM, Fishman EK. Current concepts in the diagnosis and management of renal cell carcinoma: role of multidetector ct and three-dimensional CT. Radiographics: a review publication of the Radiological Society of North America, Inc. 2001;21 Spec No:S237–54.
71. Kirkman MA, van Dellen D, Mehra S, Campbell BA, Tavakoli A, Pararajasingam R, et al. Native nephrectomy for autosomal dominant polycystic kidney disease: before or after kidney transplantation? BJU Int. 2011;108(4):590–4.
72. Lee DI, Clayman RV. Hand-assisted laparoscopic nephrectomy in autosomal dominant polycystic kidney disease. J Endourol Endourological Soc. 2004;18(4):379–82.
73. Cohen D, Timsit MO, Chretien Y, Thiounn N, Vassiliu V, Mamzer MF, et al. Place of nephrectomy in patients with autosomal dominant polycystic kidney disease waiting for renal transplantation. Progres en urologie: journal de l'Association francaise d'urologie et de la Societe francaise d'urologie. 2008;18(10):642–9.
74. Yamamoto T, Watarai Y, Kobayashi T, Matsuda Y, Tsujita M, Hiramitsu T, et al. Kidney volume changes in patients with autosomal dominant polycystic kidney disease after renal transplantation. Transplantation. 2012;93(8):794–8.
75. Ronald D, Perrone AA. Polycystic kidney disease: from bench to bedside. 1st ed. London: Future Medicine Ltd; 2013.
76. Fuller TF, Brennan TV, Feng S, Kang SM, Stock PG, Freise CE. End stage polycystic kidney disease: indications and timing of native nephrectomy relative to kidney transplantation. J Urol. 2005;174(6):2284–8.
77. Perrone RD, Ruthazer R, Terrin NC. Survival after end-stage renal disease in autosomal dominant

polycystic kidney disease: contribution of extrarenal complications to mortality. Am J Kidney Dis. 2001;38(4):777–84.
78. Li L, Szeto CC, Kwan BC, Chow KM, Leung CB, Kam-Tao LP. Peritoneal dialysis as the first-line renal replacement therapy in patients with autosomal dominant polycystic kidney disease. Am J Kidney Dis Off J Natl Kidney Found. 2011;57(6):903–7.
79. Mariani L, Bianchetti MG, Schroth G, Seiler RW. Cerebral aneurysms in patients with autosomal dominant polycystic kidney disease–to screen, to clip, to coil? Nephrol Dial Transplant Off Publ Eur Dial Transplant Assoc – Eur Ren Assoc. 1999;14(10):2319–22.
80. Xu HW, Yu SQ, Mei CL, Li MH. Screening for intracranial aneurysm in 355 patients with autosomal-dominant polycystic kidney disease. Stroke. 2011;42(1):204–6.
81. Vega C, Kwoon JV, Lavine SD. Intracranial aneurysms: current evidence and clinical practice. Am Fam Physician. 2002;66(4):601–8.
82. Schrier RW, Belz MM, Johnson AM, Kaehny WD, Hughes RL, Rubinstein D, et al. Repeat imaging for intracranial aneurysms in patients with autosomal dominant polycystic kidney disease with initially negative studies: a prospective ten-year follow-up. J Am Soc Nephrol JASN. 2004;15(4):1023–8.
83. Greving JP, Rinkel GJ, Buskens E, Algra A. Cost-effectiveness of preventive treatment of intracranial aneurysms: new data and uncertainties. Neurology. 2009;73(4):258–65.
84. Perrone RD, Malek AM, Watnick T. Vascular complications in autosomal dominant polycystic Kidney disease. Nature Rev Nephrol. 2015;11:589–98. Epub 2015 Aug 11; PMID: 26260542.
85. Hossack KF, Leddy CL, Johnson AM, Schrier RW, Gabow PA. Echocardiographic findings in autosomal dominant polycystic kidney disease. N Engl J Med. 1988;319(14):907–12.
86. Bae KT, Zhu F, Chapman AB, Torres VE, Grantham JJ, Guay-Woodford LM, et al. Magnetic resonance imaging evaluation of hepatic cysts in early autosomal-dominant polycystic kidney disease: the consortium for radiologic imaging studies of polycystic kidney disease cohort. Clin J Am Soc Nephrol CJASN. 2006;1(1):64–9.
87. Gabow PA, Johnson AM, Kaehny WD, Manco-Johnson ML, Duley IT, Everson GT. Risk factors for the development of hepatic cysts in autosomal dominant polycystic kidney disease. Hepatology. 1990;11(6):1033–7.
88. Marie C. Hogan, Tetyana V. Masyuk, Linda Page, David R. Holmes, III, Xujian Li, Eric J. Bergstralh, Maria V. Irazabal, Bohyun Kim, Bernard F. King, James F. Glockner, Nicholas F. LaRusso and Vicente E. Torres. Nephrol Dial Transplant (2012) 27: 3532–3539. doi: https://doi.org/10.1093/ndt/gfs152
89. Gevers TJ, Hol JC, Monshouwer R, Dekker HM, Wetzels JF, Drenth JP. Effect of lanreotide on polycystic liver and kidneys in autosomal dominant polycystic kidney disease: an observational trial. Liver Int. 2015;35(5):1607–14. https://doi.org/10.1111/liv.12726.
90. Chebib FT, Harmon A, Irazabal Mira MV, Jung YS, Edwards ME, Hogan MC, Kamath PS, Torres VE, Outcomes NDM. Durability of hepatic reduction after combined partial hepatectomy and cyst fenestration for massive polycystic liver disease. J Am Coll Surg. 2016;223(1):118–126.e1. https://doi.org/10.1016/j.jamcollsurg.2015.12.051. Epub 2016 Jan 14.
91. Wang MQ, Duan F, Liu FY, Wang ZJ, Song P. Treatment of symptomatic polycystic liver disease: transcatheter super-selective hepatic arterial embolization using a mixture of NBCA and iodized oil. Abdom Imaging. 2013;38(3):465–73.
92. Chandok N. Polycystic liver disease: a clinical review. Ann Hepatol. 2012;11(6):819–26.
93. Elias TJ, Bannister KM, Clarkson AR, Faull RJ. Progressive hepatic failure secondary to adult polycystic kidney disease. Aust NZ J Med. 1999;29(2):282–3.
94. Torres VE. Treatment of polycystic liver disease: one size does not fit all. Am J Kidney Dis Off J Natl Kidney Found. 2007;49(6):725–8.
95. Pirenne J, Aerts R, Yoong K, Gunson B, Koshiba T, Fourneau I, et al. Liver transplantation for polycystic liver disease. Liver Transpl. 2001;7(3):238–45.
96. Sherstha R, McKinley C, Russ P, Scherzinger A, Bronner T, Showalter R, et al. Postmenopausal estrogen therapy selectively stimulates hepatic enlargement in women with autosomal dominant polycystic kidney disease. Hepatology. 1997;26(5):1282–6.
97. Renoux C, Dell'aniello S, Garbe E, Suissa S. Transdermal and oral hormone replacement therapy and the risk of stroke: a nested case-control study. BMJ. 2010;340:c2519.
98. Jouret F, Lhommel R, Beguin C, Devuyst O, Pirson Y, Hassoun Z, et al. Positron-emission computed tomography in cyst infection diagnosis in patients with autosomal dominant polycystic kidney disease. Clin J Am Soc Nephrol CJASN. 2011;6(7):1644–50.
99. Kanaan N, Goffin E, Pirson Y, Devuyst O, Hassoun Z. Carbohydrate antigen 19-9 as a diagnostic marker for hepatic cyst infection in autosomal dominant polycystic kidney disease. Am J Kidney Dis Off J Natl Kidney Found. 2010;55(5):916–22.
100. Chauveau D, Fakhouri F, Grunfeld JP. Liver involvement in autosomal-dominant polycystic kidney disease: therapeutic dilemma. J Am Soc Nephrol JASN. 2000;11(9):1767–75.
101. de Barros BP, Nishiura JL, Heilberg IP, Kirsztajn GM. Anxiety, depression, and quality of life in patients with familial glomerulonephritis or autosomal dominant polycystic kidney disease. Jornal brasileiro de nefrologia: 'orgao oficial de Sociedades Brasileira e Latino-Americana de Nefrologia. 2011;33(2):120–8.

102. Michie S, Bobrow M, Marteau TM. Predictive genetic testing in children and adults: a study of emotional impact. J Med Genet. 2001;38(8):519–26.
103. Perez Dominguez TS, Rodriguez Perez A, Buset Rios N, Rodriguez Esparragon F, Garcia Bello MA, Perez Borges P, et al. Psychonephrology: psychological aspects in autosomal dominant polycystic kidney disease. Nefrologia. 2011;31(6):716–22.
104. Rizk D, Jurkovitz C, Veledar E, Bagby S, Baumgarten DA, Rahbari-Oskoui F, et al. Quality of life in autosomal dominant polycystic kidney disease patients not yet on dialysis. Clin J Am Soc Nephrol CJASN. 2009;4(3):560–6.
105. Vora N, Perrone R, Bianchi DW. Reproductive issues for adults with autosomal dominant polycystic kidney disease. Am J Kidney Dis Off J Natl Kidney Found. 2008;51(2):307–18.
106. Hendry WF, Rickards D, Pryor JP, Baker LR. Seminal megavesicles with adult polycystic kidney disease. Hum Reprod. 1998;13(6):1567–9.
107. Fang S, Baker HW. Male infertility and adult polycystic kidney disease are associated with necrospermia. Fertil Steril. 2003;79(3):643–4.
108. Milutinovic J, Fialkow PJ, Agodoa LY, Phillips LA, Bryant JI. Fertility and pregnancy complications in women with autosomal dominant polycystic kidney disease. Obstet Gynecol. 1983;61(5):566–70.
109. Chapman AB, Johnson AM, Gabow PA. Pregnancy outcome and its relationship to progression of renal failure in autosomal dominant polycystic kidney disease. J Am Soc Nephrol JASN. 1994;5(5):1178–85.
110. Sujansky E, Kreutzer SB, Johnson AM, Lezotte DC, Schrier RW, Gabow PA. Attitudes of at-risk and affected individuals regarding presymptomatic testing for autosomal dominant polycystic kidney disease. Am J Med Genet. 1990;35(4):510–5.
111. Tehrani AM, Farajzadegan Z, Rajabi FM, Zamani AR. Belonging to a peer support group enhance the quality of life and adherence rate in patients affected by breast cancer: a non-randomized controlled clinical trial. J Res Med Sci. 2011;16(5):658–65.

Index

B. D. Cowley, Jr., J. J. Bissler (eds.), *Polycystic Kidney Disease*,
https://doi.org/10.1007/978-1-4939-7784-0

D

E

N

O

P

MIX
Papier aus verantwortungsvollen Quellen
Paper from responsible sources
FSC® C105338

If you have any concerns about our products,
you can contact us on
ProductSafety@springernature.com

In case Publisher is established outside the EU,
the EU authorized representative is:
Springer Nature Customer Service Center GmbH
Europaplatz 3, 69115 Heidelberg, Germany

Printed by Libri Plureos GmbH
in Hamburg, Germany